# Clinical Management Notes and Case Histories in
# Cardiopulmonary Physical Therapy

W. Darlene Reid, BMR(PT), PhD
ASSOCIATE PROFESSOR
THE UNIVERSITY OF BRITISH COLUMBIA
SCHOOL OF REHABILITATION SCIENCES
VANCOUVER, BC

Frank Chung, BSc(PT), MSc
SECTION HEAD, PHYSICAL THERAPY
PHYSIOTHERAPY DEPARTMENT
BURNABY HOSPITAL
BURNABY, BC

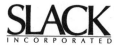
SLACK
INCORPORATED
*An innovative information, education, and management company*
6900 Grove Road • Thorofare, NJ 08086

Library of Congress Cataloging-in-Publication Data

Reid, W. Darlene.
 Clinical management notes and case histories in cardiopulmonary physical therapy / W. Darlene Reid, Frank Chung.
   p. ; cm.
 Includes bibliographical references and index.
 ISBN 1-55642-568-6 (soft bound)
 1. Cardiopulmonary system--Diseases--Physical therapy--Case studies.
 [DNLM: 1. Respiratory Tract Diseases--rehabilitation--Case Reports. 2. Heart Diseases--rehabilitation--Case Reports. 3. Physical Therapy Techniques--methods--Case Reports. WF 145 R359c 2004] I. Chung, Frank. II. Title.
 RC702.R455 2004
 616.1--dc22

                                                                                      2004006721

Printed in the United States of America.
Published by:       SLACK Incorporated
                    6900 Grove Road
                    Thorofare, NJ 08086 USA
                    Telephone: 856-848-1000
                    Fax: 856-853-5991
                    www.slackbooks.com

Contact SLACK Incorporated for more information about other books in this field or about the availability of our books from distributors outside the United States.

For permission to reprint material in another publication, contact SLACK Incorporated. Authorization to photocopy items for internal, personal, or academic use is granted by SLACK Incorporated provided that the appropriate fee is paid directly to Copyright Clearance Center. Prior to photocopying items, please contact the Copyright Clearance Center at 222 Rosewood Drive, Danvers, MA 01923 USA; phone: 978-750-8400; website: www.copyright.com; email: info@copyright.com.

For further information on CCC, check CCC Online at the following address: http://www.copyright.com.

Last digit is print number: 10   9   8   7   6   5   4   3   2   1

# DEDICATION

To my children, Janine and Jeremy, who are gifts from heaven and constantly inspire and overwhelm me with their ability to enjoy and engage in life.

Darlene Reid, BMR(PT), PhD


To Jeannie and Tiffany for their support and for providing a nourishing home environment.

Frank Chung, BSc(PT), MSc

# Contents

CARDIOPULMONARY ASSESSMENT

CARDIOPULMONARY MANAGEMENT

OVERVIEW OF MEDICAL & SURGICAL CONDITIONS & THERAPEUTIC INTERVENTIONS

SURGICAL AND MEDICAL CONDITIONS

CHRONIC RESPIRATORY CONDITIONS

# ACKNOWLEDGMENTS

**W. Darlene Reid, BMR(PT), PhD,** would like to express her sincere appreciation to colleagues and students with whom she has had the opportunity to discuss and refine concepts related to her understanding of cardiopulmonary physical therapy. Darlene would like to especially thank colleagues including Frank Chung, Judy Richardson, Sue Murphy, Pat Camp, and Michelle de Moor, who assisted in developing many of the case studies. Graduate and undergraduate students have provided invaluable input through their probing questions, which have greatly improved the clarity of the content and presentation of material in this book. Darlene would like to acknowledge the members of the Canadian Cardiorespiratory Standards and Specialization Committee for their unending inspiration to strive for better cardiopulmonary physical therapy health care and for their facilitation of a broader national and international perspective of cardiopulmonary care. Darlene is indebted to Drs. Catherine Staples and Nestor Muller for providing chest x-rays, and to Stuart Green for providing his expertise toward photographing images including all of the chest x-rays. Darlene would also like to thank Louis Walsh, who produced and assisted with many of the diagrams.

**Frank Chung, BSc(PT), MSc,** would like to express his sincere thanks to librarian Hoong Lim for providing reference materials; physical therapist Rhonda Johnston for proofreading part of the manuscript; respiratory therapists Terry Satchwill and Joanne Edwards for providing respiratory equipment for Chapter 17; clinical nurse educator Giselle Strychar for providing the medical equipment for Chapter 20; and graphic artist Hau Chee Chung for his artistic creations.

# About the Authors

**W. Darlene Reid, BMR(PT), PhD,** is an associate professor at the School of Rehabilitation Sciences, University of British Columbia, in Vancouver, British Columbia, Canada. She earned her physical therapy degree from the University of Manitoba in Winnipeg, Manitoba in 1979. She completed graduate studies in Pathology at the University of British Columbia and obtained her PhD in 1988.

Darlene teaches graduate and entry-level physiotherapy respiratory care and muscle injury, and supervises research by graduate and undergraduate students in the School of Rehabilitation Sciences, the School of Human Kinetics, and the Experimental Medicine programs at the University of British Columbia. Undergraduate courses include those related to exercise physiology and physiotherapy management of patients with cardiopulmonary conditions. Graduate teaching is related to exercise physiology, exertion-induced muscle injury, and advanced techniques in the management of cardiovascular and respiratory patients. In addition, Darlene is involved in continuing education related to these areas.

Darlene has held scholarship salary awards from the B.C. Health Research Foundation and the Killam Foundation. Her areas of research interests include respiratory muscle injury and pulmonary rehabilitation. Clinically, she has specialized in physiotherapeutic treatment for patients with acute and chronic pulmonary disease. Her clinical research has focused on therapeutic interventions directed toward the ventilatory muscles including ventilatory muscle testing, training, and rest in chronic obstructive pulmonary disease. Her most recent endeavours have been directed toward understanding different mechanisms that may contribute to diaphragm injury in animal models and evidence of diaphragm injury in humans.

Darlene has extensively published, including peer reviewed manuscripts, abstracts, review papers, and chapters. She has been a symposium speaker at a number of international conferences, including the American Thoracic Society, the combined Canadian Physiotherapy Association/American Physical Therapy Association, and the American Physical Therapy Association Combined Sections Meetings.

Darlene is a member of the Cardiorespiratory Specialization and Standards Committee and the British Columbia Lung Association Medical Advisory Board. She has served on several national and local committees related to cardiorespiratory physiotherapy as Cardiorespiratory Division Executive of the Canadian Physiotherapy Association, as Executive of the Canadian Physiotherapy Cardiorespiratory Society of Lung Association, and as the provincial coordinator of the Cardiorespiratory Physiotherapy Summit. She also has served and continues to be a reviewer of manuscripts and grants for several agencies.

**Frank Chung, BSc(PT), MSc,** graduated with a BSc(PT) degree from McGill University in Montreal, Quebec, Canada in 1981 and later obtained a MSc degree in Interdisciplinary Studies (Respiratory and Exercise Physiology) from the University of British Columbia in Vancouver, British Columbia, Canada in 1989.

Frank has taught at the School of Rehabilitation Sciences at the University of British Columbia, instructed post-graduate physical therapy courses, and published in peer-reviewed journals. He is also the list owner of a cardiorespiratory Internet interest group, CardioRespPhysio@yahoogroups.com. Frank is a member of the National Examination Test Construction and Implementation Subcommittee of the Canadian Alliance of Physiotherapy Regulatory Boards. He is also an examiner of the Canadian Physical Therapy National Examination. He works as a physical therapist at Burnaby Hospital in British Columbia, Canada.

# INTRODUCTION

*Clinical Management Notes and Case Histories in Cardiopulmonary Physical Therapy* provides an interactive learning approach to cardiopulmonary care for acute and ambulatory care patients at entry-level physical therapy. The presentation of this book is unique in that it combines 3 main components: clinical notes on assessment and management, 19 cases that show typical presentations of common pulmonary and cardiac conditions, and answer guides both for questions posed in the assessment and management chapters and for the 19 cases.

The interactive nature of the case history approach to learning engages the student and provides the opportunity to work through many of the steps of the clinical decision-making process. In addition, the cases have been carefully selected and developed over several years to illustrate a spectrum of clinical issues of which the entry-level therapist should be aware.

The active, participatory approach of learning cardiopulmonary content in the context of clinical cases immediately brings relevance to learners and it is this learning approach that they very much enjoy. Cardiopulmonary care is often complex because of the interpretation of many assessment skills and the nature of the patients cared for. Teaching in the context of a case history approach provides a greater motivation to learners because they see a "real" person benefiting from their clinical reasoning and problem solving—rather than learning information in a less contextual manner, wherein the concepts are not closely connected to a patient.

Section 1, Cardiopulmonary Assessment and Management, outlines major techniques in a brief, evidence-based manner. Interactive questions and problems are provided to reinforce basic concepts. *Cardiopulmonary Assessment* topics include: clinical decision making, chart review and interview, physical examination, interpretation of lab tests, chest radiology, pulmonary function testing, mobility and exercise testing; and EKG interpretation. *Cardiopulmonary Management* topics include adult and patient education; breathing exercises; positioning; mobilization and exercise training; airway clearance techniques; oxygen therapy; mechanical ventilation; and an overview of pulmonary, cardiac, and surgical management.

One of the major strengths of this section is its evidence-based approach. All techniques have been ranked and referenced according to levels of evidence. When careful reviews or clinical practice guidelines have not been available, the authors have provided a review of the literature for the reader. Details of this are provided in the Section 4, Appendices. For many techniques, the ratings of evidence were not obtained from a consensus of experts but rather were the interpretation of the authors.

Section 2, Case Histories, contains well-developed cases of typical presentations of pulmonary (9 cases), cardiac conditions (6 cases), and combined presentations (4 cases). Four of the cases relate to outpatient scenarios and 3 others relate to a home program or functional activity post-discharge. Each case has a history followed by several components with questions to help learners develop a therapeutic approach of deriving salient assessment factors and determining a treatment approach. Components of the case histories include some of the following: histories, descriptions and/or pictures of the physical presentation, arterial blood gas values, chest x-rays, EKG tracings, and pulmonary function reports. These cases provide a broad spectrum of examples for the learner to practice and reinforce basic information about assessment and management skills.

Section 3, Answer Guides, provides detailed information related to questions posed in the chapters on cardiopulmonary assessment and management and to questions posed in the case histories. In some cases, the answer guides provide information beyond what is required at entry level.

Section 4, Appendices, provides an overview of some of the difficulties faced by clinicians when reviewing the literature to determine best clinical practice. The appendices contain several critical reviews of the literature on areas of practice that either are contentious or have no well-established clinical guidelines.

This well-referenced, evidence-based text will provide a solid foundation for cardiopulmonary assessment and clinical management skills. The case-history approach will ensure that the learner is able to apply the information in a clinically relevant manner and facilitate development of clinical decision making and reasoning skills.

# Section 1

# Cardiopulmonary Assessment and Management

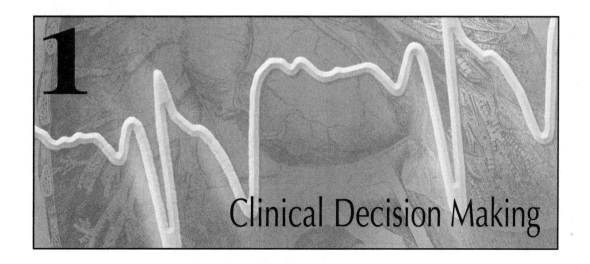

# Clinical Decision Making

## OBJECTIVES

Upon completion of this chapter, the reader should be able to:
1. Describe a clinical management pathway involving assessment, treatment goals, treatment, and reassessment
2. Define an outcome measure
3. Define levels of evidence that can be used to rate the scientific evidence supporting treatment interventions

## CLINICAL MANAGEMENT PATHWAY

The physical therapist needs to consider a *clinical management pathway* before and while assessing and treating patients with cardiovascular and respiratory disorders. One framework is shown in Figure 1-1. A thorough appreciation and understanding of the medical conditions of the patient to be treated (Chapters 18 through 20 of Section 1) will help determine the aspects of the *pathophysiology* most amenable to treatment in each patient. During the *assessment* procedures, 2 main factors need to be determined:
1. Aspects of the pathophysiology that are reversible and amenable to physical therapy
2. Other aspects of the patient that need to be treated to optimize function and to prevent complications

A *problem list* and/or *treatment goals* is generated and the patient is *treated* using best practice. Assessment is often ongoing throughout the treatment and additional measures may be taken at the end of the treatment. The physical therapist then follows the management pathway and recycles through it again (see Figure 1-1). Because of the often critical and serious nature of different cardiovascular and respiratory conditions, assessment and reassessment is tightly tied to treatment and is often the most challenging aspect of cardiopulmonary physical therapy.

## ASSESSMENT

Assessment of the respiratory and cardiovascular systems is composed of a chart review and interview, physical examination, and review of relevant lab tests and investigations (Figure 1-2). Details are in Chapters 2 through 10.

## PROBLEMS AND TREATMENT GOALS

A problem list is generated related to the pathophysiology that is reversible or is amenable to physiotherapy treatment. Table 1-1 outlines several examples of problems that might be apparent in patients with cardiopulmonary disorders. Although the pathophysiologic bases of many of these problems are distinct, the factors are

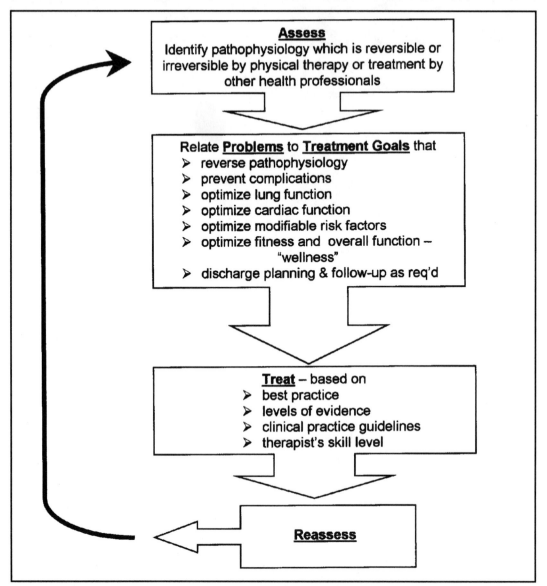

**Figure 1-1.** Cardiopulmonary physical therapy clinical management pathway.

**Figure 1-2.** Components of cardiopulmonary physical therapy assessment.

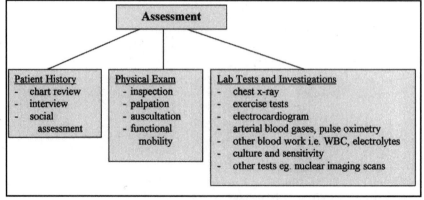

## Table 1-1

### *Potential Problems to be Addressed by Physical Therapy Interventions*

- Poor gas exchange in affected regions especially at low lung volumes ($\uparrow PaCO_2$ and $\downarrow PaO_2$)
- May desaturate with exercise/mobility
- Poor cardiovascular function
- Myocardial ischemia
- Decreased cardiac output
- Decreased oxygen transport/circulation to periphery
- Pain—incisional or trauma
- Chest or musculoskeletal or peripheral vascular pain
- Decreased mobility/poor exercise tolerance
- Decreased fitness
- Decreased strength and endurance
- Retained/increased secretions
- Recurrent infections
- Dyspnea
- Increased work of breathing
- Increased use of accessory muscles
- Deep vein thrombosis
- Ileus
- Urinary retention
- Altered cognitive status
- Altered coordination and/or balance
- Poor posture
- Decreased range of motion (ROM) of shoulder and other related joints
- Sternal limitations
- Poor nutrition
- Poor understanding of condition, care of condition, and self-management
- Decreased sense of well-being or depression
- Discharge planning needs

grouped in the table because clinically these factors are often evaluated simultaneously by using similar techniques and outcome measures. Treatment goals should be directed toward reversing pathophysiology and also toward problems related to other systems, preventing complications, improving overall wellness of the patient, and optimizing modifiable risk factors (see Figure 1-1). Treatment goals should be client-centered—especially when working with outpatients and those individuals with chronic illness. Negotiating client-centered goals will not only have a greater impact on what the client believes needs to be improved but also will facilitate compliance and long-term adherence to lifestyle changes and treatment interventions. Treatment goals are often the converse of patient problems. Thus, in many sections of this book, either treatment goals or problems will be referred to. Depending on the therapist's style of practice, most chart one or the other but not both. After the generation of a problem list or treatment goals, treatment approaches and outcomes are determined for each of these goals.

# TREATMENT USING BEST PRACTICE

Treatments are prescribed using the principles of best practice. In other words, the therapist will prescribe and carry out treatments considering the following factors:
- Those with the highest levels of scientific evidence
- Utilizing the best technique based on resources available—including time and equipment
- Prioritizing patients based on their need
- Balancing physical therapy interventions with other treatments and activities of the patient

Table 1-2

## Dean's Physiological Treatment Hierarchy for Treatment of Impaired Oxygen Transport

Premise: Position of optimal physiological function is being upright and moving

*Mobilization and Exercise*

Goal: To elicit an exercise stimulus that addresses acute, long-term, or preventative effects on the various steps in oxygen transport*

*Body Positioning*

Goal: To elicit a gravitational stimulus that simulates being upright and moving, to relieve dyspnea, to promote hemodynamic, and ventilation-perfusion effects

*Breathing Control Maneuvers*

Goal: To augment alveolar ventilation, facilitate mucociliary transport, and stimulate coughing

*Coughing Maneuvers*

Goal: To facilitate mucociliary clearance with the least effect on dynamic airway compression and adverse cardiovascular effects

*Relaxation and Energy Conservation Interventions*

Goal: To minimize the work of breathing, the work of the heart, and undue oxygen demand overall

*Range-of-Motion Exercises (Cardiopulmonary Indications)*

Goal: To stimulate alveolar ventilation and to alter its distribution

*Postural Drainage Positions*

Goal: To facilitate airway clearance using gravitational effects

*Manual Techniques*

Goal: To facilitate airway clearance in conjunction with specific body positioning

*Suctioning*

Goal: To facilitate the removal of airway secretions collected centrally

*This hierarchy is a guideline for a treatment plan. It is important to note that not all features of oxygen transport can be altered in some disease states and in some clients. A specific treatment plan should always be customized for every patient.

Modified and reprinted with permission from *Clinical Case Study Guide to Accompany Principles and Practice of Cardiopulmonary Physical Therapy,* 3rd ed., Dean E, Frownfelter D, Copyright (1996), with permission from Dr. Elizabeth Dean and Elsevier.

Chapters 11 through 20 of Section 1 outline interventions performed by physical therapists and by other health professionals. Table 1-2 shows Dean's Physiological Treatment Hierarchy for Treatment of Impaired Oxygen Transport, which provides an underlying foundation for formulating a treatment plan.[1] This hierarchy is based on the premise that getting the patient upright and moving will optimize treatment benefits. As therapists approach many patients with cardiopulmonary dysfunction, this hierarchy will provide a guideline for treatment; however, there are some exceptions and a specific treatment plan should always be customized for every patient. For example, in the intensive care unit when treating seriously ill patients, if obstruction of a bronchus

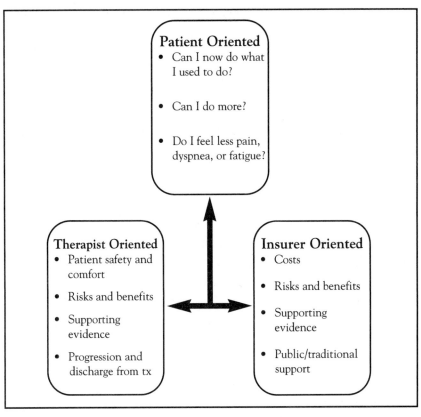

**Figure 1-3.** Reasons for outcomes.

by mucus is causing atelectasis of a lung segment or lobe, airway clearance and not mobility exercises will be the first priority of treatment.

A key determinant of treatment selection is considering *levels of evidence*. Each of the treatments outlined in this text will be rated and the scale used in this text will be as follows[2,3]:

- Grade A—Scientific evidence from well-designed and well-conducted controlled trials (randomized and nonrandomized) provide statistically significant results that consistently support the use of the treatment (and low risk of error).
- Grade B—Scientific evidence is provided by observational studies or by controlled trials with less consistent results (and moderate to high risk of error).
- Grade C—The use of the treatment is supported only by expert opinion as determined by a panel of experts; the available evidence does not provide consistent results or well-designed, controlled studies are lacking.

It is important to consider that a *lack of evidence does not necessarily mean that the treatment is not effective in a particular patient*. However, as responsible, accountable health professionals, it behooves us to always utilize the treatment with the highest level of evidence if our working environment enables this choice.

# OUTCOME MEASURES

An outcome measure is defined as a measure that has psychometric properties that enhance its ability to measure change over time in an individual or group.[4] Useful outcome measures are quantifiable, available clinically, practical, cost-effective, valid and reliable for the population/condition being tested, and should be closely associated to the problems being addressed by the physical therapy interventions.

Two important considerations for outcome measures are that:

- *Different outcomes* are relevant and *essential for all the parties involved in patient care* (Figure 1-3). These groups of individuals usually include the patient, therapist, and third-party payers. Outcomes have to be evaluated and documented in all 3 areas in order to determine if physical therapy management is effective and to sustain funding for programs.

- Outcomes vary in terms of their specificity to a problem and their evidence base.[4] *The validity of outcomes is strengthened when combined* and consistently show a change in a similar direction. For example, decreased breath sounds heard over the lower lobes on auscultation is a nonspecific finding that might reflect atelectasis or possibly decreased inspiratory effort by the patient. If this finding is combined with other findings that are consistent with this change—such as a chest x-ray that shows atelectasis in the lung bases, and a saturation of oxygen on oximetry ($SpO_2$) of 85%—the therapist can be more confident that clinically significant atelectasis is present in the patient, and the patient could benefit from cardiopulmonary physical therapy.

# REFERENCES

1. Dean E, Frownfelter D. *Clinical Case Study Guide to Accompany Principles and Practice of Cardiopulmonary Physical Therapy*. 3rd Ed. St. Louis: Mosby; 1996.
2. Wenger NK, Froelicher ES, Smith LK, et al. Cardiac rehabilitation as secondary prevention. Clinical practice guideline. *Quick Reference Guide for Clinicians*. No. 17. Rockville, MC: US Department of Health and Human Service, Agency for Health Care Policy and Research and National Heart, Lung and Blood Institute. AHCPR Pub. No. 96-0673; October 1995.
3. Sackett DL. Rules of evidence and clinical recommendations. *Can J Cardiol*. 1993;9(6):487-489.
4. Finch E, Brooks D, Stratford P, Mayo N. *Physical rehabilitation outcome measures: a guide to enhanced clinical decision making*. Canadian Physiotherapy Association. Hamilton: BC Decker Inc; 2002.

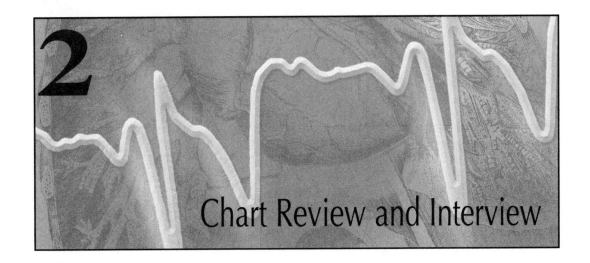

Chart Review and Interview

## OBJECTIVES

At the end of this chapter, the reader should be able to describe:
1. The different purposes of a patient interview
2. The 4 major components of an interview
3. Relevant information to be derived from a chart and an interview

A thorough chart review and focused interview are key elements of a comprehensive assessment of the patient with pulmonary and/or cardiovascular disorders. The physical therapist needs to establish an open, comfortable rapport with the patient to optimize the information derived. In addition, the therapist should have determined the purpose of the interview and possible outcomes of treatment in order to obtain essential information and to avoid extraneous questioning.

## CHART REVIEW

The chart should be carefully reviewed before the interview. Often the chart has an immense amount of information that is accurately recorded but it can also contain apparently conflicting or sparse information. The therapist needs to review the chart to derive key information relevant to physical therapy management. Depending on the manner in which this information is charted, the therapist may ask fewer questions of the patient or simply confirm information already recorded in the chart. In other cases, redundant questions may be posed to the patient because the nature of his or her answer is critical to ensure accuracy of information and/or the patient's perception of a particular issue.

## RAPPORT

Establishing and maintaining an open, comfortable rapport with patients is essential to obtain meaningful interview information and to implement an effective, ongoing physical therapy management program. The ideal setting is one that affords privacy and a minimum of distractions to both the patient and therapist. The timing of the interview should allow the patient to be prepared for questioning and to be unhurried and relaxed. The therapist position should be parallel to the patient if possible; both parties should be seated or situated in a comfortable posture for the duration of the interview. Questions should be posed in an open presentation rather than the questions being worded toward biasing the patient's response. The therapist should be listening and recording patient response in an accepting, nonjudgmental manner as reflected by facial expression, verbal acknowledgment, and body language.

Table 2-1

*Overview of Information to Be Derived From Chart Review and Interview*

- Date of birth/age
- Current or admitting diagnosis(es)

*Birth History (Important in Pediatrics)*

*Past Medical History*

Smoking
- How much?
- When?
- Currently?

Respiratory History
- Chronic
- Acute problems?
- Recent cold

Cardiovascular History
- Coronary artery disease
- Previous myocardial infarction (MI)? If so, what date?
- Previous coronary artery bypass surgery?
- Ischemic pain on exertion? ie, intermittent claudication?

Family History or Related Conditions
Cough
- Strong?
- Productive of sputum?
- Colour and consistency of sputum
- Difficulty or techniques to facilitate removal

Chest Pain
- On exertion. Angina? If so what classification?
- Other causes or associated factors

Other Conditions
- Diabetes
- Serious musculoskeletal
- Other

Allergens/Irritants

*Problems With Previous Anesthetic*

*Cognitive Status*

- Orientation to time, place, and person

*Medications*

*Laboratory Investigations*

- Eg, x-rays, blood tests, culture and sensitivity

*Risk Factors to Exercise*

- See Table 9-3 for details

*Functional History*

- Stairs
- Ambulation
- Mobility/activity
- Activities that are particularly tiring or difficult to do
- Regular exercise (type, duration, frequency, intensity)
- What limits exercise?
- Angina? ST changes? What induces angina? What alleviates angina?
- Dyspnea/shortness of breath? (At rest? At night? What level of activity? Bed flat?)
- Intermittent claudication

*Social History*

- Occupation
- Leisure activities
- Living arrangements
- Help at home

*Prior Treatment*

- Related to current respiratory and/or cardiovascular conditions
- Other ongoing health care treatments that might affect or interact with physical therapy care

*Patient Goals*

*Established Structured Questionnaires*

- Depression scores
- Health related quality of life questionnaires
- Functional status questionnaires
- Mini-mental or perceptual status
- Patient satisfaction

# PURPOSE OF INTERVIEW

A variety of questions (Table 2-1) can be posed for a thorough evaluation of the patient; however, in most clinical situations, this is not possible or warranted. The therapist's time and patient's condition may preclude

## Table 2-2

### *Purpose of Interviews in Different Clinical Settings*

- To determine client-centered goals
- To provide information
- To determine postoperative risk for pulmonary complications
- To determine patient status immediately prior to treatment
- To determine functional capacity necessary for discharge from hospital
- To facilitate patient self-management
- To determine patient satisfaction
- To determine risks and safety issues for exercise training and other physical therapy interventions
- To determine obstacles or challenges in implementing behavioral and lifestyle changes

a long interview. In addition, the chart may contain much of the key information. To ensure an efficient, informative interview the therapist needs to identify the purpose of the interview and potential outcomes of treatment to focus questioning accordingly. See Table 2-2 for some purposes of the interview in different clinical settings. For example, in an acute care setting postoperatively, the therapist should have derived most critical information from the chart and may interview the patient briefly to determine his or her current status and to maintain rapport for treatment. On the other hand, during an outpatient setting for pulmonary rehabilitation, the therapist may perform an extensive interview of all details in Table 2-1 with a major focus on the social situation and client-centered goals. This is usually performed because an extensive chart is not often available and a clear understanding of the patient's perspective is essential to begin treatments often focused on lifestyle changes of exercise training and improving self-management of their chronic respiratory condition. In summary, the physical therapist needs to have a clear perspective of the interview purpose to maximize efficiency and effectiveness in deriving information.

# FOUR MAJOR COMPONENTS OF AN INTERVIEW

The interview usually has 4 major components[1]:

1. *Opening*—when the therapist introduces him- or herself and establishes an atmosphere of empathy.
2. *Questioning*—when the therapist requests information usually by asking open-ended questions. Clarification or more information may be requested. Double or ambiguous questions and technical language should be avoided.
3. *Responding*—when the therapist clarifies or restates their interpretation of the information provided. In addition, response by silence may be appropriate to allow the therapist to observe the patient's nonverbal cues and to allow the patient to gather thoughts on a particular issue.
4. *Summarizing*—when the therapist might summarize the main points that the patient provided and also informs the patient of the next stage in the treatment plan.

# CONTENT OF THE INTERVIEW

The content of the interviewing questions can vary dramatically in different clinical settings and with different patients. Important issues to consider are:

- Purpose of the interview and potential outcomes of physical therapy treatment
- Information available from the chart, other reports, consults, and referral letters
- Current status of patient considering their physical, emotional, and psychological status
- Key information required to determine risks of treatment and ensure safe treatment is carried out
- Time available by therapist and priority of patient

For most patients, information about the main topics outlined in Table 2-1 are required by the therapist to ensure that safe, effective treatment is carried out—whether this information is derived from the interview or from other sources such as a chart and referral letter. For most individual patients, however, the therapist may delve more deeply into particular topic areas to establish the specific needs of a particular patient. In many situations, the therapist may carry out structured questionnaires or initiate additional interview processes by other health professionals to follow up on pertinent issues such as:

- Assessment by the social worker, psychologist, chaplain, or other health care professional
- Utilization of well-established, valid, health-related quality of life; functional status; or depression questionnaires
- Interview of family members, caregivers, or nursing home staff to gather more information about the home situation

# REFERENCE

1. Croft JJ. Interviewing in physical therapy. *Phys Ther*. 1980;60:1033-1036.

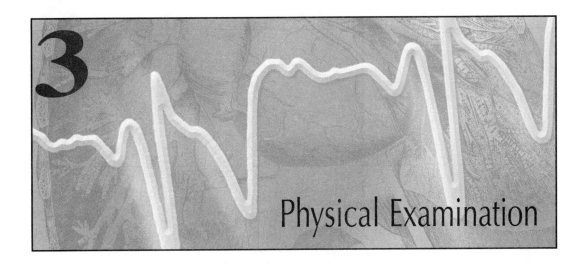

# OBJECTIVES

At the end of this chapter, the reader should be able to:
1. List and describe relevant features of the patient that should be inspected
2. Perform palpation of the chest wall and periphery
3. Describe the steps to measure vitals including radial pulse, respiratory rate, blood pressure, and oxygen saturation

# BRIEF DESCRIPTION

The physical examination consists of 4 major parts: inspecting different features of the patient for signs consistent with respiratory and/or cardiovascular disease; palpating chest wall and periphery; measuring vitals; and auscultating breath sounds. Details describing auscultating breath sounds are described in Chapter 4.

# INSPECTION

Inspection of the patient begins as soon as the therapist enters the room. Patient expression, posture, type of bed and surrounding equipment should be inspected. The therapist should focus on the following aspects of the patient.

1. General
   - Is the patient comfortable?
   - Is the patient in pain?
   - Is the patient in respiratory distress?
   - What is the build of the patient—stocky, thin, cachectic?

2. Position of the patient
   - In what position is the patient?
   - Is it a good position that will optimize recovery and minimize complications?

3. Face
   - What is the patient's expression—relaxed, anxious, distressed?
   - Is the patient awake and alert, or disoriented?
   - Are the patient's lips pink or cyanotic (bluish)?
   - Is the patient performing pursed lip breathing?
   - Is the patient breathing heavily with nostril flaring?

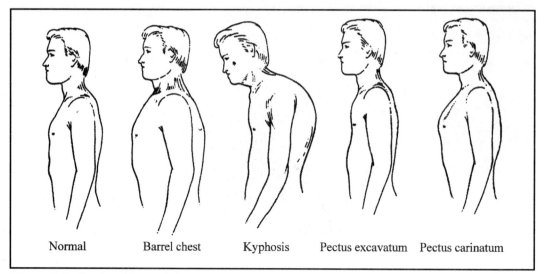

| Normal | Barrel chest | Kyphosis | Pectus excavatum | Pectus carinatum |

**Figure 3-1.** Configurations of chest wall. (Reprinted from *Textbook of Physical Diagnoses—History and Examination,* 2nd ed, Swartz MH, Copyright [1994], with permission from Elsevier.)

**Figure 3-2.** Intercostal indrawing refers to the inward movement of the intercostal spaces during inspiration. It is observed with increased inspiratory efforts especially in individuals with severe obstructive lung disease.

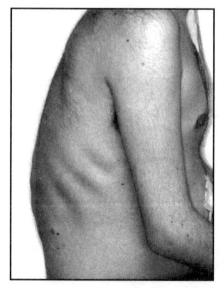

4. Neck
   - Is the patient using accessory muscles of inspiration for breathing at rest (ie, trapezius, sternocleidomastoid)?
   - Is there jugular venous distension? Distension of the jugular veins can be best observed when the patient is lying with the neck at a 45-degree angle of flexion.
5. Chest and its movement
   - What is the shape of the chest wall? See Figure 3-1. Is the chest wall symmetrical?
   - What is the pattern of breathing? Shallow or deep? Rhythmical?
   - Is there an increased effort of breathing or fatigue as shown by:
     o Indrawing—at the level of diaphragm, supraclavicular fossa, or intercostal spaces (Figure 3-2)?
     o High respiratory rate (RR)—Is the RR greater than 30 breaths per minute?
     o Asynchronous rib cage and abdominal excursion, which can be indicative of inspiratory muscle fatigue?

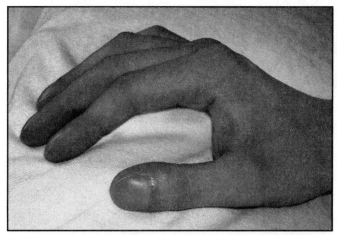

**Figure 3-3.** Clubbing of fingers occurs in individuals with severe respiratory disease. It refers to the enlargement of the distal phalanges (see thumb) and the loss of the angle at the base of the nail bed (see finger tips).

6. Skin
   - Is the skin pink and healthy or does is show pallor? Is the person sweating (diaphoretic)?
   - Does the skin have a bluish tinge (cyanosis) centrally or peripherally?
   - Are there scars or bruises?
   - Are there recent or old surgical incisions—evidence of healing or infection?
   - Are there reddened areas suggestive of prolonged pressure?
   - Are there trophic changes suggestive of arterial insufficiency? Dry, scaly skin, thick, down-turned nails, hair loss?

7. Periphery—ie, extremities
   - Is there clubbing of the fingers or toes (Figure 3-3)?
   - Is there edema? If so, how much?

8. Lines attached to the patient—look for and identify every line and lead going into or leaving the patient. Ensure they are connected properly, are not kinked, and are in a good position for their role. Chapter 20 provides more details about the lines and leads. Some of these lines and leads include:
   - Intravenous line(s)—to provide fluids and medications
   - Oxygen tube via nasal cannula or face mask
   - Feeding tube or nasogastric tube
   - Urinary catheter
   - Drainage tubes from surgical incisions, pericardial, pleural, or mediastinal cavities
   - EKG lines
   - Ear or finger probe leading to oximeter to measure oxygen saturation
   - Other lines such as central lines

# PALPATION

1. Chest wall expansion—Symmetry and amount of chest wall excursion can be assessed by having the therapist lightly place their hands on the patient's chest anteriorly or posteriorly (Figure 3-4) and then asking the patient to inspire deeply to total lung capacity. It is difficult to specifically report the magnitude of chest wall excursion using this technique. An alternative technique is to measure chest expansion using a tape measure at the level of the axilla and xiphoid. Normative values are available; however, there is a large degree of intrasubject variability even in healthy subjects. In a recent study, the standard deviation ranged from 25% to 62% in people aged 20 and older.[1]

2. Periphery—A variety of different aspects should be evaluated in the extremities depending on the admitting or referral diagnoses.

**Figure 3-4.** Evaluation of chest wall expansion. (A) Position of therapist's hands to assess the lower anterior chest wall movement. (B) Position of therapist's hands to assess the lower posterior chest wall movement.

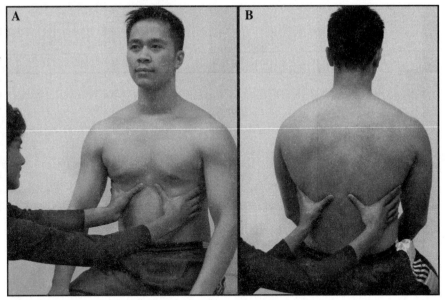

- Are the fingers and toes cold or warm to touch? This is especially important to evaluate circulation and to determine if accurate measurements will be obtained using finger probe oximetry.
- Are the ROM and strength of the limbs within normal range? This should be specifically examined if a recent surgical incision could potentially inhibit ROM. Also, this should be evaluated when the person is engaging in a regular training program.
- Does palpation elicit any joint pain?
- Is there edema and is it pitting—ie, when you gently press your finger tips in, does an indentation occur?

# MONITORING VITALS

The monitoring of vitals is important to evaluate the baseline status of the patient as well as their response to position change, mobilization, and exercise. Some measures, such as blood pressure, heart rate, and respiratory rate, are immediately responsive to the environment and internal factors of the patients. Thus, it is important that the condition of the patient and environment be considered and controlled for to provide a quiet, relaxing atmosphere if possible. Note that the heart rate (HR) and blood pressure (BP) values are often higher the first time you measure them in a client. For the patient with a respiratory condition, the monitoring of oxygen saturation ($SpO_2$) is usually essential, whereas when assessing the patient with a cardiovascular condition, a greater emphasis is placed on monitoring HR, BP, and electrocardiogram (EKG) as indicated.

1. Pulse (HR)—The heart rate provides limited information that the person is stable at rest and that they are coping with increased activity.

- In most cases the radial pulse is determined. Two or 3 fingers (not your thumb) are placed just lateral to the flexor tendons on the radial side of the wrist. Gentle pressure is applied and alleviated until the pulse is palpated and counted for 15 seconds. This value is multiplied by 4 to determine the beats per minute.
- The carotid pulse is preferred when the patient is supine or has fainted because it is easier to access and is stronger than the radial pulse. It is usually not measured in a new patient that is exercising because some individuals experience a vasovagal response and can faint when this region of the neck is palpated.
- Peripheral pulses can be palpated if peripheral arterial insufficiency is suspected but these are hard to quantify and lack reliability between clinicians.[2] Thus, Doppler ultrasound is used to obtain more accurate measures of blood pressure and circulation to the periphery.

Table 3-1

## Normal Ranges for Heart Rate, Respiration Rate, Oxygen Saturation, and Blood Pressure

| Age | Beats per minute | Breaths/min | $SpO_2$ (%) | BP |
|---|---|---|---|---|
| Infants | 120 to 160 | 30 to 60 | 100 | 74 to 100/50 to 70 |
| Adolescents | 60 to 90 | 12 to 16 | 100 | 94 to 140/62 to 88 |
| Adults | 60 to 100 | 12 to 16 | 95 to 100 | <120/<80*4 |

* See Chapter 19—Cardiovascular Condition—for more details about abnormal blood pressure and the different stages of hypertension

2. RR—Is usually assessed by observing the movement of the chest wall and/or abdomen. It is very important that the person is unaware that these measures are being taken and that the therapist does not place his or her hand on the person's chest wall or abdomen to take these measures; otherwise, the patient may consciously alter his or her RR and an inaccurate measure of RR will be obtained.

3. Saturation of Oxygen by Pulse Oximetry ($SpO_2$)—Oxygen saturation (the percentage of hemoglobin that is fully bound with oxygen) can be measured directed from the arterial blood gas sample ($SaO_2$) or indirectly using pulse oximetry by attaching a probe to the ear, finger, or various other parts of the body ($SpO_2$). There is more error in the $SpO_2$ than the $SaO_2$ measure. Very inaccurate measures will be obtained if the probe is not properly attached, when there is increased movement of the probe, and if there is poor circulation or increased pigmentation peripherally. Some oximeters have an indicator light or waveform read-out to provide confirmation of a good reading. Measurement of $SpO_2$ should be carefully done, and potential errors of measurement need to be considered and eliminated. If the palpated pulse and oximeter pulse rates match, there is a higher possibility of an accurate oximeter reading. Even when the oximeter is reading accurately, there is a ±2% to 3% error in readings between 85% and 100%. The error of measurement is larger when $SpO_2$ readings are at lower percentages.

4. BP

    • BP measurements are straightforward to do and the equipment is very inexpensive. BP is one of the simplest and most informative measures that can indicate that the person is not coping with increased exertion. In other words, if the BP drops while the activity level is increasing, it is an ominous sign that the heart is not coping with the increased workload.

    • BP is measured by positioning the bare arm, unrestricted by clothing, palm of hand facing up with the arm resting at the level of the heart. The patient should rest for 5 minutes before the measurement. The cuff of the sphygmomanometer (BP cuff) is wrapped around the upper arm of the patient with the bladder of the cuff positioned over the brachial artery approximately 2 to 3 centimeters above the crease of the elbow. Care should be taken to ensure that the tubing from the BP cuff is not rubbing on anything. The therapist places the diaphragm of the stethoscope on the antecubital (elbow) fossa. The cuff is inflated to approximately 160 mmHg (if the systolic pressure is not known) or approximately 30 mmHg above the expected systolic pressure and then the pressure is slowly released at 2 mmHg per second while listening for:

        o Systolic pressure—the first appearance of clear, repetitive, tapping sounds
        o Diastolic pressure—when the tapping sounds disappear[3]

    • If the measured pressure exceeds 140/90, it is recommended that the BP should be remeasured after a 10-minute rest period. Values of BP measured on the first clinical visit and in some situations can be higher because of increased awareness or anxiety of the patient.

    • For those patients who are hypertensive, the pressure of the cuff will need to be inflated above their systolic pressure; for most individuals, however, the peak cuff pressure should be relatively low because high pressures are uncomfortable.

    • Intra-arterial catheterization and Doppler ultrasound are used to obtain more accurate measures of blood pressure especially for those individuals with low pressures and for those in critical care.

Normal ranges for HR, RR, SPO$_2$, and BP are shown in Table 3-1.

Exercise: Draw lines on patient as listed on page 15, item 8. Now try to imagine rolling the patient over onto his or her side or standing the patient and moving them to a chair without disconnecting or pulling one of the lines out of the patient. Keeping track of all the lines and leads when moving the patient will be one of your biggest initial challenges when working in acute care.

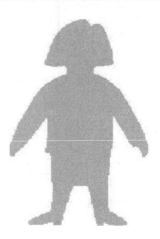

# REFERENCES

1. Kinney LaPier T. Chest wall expansion values in supine and standing across the adult lifespan. *Physical and Occupational Therapy in Geriatrics*. In press.

2. Irwin S, Tecklin JS. *Cardiopulmonary Physical Therapy*. 3rd ed. St. Louis: Mosby; 1995.

3. Campbell NRC, Abbot D, Bass M, et al. Self-measurement of blood pressure: recommendations of the Canadian coalition for high blood pressure prevention and control. *Can J Cardiol*. 1995;11(Suppl):5H-10H.

4. NIH. *Sixth report of the Joint Committee on Prevention, Detection, Evaluation, and Treatment of High Blood Pressure (JNVI), Public Health Service, National Institutes of Health, National Heart, Lung Blood Institute*. NIH Publication no 98-4080; Nov 1997.

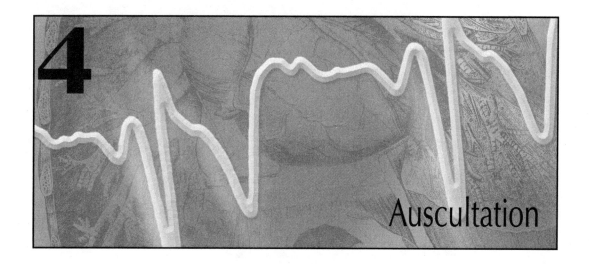

Auscultation

# OBJECTIVES

At the end of this chapter, the reader should be able to:

1. Define normal breath sounds including bronchial, bronchovesicular, and vesicular
2. Describe abnormal breath sounds
3. Describe the 2 major types of adventitious sounds and possible causes of these sounds
4. Auscultate and assess breath sounds in a patient model using appropriate technique

# NORMAL BREATH SOUNDS

Normal breath sounds (Table 4-1) are heard on auscultation over healthy lungs. There may be some variation in quality depending on the thickness and quality of chest wall tissue. Very thin people may have more bronchovesicular breath sounds whereas people with increased subcutaneous fat may have decreased breath sounds.

# ABNORMAL BREATH SOUNDS AND ADVENTITIOUS SOUNDS

Abnormal breath sounds (Table 4-2) and adventitious sounds (Table 4-3) are heard on auscultation over unhealthy regions of the lung with different pathologies. The lung pathology may be within the lung tissue or between the chest wall and lungs. Adventitious sounds are "extra" lung sounds. Crackles are discontinuous sounds—eg, fine crackles are similar to the sound that Velcro makes when it is pulled apart. Wheezes are continuous sounds like the sound made when you blow into the top of a bottle or wooden flute (see Table 4-3).

# HOW TO DO AUSCULTATION TECHNIQUE

- Explain the auscultation technique to the patient in a clear manner using laymen's terms (Table 4-4).
- If possible, position the patient in an upright position, and remove or drape clothing to facilitate easy access to anterior, lateral, and posterior auscultation points (Figure 4-1 and Table 4-5). Thorough explanation and appropriate draping is especially important when auscultating female patients.
- Instruct patient to take "deep" breaths in and out of his or her mouth and allow patient to rest periodically (after 5 to 10 breaths depending on his or her tolerance).
- While holding a stethoscope in an appropriate manner with its diaphragm against skin of chest wall, position the stethoscope diaphragm at the uppermost point anteriorly (Figure 4-1). Listen at this auscultation point for 1 complete respiratory cycle while the patient is breathing in and out of his or her mouth. Next, proceed to the contralateral side and then downward from side to side, listening for a complete respiratory cycle at each auscultation point. Auscultate 4 sites anteriorly, 2 sites laterally, and 10 sites posteriorly—usually in that order.

## Table 4-1

### *Normal Breath Sounds*

| Breath Sound | Quality/Nature | Location (in Healthy) | Respiratory Cycle |
|---|---|---|---|
| Normal or vesicular | Soft; low pitched | Most lung fields; especially peripheral | Inspiration and beginning of expiration. No pause |
| Bronchovesicular | Combination of vesicular and bronchial | Heard over main-stem bronchi especially in thin people | Inspiration and expiration. No pause |
| Bronchial | Harsh, hollow, high-pitched | Over trachea | Inspiration and expiration. Pause between inspiration and expiration |

## Table 4-2

### *Abnormal Breath Sounds*

| Breath Sound | Examples of Conditions |
|---|---|
| Bronchial | Consolidated pneumonia, lobar collapse |
| Decreased or absent | Over pleural effusion, hemothorax, pneumothorax, emphysema, contused lung, obese, elderly |

## Table 4-3

### *Adventitious Sounds*

| Term | Sound Type | Pitch | Examples of Conditions |
|---|---|---|---|
| Crackles (rales) | Discontinuous | Fine (high-pitched) | Atelectasis, interstitial pulmonary fibrosis, sometimes in healthy people |
| | | Coarse (medium or low pitched) | Retained secretions |
| Wheezes (rhonchi) | Continuous | High and/or medium-pitched; can be monophonic or polyphonic | Bronchospasm—eg, asthma, cardiogenic pulmonary edema, chronic obstructive pulmonary disease |
| | | Low-pitched; can be monophonic or polyphonic | Retained secretions in large airways |

Table 4-4

## Example of Instructions to Patient While Auscultating

- I'm going to be listening to how the air moves in and out of your lungs with my stethoscope.
- I will be placing the stethoscope in different locations on the front and back of your chest and would like you to take large breaths in and out through your mouth while I'm listening.
- If you feel light-headed, dizzy, or feel any funny sensations, let me know and I will let you rest before I continue.

**Figure 4-1.** Auscultation points anteriorly, laterally, and posteriorly. The numbering indicates the sequence of the stethescope placement.

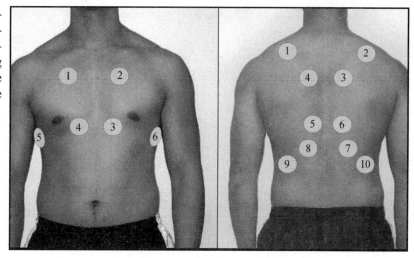

Table 4-5

## Auscultation Points and Examples of Charting

| | Anatomical landmarks | Examples of Charting |
|---|---|---|
| Four sites anteriorly | Two lateral to lower border of manubrium | ULs or upper lung fields anteriorly |
| | Two sites superior and lateral to lower end of sternum | RML or lingula, or mid lung fields anteriorly |
| Two sites laterally | Two sites laterally on mid-axillary line at approximately the fourth to fifth rib | LLs mid-axillary line |
| Ten sites posteriorly | Two sites above the midline of the scapula | Upper lung fields posteriorly |
| | Two sites lateral to spine of scapula at ~ T3 | Upper lung fields posteriorly |
| | Two sites lateral to inferior angle of scapula at ~T7 | Mid lung fields posteriorly |
| | Two sites lateral to ~ T10 | Lower lung fields posteriorly or bases |
| | Two sites slightly lower and more lateral over bases of lungs. | Lower lung fields posteriorly or bases |

Abbreviations: LLs: lower lobes; RML: right middle lobe; T3: third thoracic vertebrae; T7: seventh thoracic vertebrae; T10: tenth thoracic vertebrae; ULs: upper lobes.

- Do not:
    - o  Auscultate through clothing
    - o  Auscultate over bony areas—ie, scapula, spine
    - o  Auscultate too low over the kidneys
    - o  Allow the tubing of the stethoscope to rub against the patient, yourself, or furniture—ie, bedrails
- Do:
    - o  Auscultate low enough to hear over bases of lungs posteriorly
    - o  Listen during an entire respiratory cycle at each auscultation point
    - o  Let the patient rest after every 5 to 10 breaths
- For breath sounds and adventitious sounds, note the part of the respiratory cycle in which you hear them and where you hear them. For examples of charting, see below.

# CHARTING

- Breath sounds heard—ie, *normal* or *bronchial* is the term usually charted. Also, whether or not air entry (a/e) or breath sounds are decreased, and where the type and intensity of breath sound are heard is recorded.

    Eg: Normal breath sounds and a/e good throughout

    Eg: ↓ breath sounds over bases bilaterally

- Charting of adventitious sounds can include: whether or not they are heard, their pitch, the part of the respiratory cycle they are heard, and the location (see Table 4-1 for examples of charting locations).

    Eg: Fine end-inspiratory crackles heard over lower lung fields bilaterally

- Charting of extra pulmonary sounds (if any) can include where and in which part of the respiratory cycle they are heard. The most common extrapulmonary sound is a pleural rub, which sounds like leather rubbing together at the end of inspiration and beginning of expiration.

    Eg: End-inspiratory pleural rub heard over left lateral base

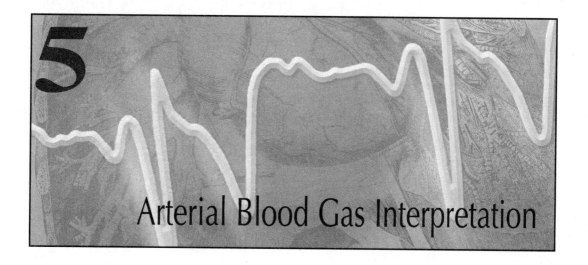

Arterial Blood Gas Interpretation

# OBJECTIVES

At the end of this chapter, the reader should be able to determine:
1. Whether arterial blood gas values are within the normal ranges
2. The presence of primary acid-base disturbances and mixed disorders when examining arterial blood gas values
3. Whether compensation has occurred when examining arterial blood gas values
4. Whether hypoventilation or other causes are the major mechanism(s) contributing to hypoxemia

# BACKGROUND

Arterial blood pH and arterial partial pressure of oxygen ($PaO_2$) need to be maintained within a relatively narrow physiologic range in order for proper function of many bodily functions including enzymes, cell function, and tissue organ function. Arterial blood gas samples provide information about 2 main issues:
1. The acid-base status of the arterial blood
2. The oxygen and carbon dioxide levels in the arterial blood

The relation between the various chemical constituents of the bicarbonate buffer system (the main blood buffer) reflects key information about other buffer systems of the blood and the function of the kidneys.

$$H^+ \ + \ \underset{\text{bicarbonate ion}}{HCO_3^-} \ \leftrightarrow \ \underset{\text{carbonic acid}}{H_2CO_3} \ \leftrightarrow \ H_2O \ + \ CO_2$$

The *law of conservation of matter*, a basic chemistry principle, states that matter is not lost or gained in a chemical reaction and equilibrium is maintained between the different products and reactants of a chemical reaction. This principle for the bicarbonate buffer system is reflected by the following equation:

$$\frac{H^+ \times HCO_3^-}{H_2CO_3} = K \text{ where K equals a constant}$$

This equation can be further modified by a log transformation, multiplying both sides by −1, and substitution of $CO_2$ for $H_2CO_3$. To account for the substitution of $CO_2$ for $H_2CO_3$ the K constant is converted to another constant. All these changes result in the:

Henderson-Hasselbach equation: $\quad pH = pK + \log \dfrac{HCO_3^-}{PaCO_2} \quad$ where $PaCO_2$ is the arterial partial pressure of carbon dioxide

The revisiting of chemistry and log transformation was necessary because it illustrates very *important practical points* to consider:

- The relationship between arterial blood pH, $HCO_3^-$, $PaCO_2$ is defined by basic chemistry principles. If one of these components changes, another one or both will change to conserve matter.
- Interpretation of arterial blood gases to determine the primary acid-base disorders and alveolar ventilation primarily involves looking at these 3 components—the arterial blood pH, $HCO_3^-$, and $PaCO_2$.
- Although the assessment of $PaO_2$ tells you about oxygenation, when interpreting arterial blood gases, examine the $PaO_2$ separately after examining the relationship between pH, $HCO_3^-$, and $PaCO_2$.

# PRIMARY DISORDERS

The primary disorders are 2 different kinds of acidoses and 2 different alkaloses. An acidosis and an alkalosis are processes that produce acid or base, respectively. Acid*emia* and alkal*emia* refer to the state of the blood; an acidemia is when the arterial blood pH is lower than the normal range and an alkalemia is when the arterial blood pH is greater than the normal range.

There are 4 primary acid-base disorders:
- Respiratory disorders—originate from the respiratory system.
  - A *respiratory acidosis* is defined as the process of producing acid ($H^+$) because of retention of $CO_2$ by a decrease in alveolar ventilation.
  - A *respiratory alkalosis* is defined as the process of reducing arterial blood acid ($H^+$) because of blowing off $CO_2$ by an increase in alveolar ventilation.
- Metabolic disorders—might be better termed nonrespiratory because not all metabolic acidoses and alkaloses arise from metabolic sources; they originate from a number of sources in the body—the main ones being the gastrointestinal system and the kidneys.
  - A *metabolic acidosis* is defined as the process of increasing acid ($H^+$) in the blood that can occur by ingestion, infusion or production of a fixed acid or by eliminating $HCO_3^-$. Examples are excessive diarrhea when $HCO_3^-$ is lost, or diabetic ketoacidosis, and lactic acidosis postcardiac arrest when $H^+$ is produced.
  - A *metabolic alkalosis* is defined as the process of reducing arterial blood acid ($H^+$) in the blood that can occur by excessive loss of fixed acids or by ingestion, infusion, or excessive renal absorption of bases— eg, $HCO_3^-$. Examples are overzealous intravenous infusion of sodium bicarbonate and excessive vomiting (which results in loss of the stomach's acidic contents).

The primary disorders occurring alone or in combination as mixed disorders are shown in Table 5-1. More examples of these primary acid-base disorders are listed in Table 5-2.

# CHANGES IN $PaO_2$ FROM AMBIENT AIR TO ARTERIAL BLOOD IN THE HEALTHY YOUNG ADULT

*Ambient Air:*
Dry inspired air is 21% oxygen resulting in a partial pressure of oxygen of                    ~160 mmHg
        (21% of atmospheric pressure at sea level  =  $0.21 \times 760 = 160$)

*Trachea:*
Hydration of inspired air results in an increase in $PH_2O$ and a decrease of the $PO_2$ to        ~150 mmHg
                                =  $0.21 \times (760 - 47)$

*Alveoli:*
Mixing of inspired air with CO2 that exchanges across the alveolar-capillary barrier results
                                in a further decrease of the $PO_2$ to      ~110 mmHg
This is termed the *alveolar partial pressure* ($PAO_2$).

*Arterial Blood:*
Incomplete diffusion of $O_2$ across the alveolar-capillary membrane results in a small drop
                                of the $PaO_2$ to      ~100 mmHg

Table 5-1

## Primary and Mixed Acid-Base Disorders

| Primary Disorders | Mixed Disorders |
|---|---|
| A. Respiratory | A. Mixed respiratory-metabolic disorders |
|   1. Acidosis |   1. Respiratory acidosis and metabolic acidosis |
|     a) Acute |   2. Respiratory acidosis and metabolic alkalosis |
|     b) Chronic |   3. Respiratory alkalosis and metabolic acidosis |
|   2. Alkalosis |   4. Respiratory alkalosis and metabolic alkalosis |
|     a) Acute | |
|     b) Chronic | B. Mixed metabolic disorders |
| |   1. Metabolic acidosis and metabolic alkalosis |
| B. Metabolic |   2. Normal plus elevated anion gap* acidosis |
|   1. Acidosis |   3. Mixed high anion gap acidosis |
|   2. Alkalosis |   4. Mixed normal anion gap acidosis |
| | |
| | C. "Triple" disorders |
| |   1. Metabolic acidosis, metabolic alkalosis, and respiratory acidosis |
| |   2. Metabolic acidosis, metabolic alkalosis, and respiratory alkalosis |

* The anion gap is an indication of the quantity of added acids and equals $[Na^+]$ - $[Cl^-]$ - $[HCO3^-]$. It is helpful in detecting mixed disorders and determining the response to therapy.[1]

# COMPENSATION

Compensation of acid-base disturbances in the blood can occur from 3 main sources. The length of time for action and extent of buffering by each of these systems varies. Acid-base buffers are solutions of 2 or more chemical compounds that prevent significant shifts in $H^+$ concentration.

1. *Buffers in body fluids* include different buffers and proteins in the blood. In the body fluids, there are 3 main buffer systems—the bicarbonate buffer, the phosphate buffer, and protein buffer.

   - The *bicarbonate buffer* (see equation below) is a relatively weak buffer chemically but a very effective buffer in the body because 2 of its components can be modified readily—$CO_2$ by the respiratory system and $HCO_3^-$ by the kidneys.

$$H^+ + HCO_3^- \leftrightarrow H_2CO_3 \leftrightarrow H_2O + CO_2$$

   - The *phosphate buffer* system is effective because its maximum buffering power occurs near the pH of blood. It is an effective intracellular buffer because of the high concentrations of intracellular phosphates.

   - *Proteins* are considered to be the most plentiful body fluid buffer.

   Buffers in body fluids can act almost immediately.

2. The *respiratory system* can modify acid-base balance by retention or blowing off of $CO_2$. The relationship between $CO_2$ and $H^+$ is shown by the equation below. Retention of $CO_2$ shifts the equation to the left producing more $H^+$. Excessive $H^+$ can be combined with $HCO_3^-$ to produce $H_2CO_3$ which can be broken down to form $H_2O$ and $CO_2$. Blowing off excessive $CO_2$ is an effective means of eliminating excessive $H^+$ in individuals with a healthy respiratory systems.

$$H^+ + HCO_3^- \leftrightarrow H_2CO_3 \leftrightarrow H_2O + CO_2$$

The respiratory system can begin buffering acid-base disturbances within minutes.

3. The *kidneys* can eliminate $H^+$ and $HCO_3^-$ or retain $H^+$ and $HCO_3^-$. The kidneys can provide very effective long-term buffering but take hours to days for their buffering capacity to be complete.

## Table 5-2

# *Causes of Primary Disorders*

### *Causes of Metabolic Alkalosis*

| *Chloride Responsive* | *Chloride Unresponsive* |
|---|---|
| Gastrointestinal Causes | Adrenal Disorders |
|   Vomiting |   Hyperaldosteronism |
|   Nasogastric suction |   Cushing syndrome |
|   Chloride-wasting diarrhea |   1) pituitary |
|   Villous adenoma—colon |   2) adrenal |
| Diuretic therapy |   3) ectopic ACTH |
| Post-hypercapnia | Exogenous Steroid |
| Carbenicillin or penicillin |   Gluco- or mineralocorticoid |
| |   Licorice ingestion |
| |   Carbenoxalone |
| | Refeeding alkalosis |
| | Alkali ingestion |

### *Causes of Respiratory Alkalosis*

| | |
|---|---|
| Anxiety | Hypoxia |
| CNS Disorders | Ventilator-induced |
|   Cerebrovascular accident | Pregnancy |
|   Tumor | Liver Insufficiency |
|   Infection | Pulmonary edema (mild) |
| Hormones-Drugs | Lung Disease |
|   Salicylates |   Restrictive disorders |
|   Catecholamines |   (early) |
|   Progesterone |   Pulmonary emboli |
|   Analeptic overdose |   Pneumonia |
| Gram negative sepsis | |

### *Causes of Metabolic Acidosis*

| *Elevated Anion Gap* | *Normal Anion Gap* |
|---|---|
| Renal failure | Hypokalemic acidosis |
| Ketoacidosis |   Renal tubular acidosis |
|   Starvation |   1) Proximal |
|   Diabetes mellitus |   2) Distal |
|   Alcohol associated |   3) Buffer deficiency |
|   Glycogenosis I |     a) Phosphate |
|   Defects in gluconeogenesis |     b) Ammonia |
| Lactic acidosis |   Diarrhea |
| |   Post-hypocapnic acidosis |
| Toxins | |
|   Methanol | Uretheral diversions |
|   Ethylene glycol |   1) Uretero-sigmoidostomy |
|   Salicylates |   2) Ileal bladder |
|   Paraldehyde |   3) Ileal ureter |
| | Normal-Hyperkalemic Acidosis |
| |   Early renal failure |
| |   Hydronephrosis |
| |   Addition of HCl |
| |   1) $NH_4Cl$ |
| |   2) Arginine—HCl |
| |   3) Lysine—HCl |
| | Sulfur toxicity |

### *Causes of Respiratory Acidosis*

| | |
|---|---|
| CNS Depression | Impaired Lung Motion |
|   Sedatives |   Pleural effusion |
|   Primary or secondary |   Pneumothorax |
|     lesions of resp. center | Acute-Chronic Lung Disease |
|     (eg. trauma, ischemia) |   Acute obstruction |
| Neuromuscular Disorders |   1) Aspiration |
|   Myopathies (eg, mus- |   2) Tumor |
|     cular dystrophies, |   3) Spasm |
|     potassium depletion) |     a) Laryngospasm |
|   Neuropathies (eg, Guillain- |     b) Bronchospasm |
|     Barré, polio) | |
| | Chronic obstructive |
| Thoracic Cage Limitation |   diseases |
|   Kyphoscoliosis | Severe pneumonia |
|   Scleroderma |   or pulmonary edema |
|   Crash injury | |
| Miscellaneous | |
|   Ventilator malfunction | |
|   Cardiopulmonary arrest | |

Abbreviations: ACTH: adrenocorticotrophic hormone; CNS: central nervous system; HCl: hydrochloric acid

Table adapted from Narins RG, Emmett M. Simple and mixed acid-base disorders: a practical approach. *Medicine.* 1980; 59(3):161-187.

Table 5-3

## Normal Ranges and Means for Arterial Blood Gas Values

| Normal Values | Range | Mean |
|---|---|---|
| pH | 7.36 to 7.44 | 7.4 |
| $PaCO_2$ | 35 to 45 | 40 mmHg |
| $HCO_3^-$ | 23 to 27 | 25 mEq/L |
| $PaO_2$ | 80 to 100 mmHg | lower when older |
| BE | −4 to +4 | 0 |

Abbreviations: BE: base excess

Table 5-4

## Primary Disorders and Compensation

| Primary Disorder | Acid-Base Disturbance | Compensation |
|---|---|---|
| Respiratory Acidosis | ↑ $PaCO_2$ | ↓ $H^+$ and/or ↑ $HCO_3^-$ |
| Respiratory Alkalosis | ↓ $PaCO_2$ | ↑ $H^+$ and ↓ $HCO_3^-$ |
| Metabolic Acidosis | ↑ $H^+$ or ↓ $HCO_3^-$ | ↓ $PaCO_2$ |
| Metabolic Alkalosis | ↓ $H^+$ or ↑ $HCO_3^-$ | ↑ $PaCO_2$ |

Abbreviations: ↓ : decrease; ↑ : increase

# CAUSES OF HYPOXEMIA

Hypoxemia refers to a decreased oxygen level in arterial blood whereas hypoxia refers to a decreased oxygen level in tissue. The 4 main causes of hypoxemia include: alveolar hypoventilation, diffusion impairment, shunt, and ventilation-perfusion mismatching in the lungs. A fifth cause that can be very relevant to people with moderate to severe chronic lung disease is a decreased inspired oxygen concentration that can occur at higher altitudes or during a plane flight. When assessing arterial blood gases it is important to keep in mind that healthy younger adults have a $PaO_2$ of 100 mmHg, whereas older adults have a progressively lower $PaO_2$; a normal $PaO_2$ for a healthy 70- to 80-year-old is approximately 75 to 80 mmHg.

# APPROACH TO ARTERIAL BLOOD GAS INTERPRETATION

1. Identify whether or not each parameter is within the normal range. If the value is outside the normal range, determine by how much (determine difference from mean), and what direction. See Table 5-3 for normal values.
2. Determine the primary process and whether compensation or mixed disorders are present. Do the directional changes match any of the patterns shown for the primary disorders (Table 5-4)? Check the pH first, $PaCO_2$, then $HCO_3^-$, and $PaO_2$ last.
3. Refine your decision.
   - Determine whether compensation has occurred. If the change in $HCO_3^-$ is greater or less than expected for an acute disorder, 2 disorders or compensation may be present. See first Rule of Thumb (Table 5-5).

Table 5-5

## Rules of Thumb and Points to Consider When Refining ABG Diagnoses

### Two Rules of Thumb

1. Acute respiratory acidosis and alkalosis—relation between plasma bicarbonate ion and $PaCO_2$
   - *During an acute respiratory acidosis*—an increase in $PaCO_2$ of 10 mmHg results in the $HCO_3^-$ increasing 1 mEq/L
   - *During an acute respiratory alkalosis*—a decrease in $PaCO_2$ of 10 mmHg results in the $HCO_3^-$ decreasing 2 mEq/L

If the change in $HCO_3^-$ is greater, then compensation has occurred.
   - Generally, in order to *differentiate between acute and chronic respiratory acidosis*, if the $HCO_3^-$ is greater than 30 mEq/L, then a chronic respiratory acidosis is present.

2. Is hypoventilation (decreased alveolar ventilation) the major mechanism for hypoxemia?
   - If *hypoventilation* is the major mechanism for *hypoxemia*, the $PaO_2$ should only be decreased 1 mmHg for every 1 mm Hg increase in $PaCO_2$. If there is a greater decrease in the $PaO_2$, there must be other causes for the hypoxemia—ie, ventilation-perfusion mismatch, shunt, and/or diffusion impairment.

### Two Points to Consider

1. *Chronic or compensated metabolic acidosis and alkalosis*—should happen fairly quickly via changes in ventilation by the respiratory system. The $PaCO_2$ should move in the same direction as the pH. If compensation has occurred, the $PaCO_2$ should approximate the 2 numbers to the right of the decimal of the pH—eg, if pH is 7.3 then the $PaCO_2$ should be 30.[1]
2. *Physiological compensation never returns the pH to the normal range except in a respiratory alkalosis.* If the pH is normal and 1 disorder has been identified that is not a respiratory alkalosis, look for another.

---

- There are 4 major causes of hypoxemia. The second rule of thumb will provide some support to whether a lower $PaO_2$ is due to less alveolar ventilation or other causes of lung pathology—ie, diffusion impairment, ventilation-perfusion mismatch, and/or shunt
- Points to consider (see Table 5-5) provide 2 final checks to ascertain if your hunch about the arterial blood gas disorder is correct.

# OXIMETRY AND SATURATION OF OXYGEN

$SaO_2$ is the percent of hemoglobin that is fully bound to oxygen, as measured from an arterial blood sample. A pulse oximeter can estimate the $SaO_2$ by examining the different light absorption of oxyhemoglobin and deoxyhemoglobin and this estimate is termed the $SpO_2$. Widespread use of oximetry has resulted in the $SpO_2$ being used extensively to estimate arterial oxygenation levels. It is essential to note that $SpO_2 \neq PaO_2$. This is the most important point of this chapter so it will be repeated. $SaO_2 \neq PaO_2$. Examine an oxygen dissociation curve (Figure 5-1—$PaO_2$ versus $SaO_2$ plot) carefully and complete Table 5-6. Memorize the last 3 rows of this table and *never confuse $SpO_2$ with $PaO_2$.* A $PaO_2$ of 55 mmHg is usually the absolute cut-off for discontinuing exercise whereas if one confused this with a cut-off of a $SpO_2$ of 55%, this would correspond to the patient continuing to exercise until a $PaO_2$ of 30 to 40 mmHg—*a very grave error indeed.*

Table 5-7 shows the acceptable and poor arterial blood gas values. Another point to keep in mind is that if the arterial blood gas values deteriorate quickly, it is usually more serious for the patient than if the arterial blood gases slowly deteriorate over weeks or months.

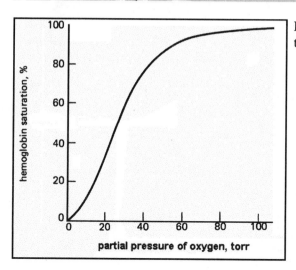

**Figure 5-1.** Matching values of oxygen saturation and arterial partial pressure of oxygen.

Table 5-6

## Matching Values of Oxygen Saturation and Arterial Partial Pressure of Oxygen

Complete the table using the oxygen-dissociation curve in Figure 5-1. These are the values one would expect with a normal body temperature and pH. If the temperature were higher and the pH were lower, the $SaO_2$ would be lower for a given $PaO_2$.

Note: $SaO_2 \neq PaO_2$

| $SaO_2$ (%) | $PaO_2$ (mmHg) |
|---|---|
| 75 | |
| 83 | |
| 85 | |
| 89 | |
| 93 | |

Table 5-7

## Acceptable and Poor Arterial Blood Gas Values

| | pH | $PaCO_2$ (mmHg) | $HCO_3^-$ (mEq/L) | $SpO_2$ (%) |
|---|---|---|---|---|
| Very Poor | 7.0 | 80 | 5 | 85 |
| Poor | 7.2 | 60 | 15 | 90 |
| Acceptable ↔ Normal | 7.4 | 40 | 25 | 95 |
| Poor | 7.6 | | 35 | |
| Very Poor | 7.8 | | 45 | |

# REFERENCES

1. Halperin ML, Goldstein MB. *Fluid, Electrolyte, and Acid-Base Physiology. A Problem-Based Approach.* Philadelphia: WB Saunders Co; 1999.
2. Narins RG, Emmett M. Simple and mixed acid-base disorders: a practical approach. *Medicine.* 1980; 59(3):161-187.

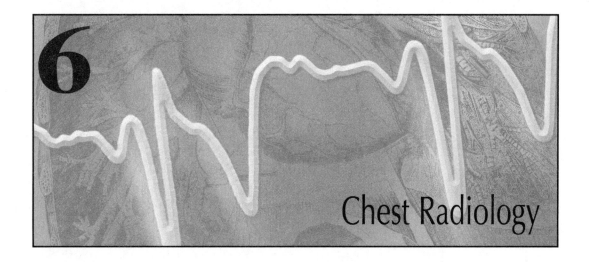

**Chest Radiology**

## OBJECTIVES

Upon completion of this chapter, the reader should be able to:
1. List factors that affect the opacity and lucency of a normal chest x-ray
2. List the common projection views and how anatomical structures might be affected by different views
3. Develop a systematic approach for observing a normal chest x-ray
4. Define major signs of lung pathology on a chest x-ray including: atelectasis; space-occupying lesions; silhouette sign; and airspace, interstitial, or vascular patterns

## RADIOLUCENCY AND OPACITY

The density of different body tissues determines radiolucency and opacity. Structures that are more dense do not allow as many x-rays to pass through the body to penetrate the chest x-ray plate. This results in more dense structures appearing more radio-opaque or white. In contrast, less dense tissue allows more x-rays to pass through the body to penetrate the chest x-ray plate and appear blacker.

### Exercise

Place a piece of gauze on an overhead projector and lay a metal object beside it (paper clip or bracelet). One could also place a piece of gauze or paper clip in path of light from a small lamp. Which object is denser? Which object allows more light to pass through it and which object blocks more of the light?

Structures that can be observed on a chest x-ray issues are shown in Figure 6-1, from the least dense (radiolucent) to the most dense (radio-opaque). Normal aerated lung tissue allows more x-rays to pass through to the x-ray plate and thus appears blacker or radiolucent. In contrast, bone absorbs more x-rays and appears whiter or radio-opaque. Metal objects appear the most radio-opaque.

An overexposed chest x-ray, which has absorbed more x-rays, is more radiolucent relative to normal exposure. An underexposed chest x-ray that has absorbed fewer x-rays is more radio-opaque relative to normal exposure.

## CHEST X-RAY VIEWS OR PROJECTIONS

The most common views are posterior-anteriors and lateral projections:
1. *Posterior-anterior (PA)*—For the PA view, the plate is anterior and x-rays penetrate from posterior to anteriorly. This gives maximum clarity of anterior structures and the anterior structures will not be magnified relative to an anterior-posterior (AP) view. When is a PA chest x-ray usually taken?
2. *Lateral*—The plate is in contact with the left side of the thorax and the x-rays penetrate from right to left. When are a lateral and a PA chest x-ray taken?

**Figure 6-1.** Density of tissue and radio-opacity.

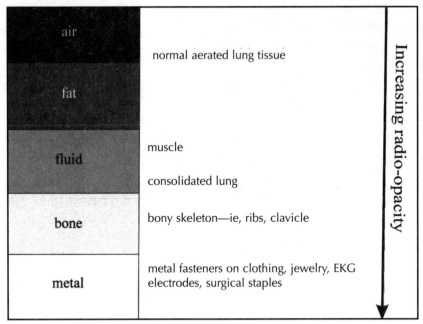

PA and lateral views are the most common but an AP is usually done when a portable x-ray is required of a patient on bed rest. This does not usually show some thoracic structures as clearly compared to a PA because of the direction of x-ray penetration and the inability to position the patient in an upright and symmetrical fashion. The plate is behind the person's back and the x-rays penetrate from front to back. The heart can appear enlarged and its outline will be softer because the heart is farther away from the x-ray plate.

## Exercise

Place an object (your hand or pen) in front of a light source and observe the size of the shadow cast. Move the object closer toward the light source. What happens to the size of the shadow of the object when it is moved closer to the light source and farther away from the surface where the shadow is reflected? What happens to the clarity of the shadow? Are the edges of the shadow crisper or less crisp as it moves further from the surface where it is reflected? Similarly when the structures are close to the x-ray plate, their outlines will appear crisper—ie, the heart shadow will be crisper in the PA than the AP because the heart is closer to the x-ray plate in the PA.

The *lateral decubitus* x-ray, a less common view, is taken when the person is lying on his or her side. Fluid shifts to the lowermost region. Thus, if a pleural effusion is suspected, an x-ray might be taken in the upright and lateral decubitus positions. In the upright position, fluid will tend to collect at the bases of the lungs and thus increased radio-opacity will be apparent at the bases. In the lateral decubitus position, fluid will tend to collect at the lower most borders of the lung and thus, increased radio-opacity will be apparent laterally in the lower-most lung.

# A SYSTEMATIC APPROACH TO
# ASSESSMENT OF CHEST X-RAYS

Identify the following features on normal chest x-ray (Figure 6-2).
1. Identify details of the film—patient's name, age, date film was taken, patient's position, view of film (PA, AP, lateral or other), orientate the film properly on screen (note right versus left or posterior versus anterior). Note whether various lines or leads are inserted or crossing the chest—eg, endotracheal tube, nasogastric tube, EKG leads, and central lines.

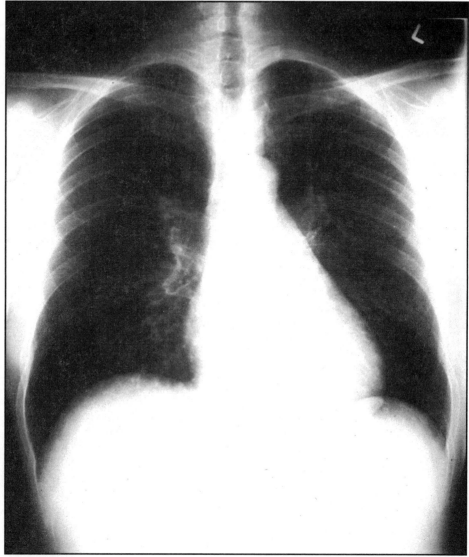

**Figure 6-2.** Normal chest x-ray.

2. Assess quality of film.
   - *Exposure*—Can you see the intervertebral spaces through the shadow of the trachea? If the chest x-ray has normal exposure, the intervertebral spaces should be apparent superimposed on the shadow of the trachea and are much less apparent superimposed on the shadow of the heart. If the intervertebral spaces are clearly apparent superimposed on the shadow of the heart, the film is overexposed (or too black). If the intervertebral spaces are not apparent superimposed on the shadow of the trachea and heart, the film is underexposed (too white).
   - *Centering and symmetry of thorax*—The sternoclavicular joints should be an equal distance from the spines of the thoracic vertebrae. The clavicles should be level and symmetrical.
   - *Inspiratory volume or effort*—The anterior end of the sixth rib should clear or just bisect the diaphragm on the right side. If more ribs are apparent above the hemi-diaphragm, the inspiratory volume is large or the patient is hyperinflated. If fewer ribs are apparent above the hemidiaphragm, the inspiratory volume is small or the patient has restricted lung volumes.

3. Assess the specific features related to the patient's condition.
   - *Bony skeleton*—Look at the position of clavicles, scapulae, and ribs. Are the scapulae retracted off the lung fields? Are the ribs close together? Far apart? More horizontal than usual? Are there any fractures present?
   - *Soft tissues*
     - o *Heart*—The mediastinal shadow should be slightly to the left of center and in contact with the diaphragm. The cardiothoracic index is the ratio of the width of the heart to the width of the chest. The cardiothoracic index should be about one-third to one-half. Look for the aortic arch, also known as the aortic knob, to the left of the midline. A cardiophrenic angle is the intersection of the vertical curvature of the heart shadow and the horizontal curvature of the hemidiaphragm. Look for sharp cardiophrenic angles on the right and left side of the heart.
     - o *Hilum*—Normally, the hilum is 1 to 2 cm higher on the left than on the right side of the mediastinum. What does it consist of?
     - o *Diaphragm*—The right hemidiaphragm is higher (because the liver is beneath it). The left side can have gas bubbles beneath it because of gas in the stomach. A costophrenic angle is the intersection between the lateral chest wall and the diaphragm. Costophrenic angles should be deep (an acute angle) and sharply defined. Locate the right and left costophrenic angles.
     - o *Trachea*—The shadow of the trachea should be in the midline. It is a vertical radiolucent (black) shadow located over the cervical spinous processes that extends inferiorly below the clavicles. If an endotracheal tube is in place, its distal tip should be at the level of the clavicular heads.
     - o *Breast shadows*—Breast shadows in females should be identified. These are semi-circular shadows observed over the lungs fields and lateral aspects of the chest wall. They can be located lower than expected on heavier or older female patients.
     - o *Subcutaneous tissue*—Look for subcutaneous emphysema or other unusual features (swelling, fibromas, obesity).
   - *Lung fields and boundaries*
     - o Check the *boundaries of lung* to ensure that they are in contact with the chest wall and diaphragm. Vascular markings should be faint and extend out in a branch-like manner to the periphery of the lung fields. The lung fields should not be completely radiolucent or black but usually have vascular markings that extend from the mediastinum and become progressively more faint toward the periphery.
     - o Does there appear to be any *fluid* or *air* present? Air will be black; fluid will be white.
     - o Is there *pleural thickening*? Look along the periphery of the lung fields for this feature.
     - o Is there a homogeneous density throughout the lungs or is there *increased opacity* or *lucency*?
     - o Can you see the horizontal (on the right side only) or oblique (can be observed on the left and right side) fissures? If so, are they in their normal position? These fissures are only seen with pathology.
     - o Is there *volume loss*?
     - o Is there an *airspace* or an *interstitial* pattern (see explanations below under Pathological Features)?
     - o Can you see an *air-fluid level* or an *air bronchogram* (see explanations under Pathological Features)?
     - o Are the *vascular markings* increased?
     - o Is the *silhouette sign* present or absent? If absent, locate (see explanations under Pathological Features).

# PATHOLOGICAL FEATURES

The silhouette sign (Table 6-1 and Figure 6-3) is the profile of soft tissues superimposed on the lung fields. The silhouette sign is lost when lung pathology is directly adjacent to a soft tissue structure because the density of atelectatic or pneumonic lungs is similarly dense to the soft tissues. Consolidation or collapse density is similar to that of the heart or muscle. If these 2 tissues are in the same plane, the image of the collapsed lung will become confluent with the heart or diaphragm and their respective borders will become obliterated. Its absence is indicative of airspace disease or fluid-occupying lesions.

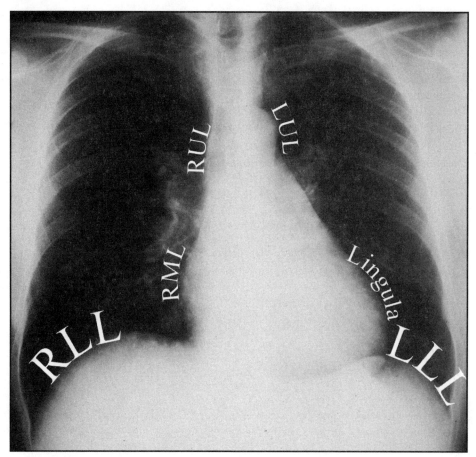

**Figure 6-3.** The silhouette sign.

***

Table 6-1

## *The Silhouette Sign*

| *Shadow of Soft Tissue Structure Lost* | *Location of Lung Pathology* |
| --- | --- |
| Ascending aorta | Right upper lobe |
| Aortic arch | Left upper lobe |
| Upper left heart border | Left upper lobe |
| Lower right heart border | Right middle lobe |
| Lower left heart border | Lingula |
| Right hemi-diaphragm | Right lower lobe |
| Left hemi-diaphragm | Left lower lobe |

Identifying the outline of the soft tissue structure that is no longer observable can indicate the location of lung pathology.

# ATELECTASIS

Soft tissue structures will move toward regions of lung collapse or atelectasis. Atelectasis can be reflected by the following changes on the chest x-ray:

1. Fissures will be outlined by collapsed lung. The horizontal fissure will move upward and the oblique fissures will move downward.
2. The hemi-diaphragm will be elevated on the side of collapse.
3. The trachea, mediastinum, and/or hilar shadows will deviate toward the side of collapse.
4. There will be increased density of the collapsed lobe or segment.
5. There will be compensatory aeration of lung that is not collapsed.

## Space-Occupying Lesions

Space-occupying lesions will result in movement away from the pleural effusion, pneumothorax, or hemothorax. Changes in position will shift the pleural effusion to the dependent (lowermost) region of the lung.

## Three Patterns of Disease on Lung Fields

1. *Airspace or alveolar pattern* is caused by pathology that fills the airspaces or alveoli and thus, the increased opacity is more "fluffy" in appearance. Fluffy is a relative term so don't imagine fluffy white clouds when you're looking for an airspace or alveolar pattern.
2. *Interstitial pattern* is caused by pathology in the interstitial space and thus, the increased opacity is more "netlike" in appearance.
3. *Vascular pattern* is caused by the pulmonary vascular tree being engorged and thus, the increased opacity radiates from the hilum in a branching manner.

## Other Signs of Lung Pathology

- *Air-fluid level* usually results from liquefaction of an abscess. Connective tissue "scarring," which appears as a white ring on the chest x-ray, can surround the abscess. The liquid in the lowermost part of the abscess will appear white with a flat horizontal line across the middle region of the abscess.
- *Air bronchogram* is shown as a radiolucent (black shadow) of a relatively large airway against radio-opaque (white) consolidated lung tissue.

## Other Abnormal Features

Subcutaneous emphysema is pockets of air in the subcutaneous tissue that occurs in some patients after surgery or major trauma. Small radiolucent (black) pockets of air are apparent on the more radio-opaque (white) subcutaneous tissue.

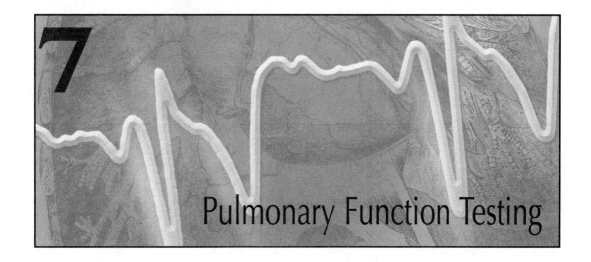

# Pulmonary Function Testing

## OBJECTIVES

Upon completion of this chapter, the reader should be able to:
1. Define lung volumes and lung capacities
2. Define spirometric values ($FEV_1$, FVC, and $FEV_1$/FVC ratio)
3. Describe how lung volumes, lung capacities, and spirometric values vary in obstructive and restrictive lung diseases

The most common tests of lung function are spirometric and lung volume measures. Abbreviations are used for almost all parameters of lung function. Be sure to know what the abbreviation is short for in addition to understanding the definition.

## SPIROMETRY—FORCED EXPIRATORY VOLUMES

For performance of the test, the subject wears nose clips and is positioned in a standard position (either sitting or standing). Following a maximum inspiration, the subject performs a maximal expiration as quickly and forcefully as possible. Three main measures are determined from this test:
1. *Forced Vital Capacity (FVC)* is the total volume of air exhaled with a maximal forced expiratory effort after a full inspiration.
2. *Forced expiratory volume in one second ($FEV_1$)* is the volume of air expired during the first second of a forced vital capacity maneuver.
3. *Ratio of $FEV_1$/FVC ($FEV_1$/FVC)*—The normal value for this ratio is 80%. In other words, most young healthy adults can forcibly blow out 80% of their vital capacity within the first second of expiration.

Figure 7-1 illustrates a spirometric tracing with the measures of $FEV_1$ and FVC. Other measures can be derived from a forced expiratory maneuver, including:
- The peak expiratory flow rate (PEFR), which is the highest flow rate obtained during a forced expiratory maneuver. An estimate of PEFR can be obtained with an inexpensive hand-held flow meter and can be used for home-monitoring of asthma in adults and children.
- The forced expiratory flow from 25% to 75% of the vital capacity ($FEF_{25-75}$) is the average flow rate during this middle half of the forced expiratory vital capacity (see Figure 7-1).

Both the PEFR and $FEF_{25-75}$ have higher coefficients of variation for repeated measures compared to the $FEV_1$ and FVC measures.[1]

## LUNG VOLUMES AND CAPACITIES

Measurement of lung volumes is the second most common pulmonary function test performed. More sophisticated testing equipment is required in order to measure the amount of air remaining in the lungs after a max-

**Figure 7-1.** Spiromet-ric tracing of a healthy 70-kg man. The volumes measured for $FEV_1$ and FVC are shown. $FEF_{25-75}$ is the forced expiratory flow from 25% to 75% of the vital capacity or flow rate during the middle half of the forced vital capacity as shown by the large bracket. The $FEF_{25-75}$ would be the slope of the curve in this part of the maneuver.

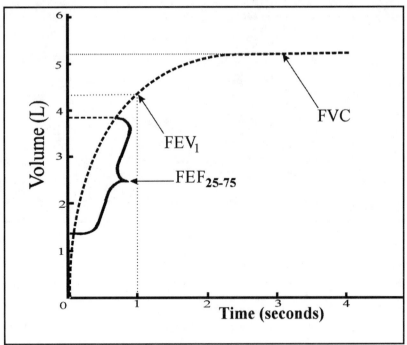

imal expiration. Air remaining in the lung can be evaluated using a helium dilution technique or by pressure plethysmography. Both of these techniques require a significant amount of specialized measuring apparatus.

This pulmonary function test is performed by having the participant wear nose clips while sitting in a plethysmograph or connected to a measuring device that uses helium dilution. The participant breathes in and out normally, and then takes a large inspiration, followed by a relaxed full expiration. In contrast to spirometric measures, the participant is asked to do maximal expiration in an unforced manner.

Four lung volumes and 4 lung capacities are derived from the maneuvers.

## Lung Volumes

Lung volumes cannot be further subdivided and lung capacities consist of a combination of 2 or more standard lung volumes.

1. *Tidal volume (TV or VT)* is the volume of air inhaled or exhaled during breathing. This refers to breathing at rest or during situations when breathing is increased, such as during exercise.
2. *Inspiratory reserve volume (IRV)* is the maximum volume of air that can be inhaled to total lung capacity over and above the tidal volume.
3. *Expiratory reserve volume (ERV)* is the maximum volume of air that can be exhaled from the end-expiratory level or from functional residual capacity (FRC) to residual volume.
4. *Residual volume (RV)* is the volume of air remaining in the lungs after a maximal expiration. RV = total lung capacity (TLC) – VC.

## Lung Capacities

Lung capacities are comprised of more than one lung volume.

1. *Inspiratory capacity (IC)* is the maximal volume of air that can be inhaled. In other words, IC is the difference between TLC and FRC. IC = TLC – FRC. It is also the sum of VT and IRV.
2. *Functional residual capacity (FRC)* is the volume of air remaining in the lungs at the end of an ordinary expiration, ie, at the resting level or end-expiratory level. FRC = RV + ERV.
3. *Vital Capacity (VC)* is the maximum volume of air that can be expelled after a maximum inspiration—ie, from TLC to residual volume. VC = TLC – RV. VC is also the sum of ERV + VT + IRV.
4. *TLC* is the total amount of air in the lungs after a maximal inspiration. It is the sum of all lung volumes. TLC is the sum of RV + ERV + VT + IRV.

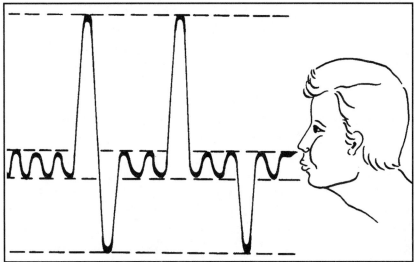

**Figure 7-2.** Tracing of lung volumes and capacities. (Reprinted from *Principles and Practice of Cardiopulmonary Physical Therapy*, 3rd ed., Dean E, Frownfelter D. Copyright [1996] with permission from Elsevier.)

Table 7-1

### Force Expiratory Values and Lung Volumes in Restrictive and Obstructive Lung Disorders

| Interpretation | FVC | FEV1 | FEV$_1$/ FVC ratio | RV | TLC |
|---|---|---|---|---|---|
| Airway obstruction | normal or low | low | low | high | high |
| Lung restriction | low | normal or low | normal or high | normal or low | low |
| Both obstruction and restriction | low | low | low | variable | variable |

# CHANGES IN SPIROMETRY AND LUNG VOLUMES IN VENTILATORY IMPAIRMENT

Two major patterns of ventilatory impairment can be shown by these measures of pulmonary function—an *obstructive* pattern characterized by airways obstruction and a *restrictive* pattern characterized by stiff lungs and/or a stiff chest wall. The main changes in spirometry and lung volumes are shown in Table 7-1.

Many other pulmonary function tests can be performed for clinical and research purposes. The reader is referred to the reference list for description of these tests.

# EXERCISES

1. Figure 7-1 shows a spirometric tracing for a healthy man. Draw in a tracing for a similar sized man with severe obstructive lung disease and a tracing for a man with severe restrictive lung disease.

2. Figure 7-2 (from left to right) shows the tracing when lung volumes and capacities are measured. Label the different lung volumes and lung capacities on this tracing.

# REFERENCES

1. Fraser RG, Paré JA, Paré PD, Fraser RS, Genereux GP. *Diagnosis of Diseases of the Chest*. Philadelphia: WB Saunders; 1988;431.

# BIBLIOGRAPHY

Cherniack RM. *Pulmonary Function Testing*. 2nd ed. Philadelphia: WB Saunders; 1992.

Hughes JMB, Pride NB. *Lung Function Tests: Physiological Principles and Clinical Applications*. London: WB Saunders; 1999.

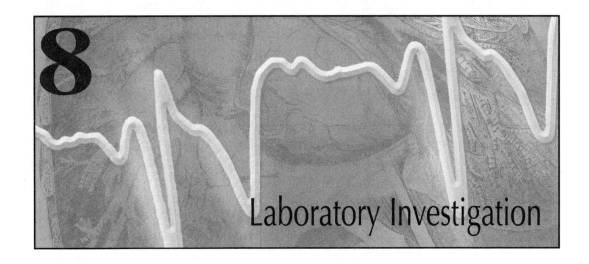

**8**

# Laboratory Investigation

## OBJECTIVES

Upon completion of this chapter, the reader should be able to describe:
1. Laboratory investigations for cardiovascular disease
2. Laboratory investigations for pulmonary disease
3. Laboratory hematological investigations and their clinical implications
4. Basic chemistry investigations and their clinical implications
5. Laboratory investigations for liver disease
6. Laboratory investigations for renal disease
7. Laboratory investigations for endocrine disorders and clinical presentations

This chapter outlines some of the common laboratory investigations frequently used on cardiopulmonary patients and their clinical implications. Other common laboratory investigations such as hematology; basic chemistry; and tests for liver, renal, and endocrine functions are also discussed.

## COMMON LABORATORY INVESTIGATION OF CARDIOVASCULAR DISEASE

Common laboratory investigations that are frequently used to determine the diagnosis and management of cardiovascular disease are enzyme tests for acute myocardial infarction (AMI),[1-5] lipid profiles for management of coronary artery disease,[6-11] and monitoring of clotting factors.

To diagnose AMI, blood samples are obtained promptly after the onset of symptoms and repeated at appropriate intervals (Table 8-1A). A series of elevated creatine kinase myocardial bound (CK-MB) or troponin I is indicative of an AMI (Table 8-1B).[1,2,4,5]

In patients with coronary artery disease (CAD), increased serum levels of low-density lipoprotein cholesterol (LDL-C), decreased high-density lipoprotein cholesterol (HDL-C), and high cholesterol/HDL-C ratio are associated with an increased risk for developing CAD (Table 8-2A).[6-11] Other risk factors for CAD are age, family history, smoking, hypertension, and diabetes mellitus.

C-reactive protein (CRP), a systemic marker of inflammation and the acute phase response, is also a powerful predictor of cardiovascular risk. A high concentration of CRP is highly correlated with the incidences of cardiovascular endpoints such as AMI, stroke, progression of peripheral vascular disease, and mortality[12-14] (Table 8-2B).

There are medical conditions that require anticoagulation therapy:
- In diseases such as pulmonary emboli and deep vein thrombosis
- For prevention of clotting—eg, postsurgical immobility, total knee arthroplasty, atrial fibrillation, and those patients with mechanical heart valves

## Table 8-1A

### *Variations of Enzyme Concentrations Over Time in the Detection of an Acute Myocardial Infarction*

| Enzyme | Rise | Peak | Normalization |
|---|---|---|---|
| CK12 hrs | 36 to 72 hrs | 3 to 5 days | — |
| CK-MB | 4 to 8 hrs | 24 hrs | 3 days |
| Troponin I | 3 hrs | 14 to 18 hrs | Remains elevated for 5 to 7 days |

## Table 8-1B

### *Example of a Laboratory Investigation Report of an AMI*

#### BIOCHEMICAL INVESTIGATION FOR AMI

** A single negative CK-MB or Troponin does not exclude a diagnosis of MI. **
**** Interpretive comments may not apply immediately after cardiac surgery. ****

| Test | Result | Reference |
|---|---|---|
| CK | 600 | <165 U/L |
| CK-MB | 15 | <2.5 |
| Troponin I | 20 | <del>&lt;0.6 µg/L</del> 0.00 |

Abbreviations: CK: creatine kinase; CK-MB: creatine kinase myocardial bound

## Table 8-2A

### *Example of a Laboratory Investigation Report of a Lipid Profile*

#### LIPID PROFILE

A cholesterol/HDL-C ratio of 5.0 in males and 4.4 in females is associated with average risk.
Higher ratios are associated with increased risk of CAD.
For patients with CAD, the desirable range for LDL-Cholesterol is lower than in the general population.
In CAD patients an LDL-Cholesterol level of less than 2.6 mmol/L is suggested.

| Test | Result | Reference |
|---|---|---|
| LDL | 4.0 | 1.5-3.4 mmol/L |
| HDL | 0.7 | >0.9 mmol/L |
| Triglyceride | 1.4 | <2.3 mmol/L |
| Cholesterol | 6 | 2.0 to 5.2 mmol/L |

---

Table 8-2B

### Example of a Laboratory Investigation Report of C-Reactive Protein and Its Reference Range

C-REACTIVE PROTEIN

| Test | Result | Reference |
|------|--------|-----------|
| CRP | 52.0 | 0.2 to 7.5 mg/L |

Abbreviation: CRP: C-reactive protein

---

Table 8-3

### Example of a Laboratory Report Showing Common Parameters Used to Monitor Anticoagulation Therapy

ROUTINE COAGULATION
THERAPEUTIC RANGES: ** INR **
Mechanical Heart Valves 2.5 to 3.5
All other indications 2.0 to 3.0
** aPTT ** (Heparin Therapy) 60 to 85 sec

| Test | Result | Reference |
|------|--------|-----------|
| INR | 1.5 | 0.8 to 1.2 |
| aPTT | 64 | 22 to 33 sec |

Abbreviations: aPTT: activated partial thromboplastin time; INR: international normalized unit
Note if the INR and aPTT is greater than the upper reference limit, the blood is clotting slower than normal.

---

The level of blood coagulation is closely monitored and the medication is titrated to therapeutic levels to maintain clotting factors within a clinically acceptable range (Table 8-3).

# COMMON LABORATORY INVESTIGATION OF PULMONARY DISEASES

Common laboratory investigations that are frequently ordered to help in the diagnosis and management of pulmonary disease include sputum and microbiology procedures to determine the presence and type of pulmonary infections.

In patients with respiratory disease, sputum color may vary from time to time. Sometimes, a specific sputum color might be suggestive of a particular disease (Table 8-4). However *sputum culture and sensitivity is required* to obtain a definitive diagnosis. In COPD patients, the presence of green (purulent) sputum was 94.4% sensitive and 77.0% specific for a high bacterial load and indicates a clear subset of patients that are likely to benefit from antibiotic therapy.[15] Patients who produced white (mucoid) sputum during the acute exacerbation improved without antibiotic therapy, and sputum characteristics remained the same even when the patients had returned to their stable clinical state.[15]

Clinical microbiology procedures are frequently used to isolate, identify, and cultivate bacteria, fungi, and viral specimens to allow appropriate use of medication for the treatment of pneumonia (Table 8-5). Gram stain-

Table 8-4

## Sputum Color in Different Diseases

| Sputum Color | Likely conditions |
|---|---|
| Anchovy-paste (dark brown) | Amoebic liver abscess rupture into bronchus |
| Green with sweet smell | Pseudomonas infection |
| Milky | Bronchoalveolar carcinoma |
| Mucopurulent | Bronchiectasis |
| Red current jelly | Klebsiella pneumoniae |
| Red pigment | Serratia marcescens; rifampin overdose |
| Rusty | Lobar pneumonia |
| White and mucoid without pus | Asthma |
| Yellow | Jaundice |

Table 8-5

## Classification of Bacterial Pneumonias

| Organism | Conditions |
|---|---|
| GRAM POSITIVE | |
| Streptococcus pneumonia | Community-acquired pneumonia |
| Staphylococcus aureus | Nosocomial. Associated with trauma, tracheostomy, or age |
| Streptococcus pyognes (Group A) | Uncommon, frequently with rapid progression |
| Streptococcus agalactiae (Group B) | Neonates and immunocompromised patients |
| GRAM NEGATIVE | |
| Haemophilus influenzae | Community-acquired. Associated with pediatrics, chronic lung disease, cystic fibrosis patients |
| Moraxella (Branhamella) catarrhalis | Associated with patients with underlying disease and nosocomial infection |
| Enterobacteriaceae (eg, Klebsiella, Escherichia coli, and Serratia) | Nosocomial |
| Pseudomonas aeruginosa | Nosocomial |
| Acinetobacter | Nosocomial |
| Anaerobes (eg, peptostreptococcus, actinomyces, fusobacterrium, bacteroides) | Nosocomial. Associated with aspiration, necrotizing pneumonias as well as lung abscess |

ing uses a staining technique to determine cell composition and visualize cell morphology. It allows rapid presumptive diagnosis of different bacterial infections. Acid-fast is another common cell wall staining technique used to identify mycobacteria (eg, tuberculosis). Direct immunofluorescent microscopy or DNA probes are required to identify *Legionella pneumophila*.

Once sputum specimens are cultured and isolated to identify the specific pathogen, different antibiotics are added to the culture media to determine their sensitivity. An example of a culture and sensitivity report is shown in Table 8-6.

Table 8-6

*Example of a Sputum Culture and Sensitivity (C&S) Report*

SPUTUM C & S

| Procedure | Result |
|---|---|
| Gram Stain | +3 Polymorphs |
| | Debris |

*SPUTUM Culture Final*

+2 *P. aeruginosa*
+2 *Candida albicans*
Yeast may be present in the respiratory tract but is rarely a cause of pneumonia.

*P. Aeruginosa*

| | Rx | Average Adult Dose |
|---|---|---|
| Ciprofloxacin | S | 400 mg q12h |
| Gentamicin | R | 100 mg q12h |
| Timentin | S | 3.1 g q4h |

Abbreviations: mg: milligram; q4h: every 4 hours; q12h: every 12 hours; R: Resistant; Rx: treatment reaction; S: sensitive.

# COMMON HEMATOLOGICAL LABORATORY EXAMINATIONS

A large number of hematological investigations are frequently ordered to assist in the diagnosis and management of different cardiopulmonary diseases. The reference range and clinical implications of abnormal findings are summarized in Table 8-7. Bacterial infection is usually associated with increased neutrophils whereas a viral infection is usually associated with an increase in lymphocytes and monocytes.

Disseminated intravascular coagulopathy (DIC) is characterized by a decrease in platelets (PLT) and a rise in activated partial thromboplastin time (aPTT), and is confirmed by an increase in fibrin split products (FSPs). DIC may be secondary to sepsis, cancer, or chronic inflammatory disease. Microemboli formation with widespread tissue ischemia and infarct leading to multi-organ failure is common in DIC if left untreated.

# OTHER COMMON LABORATORY EXAMINATIONS: BASIC CHEMISTRY

Common blood work that is routinely ordered to help in the diagnosis and management of cardiopulmonary disease includes tests to determine information about electrolyte and fluid balance in patients as shown in Table 8-8. Any significant deviation outside the normal range can cause deleterious effects in the physiological function of the body.

# COMMON LABORATORY INVESTIGATIONS OF LIVER DISEASE

Common laboratory investigations that are frequently ordered to help in the diagnosis and management of liver disease include measuring the enzyme levels of 2 marker protein transferases and ammonia levels.

Excessive alcohol use, intravenous drug use, and infection are common causes of liver disease resulting in elevated liver enzymes (Table 8-9). The enzymes levels are useful in monitoring the progress of the disease and response to treatment.

Table 8-7

## Common Laboratory Hematological Values and Clinical Implications

| | Reference Range | Increased In | Decreased In |
|---|---|---|---|
| Hemoglobin (Hb) | 135 to 180 g/L | Sickle cell disease; hemo-concentration; transfusion; COPD; acclimatization to high altitude | Blood loss; hemodilution; liver disease; iron deficiency anemia |
| Red blood cell count (RBC) | 4.30 to 5.90 x 1012/L | Megaloblastic anemia; pernicious anemia; fish tapeworm infestation; liver disease; alcohol intoxication. | Iron deficiency; lead poisoning; chronic inflammation |
| Mean corpuscular volume (MCV) | 80 to 100 Fl | Macrocytic anemias; chronic alcoholism | Microcytic anemias; marked leukocytosis |
| Platelet (PLT) | 150 to 400 x109/L | Malignancy; post surgery; RA; acute infection; cardiac disease; liver cirrhosis | *Causes of thrombocytopenia:* Drugs (eg, gold, sulfonamides, chemotherapeutic agents, penicillins, beta-blockers, calcium channel blockers, quinidine); hereditary; DIC *Common physical signs:* Petechiae (pin point hemorrhage); ecchymoses (multiple small superficial bruises) |
| White blood cell count (WBC) | 4.0 to 11.0 x109/L | Infection; leukemia | Marrow failure; gram negative sepsis |
| Neutrophils (participates in acute inflammation) | 2.0 to 8.0 x109/L | Neutrophilia (which can be associated with a *shift to the left*[1]): Acute infection; inflammation (eg, vasculitis, acute gout, eclampsia); poisoning (eg, chemicals, venoms); exercise; emotional stress; tissue necrosis; medications (eg, histamine, steroid); acute hemorrhage | Neutropenia: Overwhelming bacterial infection; viral infection; drugs (eg, sulfonamides, antibiotics, analgesia, marrow depressants); ionizing radiation; hematopoietic diseases; anaphylactic shock; lupus |
| Eosinophils (participates in helminthic infection and allergic responses) | 0.0 to 0.7 x109/L | Allergic diseases (eg, asthma, hay fever, drug therapy); parasitic infestation; collagen-vascular disease (eg, RA, SLE, scleroderma); hematopoietic diseases | |
| Basophils (participates in allergic response) | 0.0 to 0.2 x109/L | Some leukemias; polycythemia; post-splenectomy; chicken pox; smallpox; Hodgkin's disease | Hyperthyroidism; pregnancy; acute phase of infections; immediately postradiation; chemotherapy; glucocorticoid treatment |
| Lymphocytes (produces antibodies and regulates immune response) | 1.0 to 4.0 x109/L | *Lymphocytosis:* viral infections; chronic inflammatory bowel diseases; lymphatic leukemia | *Lymphocytopenia:* Radiation or chemotherapy treatment; corticosteroids use; decrease production in diseases such as AIDS; malignancy; SLE; renal failure; myasthenia gravis |

Table 8-7 (continued)

## *Common Laboratory Hematological Values and Clinical Implications*

| | Reference Range | Increased In | Decreased In |
|---|---|---|---|
| Monocytes (participates in inflammation, repair and regenerative responses) | 0.0 to 0.8 x109/L | Infections (eg, bacteria endocarditis, TB, malaria, typhus); some leukemias; malignant lymphomas; post splenectomy; auto-immune disease (eg, RA, SLE, sarcoidosis, ulcerative colitis) | |

Abbreviations: AIDS: acquired immune deficiency syndrome; RA: rheumatoid arthritis; SLE: systemic lupus erythematosous; TB: tuberculosis.

[1]The term "shift to the left" is frequently used to characterize an increase in immature or band-cell forms of neutrophils in the differential white blood cell count

Table 8-8

## *Common Basic Chemistry Report and Clinical Implications.*

| | Reference Range | Increased In | Decreased In |
|---|---|---|---|
| Sodium | 135 to 145 mmol/L | Dehydration | Overhydration |
| Potassium | 3.5 to 5.0 mmol/L | Renal retention; redistribution-acute acidosis; decrease insulin; drugs (eg, succinylcholine, excess of digitalis); increased ingestion | Excess renal secretion; drugs (eg, diuretics, aldosterone, high doses of cortisone); vomiting; diarrhea; excessive sweating; severe burns; draining wound; intra- and extra-cellular shift |
| Chloride | 98 to 108 mmol/L | Hyperchloremic metabolic acidosis; respiratory alkalosis; drugs (eg, IV saline, steroids, salicylate intoxication); diabetes insipidus | Prolonged vomiting and suction; chronic respiratory acidosis; salt losing renal disease; primary aldosteronism |
| Calcium | 2.1 to 2.6 mmol/L | Hyperparathyroidism; Hyperthyroidism; neoplasms; granulomatous diseases | Hypoparathyroidism; chronic use of anticonvulsant drugs; obstructive jaundice; renal failure |
| Magnesium | 0.7 to 1.2 mmol/L | Ingestion (eg, antacids, enemas, parental nutrition); renal failure; diabetic coma; hypothyroidism | Renal problem; drugs (eg, furosemide, thiazides, gentamicin, tobramycin, cyclosporine, amphotericin B, aminoglycosides); acute alcoholism; starvation; hyperthyroidism; severe burn; sepsis |

Table 8-9

### Common Laboratory Tests for Liver and Clinical Implications

|  | Reference Range | Increased In | Decreased In |
|---|---|---|---|
| ALT | <50 U/L | Liver diseases | Acute viral hepatitis |
| AST | <36 U/L | Liver diseases; AMI; musculoskeletal trauma; surgery and intramuscular injections | Azotemia; chronic hemodialysis; diabetic ketoacidosis |
| Ammonia | <40 mmol/L | Severe liver disease | Renal failure |

Abbreviations: ALT: alanine aminotransferase; AST: aspartate aminotransferase; U/L international unit of enzyme activity per liter.

Table 8-10

### Clinical Implications for Laboratory Investigations for Renal Disease and an Example of an Urinalysis Report

|  | Reference Range | Increased In | Decreased In |
|---|---|---|---|
| Urea | 2 to 9 mmol/L | Impaired kidney function | Severe liver damage; malnutrition; anabolic hormones; low protein and high carbohydrate diet; celiac disease |
| Creatinine | 30 to 130 μmol/L | Impaired kidney function; ingestion of creatinine (roast meat) |  |

URINALYSIS REPORT

| Test | Result | Reference |
|---|---|---|
| Appearance | Clear |  |
| Color | Straw |  |
| pH | 5.0 | 5 to 7 |
| Leukocyte | Negative | Negative |
| Urine nitrites | Negative | Negative |
| Protein | Negative | Negative g/L |
| Glucose | Negative | Negative mmol/L |
| Ketones | Negative | Negative |
| Blood | Moderate | Negative |
| Urine volume | 20 ml |  |

# COMMON LABORATORY INVESTIGATIONS FOR RENAL DISEASE

Common laboratory investigations that are frequently ordered to help in the diagnosis and management of renal disease include checking for levels of urea, creatinine, its pH, and the presence of components not usually present in urine.

Normal renal function is required to maintain acid-base, fluid and electrolyte balance. Table 8-10 shows some common laboratory tests used for diagnosis of renal disease. Additional tests such as creatinine clearance, which involves a 24-hour urine collection and urine analysis, is also commonly done.

Table 8-11

## Common Laboratory Tests for Endocrine Disorders and Clinical Implications

| Test | Change | Conditions | Clinical presentation |
|------|--------|------------|------------------------|
| Total thyroxine (T4) and Triiodothyronine (T3) | Increased | Hyperthyroidism | Tachycardia; hyper-reflexia; anxiety; tremor; weight loss; weakness |
| | Decreased | Hypothyroidism | Bradycardia; hypertension; fatigue; lethargy; hypo-reflexia; weakness; joint pain |
| Parathyroid (PTH) | Increased | Hyperparathyroidism | Psychosis; anorexia; constipation; weight loss; abdominal pain; pathological fractures; kidney stones |
| | Decreased | Hypoparathyroidism | Paresthesia; hair loss; weakness |
| Random glucose | >6.1 mmol/L | Hyperglycemia/ diabetes | Polyuria; polydipsia; polyphagia, weight loss |

# COMMON LABORATORY EXAMINATIONS ASSOCIATED WITH ENDOCRINE DISORDERS

Common laboratory investigations that are frequently ordered to help in the diagnosis and management of cardiopulmonary disease with atypical presentations can include investigation of endocrine disorders.

Thyroid problems and diabetes are common in the elderly and especially those with cardiovascular disease. These endocrine disorders can further impair the neuromuscular function of these patients (Table 8-11).

# REFERENCES

1. Adams JE, Bodor GS, Davila-Roman VG, et al. Cardiac troponin I: a marker with high specificity for cardiac injury. *Circulation*. 1993;88:101-106.

2. Bahit MC, Criger DA, Ohman EM, et al. Thresholds for the electrocardiographic change range of biochemical markers of acute myocardial infarction (GUSTO-IIa data). *Am J Cardiol*. 2002;90:233-237.

3. Ferguson JL, Beckett GJ, Stoddart M, et al. Myocardial infarction redefined: the new ACC/ESC definition, based on cardiac troponin, increases the apparent incidence of infarction. *Heart*. 2002;88:343-347.

4. Hamm CW. New serum markers for acute myocardial infarction. *N Eng J Med*. 1994;331:607-608.

5. Meier MA, Al-Badr WH, Cooper JV, et al. The new definition of myocardial infarction. Diagnostic and prognostic implications in patients with acute coronary syndromes. *Arch Intern Med*. 2002;162:1585-1589.

6. Ballantyne CM, Rangaraj GR. The evolving role of high-density lipoprotein in reducing cardiovascular risk. *Prev Cardiol*. 2001;4:65-72.

7. Brown WV. Cholesterol lowering in atherosclerosis. *Am J Cardiol*. 2000;86:29H-34H.

8. Fedder DO, Koro CE, L'Italien GJ. New National Cholesterol Education Program III guidelines for primary prevention lipid-lowering drug therapy: projected impact on the size, sex, and age distribution of the treatment-eligible population. *Circulation*. 2002;105:152-156.

9. Jones PH. Lipid-lowering treatment in coronary artery disease: how low should cholesterol go? *Drugs*. 2000;59:1127-1135.

10. Ito MK, Delucca GM, Aldridge MA. The relationship between low-density lipoprotein cholesterol goal attainment and prevention of coronary heart disease—related events. *J Cardiovasc Pharmacol Ther*. 2001;6:129-135.

11. Robinson JG, Boland LL, McGovern PG, et al. A comparison of NCEP and absolute risk stratification methods for lipid-lowering therapy in middle-aged adults: the ARIC study. *Prev Cardiol.* 2001;4:148-157.

12. Koenig W, Pepys MB. C-reactive protein risk prediction: low specificity, high sensitivity. *Ann Intern Med.* 2002;136:550-552.

13. Mosca L. C-reactive protein—to screen or not to screen? *N Engl J Med.* 2002:347;1615-1617.

14. Ridker PM, Rifai N, Rose L, et al. Comparison of C-reactive protein and low-density lipoprotein cholesterol levels in the prediction of first cardiovascular events. *N Eng J Med.* 2002:347;1557-1565.

15. Stockley RA, O'Brien C, Pye A, et al. Relationship of sputum color to nature and outpatient management of acute exacerbations of COPD. *Chest.* 2000;117:1638-1645.

# BIBLIOGRAPHY

Henry JB. *Clinical Diagnosis and Management by Laboratory Methods.* Philadelphia: WB Saunders; 1996.

Koepke JA. *Practical Laboratory Hematology.* New York: Churchill Livingstone; 1991.

Lab Tests Online. 2001-2004. American Association for Clinical Chemistry. http://www.labtestsonline.org. Accessed April 27, 2004.

Pagana KD, Pagana TJ. *Diagnostic and Laboratory Test Reference.* St. Louis: Mosby; 2001.

Tilton RC, Balows A, Hohnadel DC, et al. *Clinical Laboratory Medicine.* St. Louis: Mosby-Year Book; 1992.

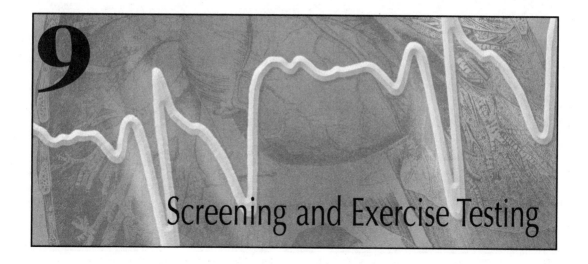

# OBJECTIVES

After this chapter, the reader should be able to:
1. Identify *patients at risk* for problems during exercise, and outline the level of monitoring and supervision procedures for exercising these patients
2. List absolute and relative contraindications to exercise for an individual
3. Describe different exercise testing designs
4. List indications for stopping exercise and exertional activities

# RATIONALE

Many principles defined for exercise prescription for healthy people apply to patients. For outpatients and especially inpatients, the complexity and acuteness of their conditions may require considerable caution by the physical therapist to ensure that the exercise is both *effective* and *safe*. In order to prescribe an exercise program, the physical therapist needs to determine the *training safety zone* that is limited by (Figure 9-1):
- Minimum intensity to provide an *effective training* program
- Maximum intensity that shouldn't be exceeded to ensure *safe training*

The minimum intensity is determined by:
- The level that will induce a physiologic training response, induce improvement in neuromuscular coordination, balance, motor learning, and self-confidence
- The level that the patient is comfortable training because of fear or discomfort with exercising

The maximum intensity is determined by how safely the patient can exercise at a higher intensity. The determination of this intensity may be very straightforward or it may be based on a variety of factors for each patient. For example, a young adult patient may exercise to maximal intensity with only 1 limiting factor such as the pain associated with an orthopedic problem. On the other hand, a 73-year-old woman in a pulmonary rehabilitation program may have her maximal intensity limited by a number of factors such as:
- The exercise intensity that she desaturates below 87%
- The exercise intensity that causes angina
- The exercise intensity that causes significant ST depression
- Arthritis and back pain
- Fatigue and general well being on a given day

Further, the level of exercise that could potentially induce one of these untoward responses can vary from day-to-day. The minimum and maximum intensities can be very complicated in estimating because of the various pathologies that a patient may have and because target exercise based on age-predicted HR is meaningless

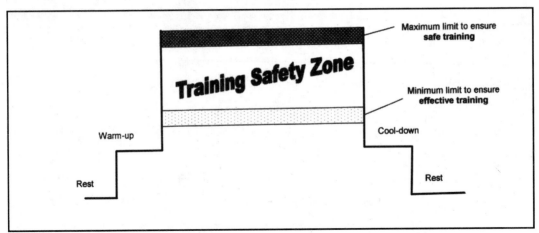

**Figure 9-1.** The training safety zone. The physical therapist needs to prescribe exercise to target a training safety zone. This ensures that the exercise prescribed is below the upper limit that could potentially elicit an untoward response and above the lower limit that would induce a training response (see text). Both the upper and lower limits are ranges because the patient's health conditions and related exercise response can vary on a daily basis.

for many patients.[1] Many of the patients who we treat need to exercise at a lower HR than their age-predicted HR. In addition, deriving the age-predicted HR is not very specific; the 95% confidence interval for an age-predicted HR is 40 to 60 beats per minute.[1]

Exercise testing in some form is usually essential in order to determine the maximum and minimum limits for the training-safety zone. Often exercise testing is not performed in the clinical setting; in this situation, the therapist usually has to expend additional efforts monitoring and adjusting an ineffective or overly aggressive training protocol during training sessions to define the appropriate training intensity.

# SCREENING FOR EXERCISE RISK
# AND CONTRAINDICATIONS TO EXERCISE

Before exercise testing or evaluation, all patients need to be screened to determine their risk(s) when performing exercise. Tables 9-1 and 9-2 list contraindications and precautions to exercise. The patient should be thoroughly evaluated to determine if there are any underlying conditions that are contraindications and/or precautions to exercise.[2] Often this information is not available for many patients. In this situation, the "Exercise Screening Questionnaire Using ACSM Criteria" (Table 9-3) is an up-to-date comprehensive screening tool for this purpose.[3] Depending on how patients answer these questions and the complexity of their underlying health conditions, this questionnaire should be supplemented with additional questions. The response to this questionnaire will assist the therapist to determine if the patient is:

- Low risk (young, and no more than 1 risk factor): Can do maximal testing or enter a vigorous exercise program
- Moderate risk (older, 2 or more risk factors): Can do submaximal testing or enter a moderate exercise program
- High risk (one or more symptoms, or disease): Can do no testing without a physician present; can enter no program without physician referral

Table 9-1

## *Contraindications to Exercise*

### *Absolute Contraindications*

- Acute myocardial infarction (EKG, enzymes)
- Unstable angina
- Serious arrhythmias (brady- and tachy-dysrhythmias, SSS, multifocal PVCs, second- or third-degree heart block, uncontrolled ventricular arrhythmia, atrial dysrhythmia that compromises cardiac function)
- Acute pericarditis, endocarditis, myocarditis
- Uncompensated or uncontrolled heart failure, severe aortic stenosis
- Severe left ventricular dysfunction
- Acute pulmonary embolism or infarction
- Aneurysm of the heart or aorta
- Uncontrolled systemic hypertension
- Uncontrolled asthma
- Acute thrombophlebitis or deep venous thrombosis
- Intracranial pressure >20 mmHg

### *Relative Contraindications*

- Significant arterial hypertension (resting diastolic >110 mmHg or systolic >200 mmHg)
- Pulmonary hypertension
- Brady- or tachyarrhythmias
- Moderate valvular disease
- Uncontrolled metabolic disease (eg, diabetes, thyrotoxicosis, or myxedema)
- Oxygen saturation <85% on room air
- Unstable asthma
- Diabetic patient with autonomic denervation of the heart

### *Contraindications (With Cancer and Diabetes)*

- Vomiting within previous 24 to 36 hours
- Severe diarrhea within previous 24 to 36 hours
- IV chemotherapy within previous 24 hours
- Activity that may traumatize the feet in the presence of peripheral neuropathy or microangiopathy
- Systolic pressure >180 mmHg in the presence of proliferative retinopathy
- Uncontrolled blood glucose; blood glucose should be within or near normal range
- Hematocrit <25%
- Hemoglobin <8 g/dL
- White blood count <500/mm with fever
- Platelet count <5000/mm$^3$

### *Vague Contraindications*

- Acute or serious noncardiac disorders
- Patient not able to understand instructions (delirium, dementia)
- Severe physical handicap or disability
- Psychiatric disease
- Noncompliant patient
- Neuromuscular, musculoskeletal, or rheumatoid disorders that are exacerbated by exercises
- Other conditions that could be aggravated by exercise

Abbreviations: PVC: premature ventricular contraction; SSS: sick sinus syndrome.

Adapted from Olivier FL. Suggested guidelines for use of exercise with adults in acute care setting. *Physiother Can.* 1998;152:127-136, with permission from BC Decker.

Table 9-2

## Precautions to Exercise

### Precautions

- Hematocrit >25%
- Hemoglobin 8 to 10 g/dL
- White blood count >500/mm$^3$
- Platelet count 5000 to 10000/mm$^3$
- A drop in skin temperature, cool and light perspiration, and peripheral cyanosis
- Lightheadedness or vertigo
- A drop in systolic pressure (>20 mmHg) or below pre-exercise level
- A rise in systolic blood pressure to >250 mmHg or of diastolic pressure to >120 mmHg
- Confusion, nausea, muscle cramping, headache, visual disturbances, cyanosis, or vomiting
- Acute infection with fever and elevated white blood count
- coronary artery disease with cardiomyopathies, valvular heart disease, abnormal exercise test, previous cardiac arrest, complex ventricular arrhythmias, three-vessel disease or left main disease or ejection fraction less than 30%
- Post-exercise heart rate within 20 beats/min of resting rate
- Post-exercise systolic pressure within 15 mmHg of resting pressure
- Abnormal (serum) electrolyte values: calcium <6.5 or >13.5 mg/dL, magnesium <0.5 or >4.5 mg/dL, phosphorus <1.0 mg/dL, potassium <3.0 >6.0 mEq/L, sodium <125 or >155 mEq/L
- Systolic blood pressure <90 mmHg or central venous pressure <5 mmHg
- Heart rates <30 to 35/min and >150 to 180/min may cause syncope. Similarly, respiratory rate above 40 breaths per minute leads to fatigue and respiratory failure
- Uncompensated arterial blood gases: pH <7.34 or >7.46, carbon dioxide <35 mEq/L or >45 mEq/L, partial pressure of oxygen <80 mmHg
- Use of medication necessitating continuous cardiac monitoring: adenosine, bretylium tosylate, esmolol HCl, isoproterenol HCl, lidocaine HCl, magnesium sulphite, metoprolol, nitroglycerin, nitroprusside sodium, norepinepherine bitartrate, phenytoin sodium, procainamide HCl and verapamil HCl
- Presence of an intra-aortic balloon pump or temporary pacemaker

### Suggested Precautions

- Lack of cooperation
- Fever (oral temperature >37.7°C or >99.8°F)
- Blood glucose <40 or >500 mg/dL
- Respiratory rate >30 breaths/min
- Medications may require cardiac monitoring: alteplase, amphotericin B, amrinone lactate, atropine, calcium chloride, digoxin, disopyramide, dobutamine HCl, dopamine HCl, epinephrine, labetalol, mexiletine HCl, moricizine, propafenone, propranolol, quinidine, tocainide HCl
- Occasional premature ventricular contractions do not absolutely contraindicate exercise testing
- Poorly controlled diabetes or other metabolic disorders
- Epilepsy
- Acute cerebrovascular disease
- Poorly controlled respiratory failure
- Excessive muscle soreness or fatigue that is residual from last exercise or activity session

Adapted from Olivier FL. Suggested guidelines for use of exercise with adults in acute care setting. *Physiother Can.* 1998;152:127-136 with permission from BC Decker.

Table 9-3

## Exercise Screening Questionnaire Using ACSM Criteria

Name _____Sex ___ Date _____

I. *Risk factors (2 or more places individual at moderate risk)*

____ 1. Have any of your brothers or sisters had a heart attack, before the age of 55 (male relatives) or 65 (female relatives)?

____ 2. Have you smoked cigarettes in the past 6 months?

____ 3. What is your usual BP (>140/90)? Do you take BP medication?

____ 4. What is your LDL cholesterol? If you don't know your LDL, what is your total cholesterol? What is your HDL cholesterol? [Either LDL >130 (use total cholesterol >200 if LDL not known) OR HDL <35 is a risk. Note: HDL >60 is a "negative" risk factor.]

____ 5. What is your fasting glucose (>110)?

____ 6. What is your height and weight (BMI >30)? Also, what is your waist girth (>100 cm)?

____ 7. Do you get at least 30 minutes of moderate physical activity most days of the week (or its equivalent)?

II. *Symptoms (1 or more places individual at high risk)*

____ 1. Do you ever have pain or discomfort in your chest or surrounding areas? (ie, ischemia)

____ 2. Do you ever feel faint or dizzy (other than when sitting up rapidly)?

____ 3. Do you find it difficult to breathe when you are lying down or sleeping?

____ 4. Do your ankles ever become swollen (other than after a long period of standing)?

____ 5. Do you ever have heart palpitations, or an unusual period of rapid heart rate?

____ 6. Do you ever experience pain in your legs (ie, intermittent claudication)?

____ 7. Has a physician ever said you have a heart murmur? (Has he/she said it is OK, and safe for you to exercise?)

____ 8. Do you feel unusually fatigued or find it difficult to breathe with usual activities?

III. *Other*

____ 1. How old are you? (Men >45, women >55 are at moderate risk.)

____ 2. Do you have any of the following diseases: heart disease, peripheral vascular disease, cerebrovascular disease, COPD (emphysema or chronic bronchitis), asthma, interstitial lung disease, cystic fibrosis, diabetes mellitus, thyroid disorder, renal disease, or liver disease? (Yes, to any disease places individual at high risk.)

____ 3. Do you have any bone or joint problems, such as arthritis or a past injury that might get worse with exercise? (Exercise testing may need to be delayed or modified.)

____ 4. Do you have a cold or flu, or any other infection? (Exercise testing must be delayed.)

____ 5. Are you pregnant? (Exercise testing may need to be delayed or modified.)

____ 6. Do you have any other problem that might make it difficult for you to do strenuous exercise?

*Interpretation*

*Low risk (young, and no more than 1 risk factor):* can do maximal testing or enter a vigorous exercise program. *Moderate risk (older, or 2 or more risk factors):* can do submaximal testing or enter a moderate exercise program. *High risk (1 or more symptoms, or disease):* can do no testing without physician presence; can enter no program without physician referral.

Reprinted from Swain DP, Leutholz BC. *Exercise Prescription. A Case Study Approach to the ACSM Guidelines.* Champaign, IL: Human Kinetics; 2002;3-4 with permission.

Adapted with permission from Franklin BA. *ACSM's Guidelines for Exercise Testing and Prescription.* 6th ed. Philadelphia: Lippincott Williams & Wilkins; 2000.

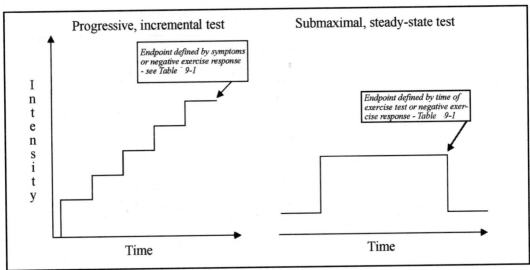

Figure 9-2. Format of progressive, incremental, and submaximal steady-state exercise tests.

# Determination of Exercise Test
## or Exercise Evaluation Procedure

After ensuring that the patient is medically stable and screening them for risks to exercise, the most cost-effective exercise evaluation procedure must be determined. For some patients such as those post-MI, the only option will be a fully monitored, physician-supervised stress test. In other cases, such as a 21-year-old adult with no risk factors, the person may perform the first session of his or her training protocol with only minimal monitoring of their subjective response by the physical therapist. Exercise tests can be a submaximal test or a progressive, incremental test to the symptom-limited maximum (Figure 9-2). The maximal, incremental test may provide more information about the patient's anaerobic exercise response. It is usually much more stressful, however, and the information gained may not warrant the risks of a negative exercise response. On the other hand, submaximal testing is less stressful and may more closely parallel the response of the patient to activities of daily living.[4,5] Different types of tests can provide very different information. For example, a submaximal test will not indicate how an individual will respond to maximal exercise and may not elicit any untoward signs and symptoms indicative of a poor exercise response at maximal or near-maximal intensities.

### Progressive, Incremental Exercise Tests

There are a variety of exercise protocols that can be used when performing an incremental exercise test (Figure 9-3).[6] From a clinical perspective, there are 3 main types of incremental exercise tests used:

1. *Cardiac stress testing* is a rapidly progressing incremental test used to assess the presence and severity of CAD. This is usually performed on a treadmill; however, it can be carried out on a cycle ergometer. The patient is connected to an EKG and a rhythm strip is recorded. A complete 12-lead EKG is taken at frequent intervals. Every 2 to 3 minutes, the speed and incline of the treadmill is increased until the patient:
   - Reaches their age-predicted heart rate or the maximum stage of the exercise test
   - Has symptoms supervene or significant changes on the EKG occur
   - Cannot continue for other reasons

In addition to assessing the presence of cardiac disease, the stress test can help determine the probable outcome of the patient's illness and identify subjects that could improve with interventions.[7]

| Functional Class | Clinical Status | $O_2$ Cost ml/kg/min | METs | Bicycle Ergometer (1 watt = 6 KPDS; for 70 kg body weight) KPDS | Bruce (3 min stages) MPH | Bruce %GR | Kattus MPH | Kattus %GR | Balke Ware (% grad at 3.3 MPH, 1-min stages) | Ellestad (3/2/3-min stages) MPH | Ellestad %GR | USAFSAM (2 or 3 min stages) MPH | USAFSAM %GR | "Slow" USAFSAM MPH | "Slow" USAFSAM %GR | McHenry MPH | McHenry %GR | Stanford % grade at 3 MPH | Stanford % grade at 2 MPH | METs |
|---|---|---|---|---|---|---|---|---|---|---|---|---|---|---|---|---|---|---|---|---|
| | | | | | 5.5 | 20 | | | | | | | | | | | | | | |
| Normal and I | Healthy, dependent on age, activity | 56.0 | 16 | | 5.0 | 18 | | | 26, 25 | 6 | 15 | | | | | | | | | 16 |
| | | 52.5 | 15 | | | | | | 24, 23 | | | 3.3 | 25 | | | | | | | 15 |
| | | 49.0 | 14 | | | | 4 | 22 | 22, 21 | 5 | 15 | | | | | | | | | 14 |
| | | 45.5 | 13 | 1500 | 4.2 | 16 | | | 20, 19 | | | 3.3 | 20 | | | 3.3 | 21 | | | 13 |
| | | 42.0 | 12 | 1350 | | | 4 | 18 | 18, 17 | | | | | | | 3.3 | 18 | 22.5 | | 12 |
| | Sedentary healthy | 38.5 | 11 | 1200 | | | | | 16, 15 | 5 | 10 | | | | | | | 20.0 | | 11 |
| | | 35.0 | 10 | 1050 | 3.4 | 14 | 4 | 14 | 14, 13 | | | 3.3 | 15 | 2 | 25 | 3.3 | 15 | 17.5 | | 10 |
| | | 31.5 | 9 | 900 | | | 4 | 10 | 12, 11 | | | | | | | 3.3 | 12 | 15.0 | | 9 |
| | Limited | 28.0 | 8 | 750 | | | | | 10, 9 | 4 | 10 | 3.3 | 10 | 2 | 20 | | | 12.5 | | 8 |
| | Symptomatic | 24.5 | 7 | | 2.5 | 12 | 3 | 10 | 8, 7 | 3 | 10 | | | 2 | 15 | 3.3 | 9 | 10.0 | 17.5 | 7 |
| II | | 21.0 | 6 | 600 | | | | | 6, 5 | | | 3.3 | 5 | | | 3.3 | 6 | 7.5 | 14 | 6 |
| | | 17.5 | 5 | 450 | 1.7 | 10 | 2 | 10 | 4, 3 | 1.7 | 10 | | | 2 | 10 | | | 5.0 | 10.5 | 5 |
| III | | 14.0 | 4 | 300 | | | | | 2, 1 | | | 3.3 | 0 | 2 | 5 | | | 2.5 | 7 | 4 |
| | | 10.5 | 3 | | 1.7 | 5 | | | | | | | | | | 2.0 | 3 | 0.0 | 3.5 | 3 |
| | | 7.0 | 2 | 150 | 1.7 | 0 | | | | | | 2.0 | 0 | 2 | 0 | | | | | 2 |
| IV | | 3.5 | 1 | | | | | | | | | | | | | | | | | 1 |

**Figure 9-3.** Different protocols of progressive incremental exercise tests. Different protocols can be used for the bicycle ergometer and treadmill tests. Note: how the increments, and first and last stages compare to indicators of functional class, clinical status, oxygen cost and MET level. (Reprinted from Froelicher VF, Myers J, Follansbee WP, Labovitz AJ. *Exercise and the Heart*. St. Louis: Mosby; 1993 with permission.)

2. *Cardiopulmonary exercise test* focuses on both the cardiovascular and pulmonary response to exercise. The patient can be monitored with a 3- or 12-lead EKG and ventilatory parameters are measured by having the patient breathe in and out of a mouthpiece connected to apparatus that measures flow rates and/or expired volumes in order to perform ventilatory expired gas analysis. By performing ventilatory expired gas analysis in addition to the EKG, the pattern of breathing, oxygen consumption, and EKG rhythm can be assessed concurrently during the same exercise test. The ventilatory expired gas analysis can provide information about dead space ventilation, alveolar ventilation, total ventilation, frequency of breathing, and tidal volume, which is often plotted in graphical format against normative values.[8] This analysis of the expired gases is useful for diagnostic purposes in both cardiac and pulmonary disease. The cardiopulmonary exercise test provides information about:

- Exercise responses that are related to pulmonary disease such as COPD or restrictive lung disease. For example, is the patient ventilatory limited during exercise? Do they desaturate? Do they show a metabolic acidosis?

- Possible elevation of the oxygen-consumption work rate. This could be due to poor exercise technique or obesity—both of which are modifiable.

- The presence of an elevated minute ventilation: carbon dioxide production which is linked to ventilation: perfusion mismatch in heart failure patients.[9] This may also indicate a poorer prognosis.[10]

- Evidence of other pathologies limiting exercise such as cardiac disease.

- An estimate of the proportionate contribution of the patient's anaerobic, pulmonary, and cardiac responses to exercise limitation.

3. Exercise test to detect exercise-induced asthma

Further details about various protocols are provided by Froelicher et al[6] and Noonan and Dean.[5]

### Submaximal Exercise Test

Submaximal exercise tests can be single-stage or multi-stage to a predetermined end-point—ie, percentage of age-predicted maximal HR. The most common submaximal test is the 6-minute walk test. Other variants of this test are the 2-min and 12-min walk tests. This test should be considered complementary to and not a replacement of the cardiopulmonary exercise test because extensive monitoring of ventilation and EKG cannot be performed during the walk-test. Thus, diagnosis of the specific cause of exercise limitation cannot be determined.[4] Results from the 6-minute walk test, however, are highly correlated to the endpoint of cardiopulmonary testing (r = 0.73)[4] and of equal importance, are better correlated to quality of life than peak oxygen uptake.[4] Because this test is apparently simple to perform, it is often carried out in an invalid manner. The therapist is strongly encouraged to follow the guidelines for the 6-minute walk test as provided in a statement by the American Thoracic Society.[4] An example of a 6-minute walk test record form is shown in Figure 9-4.[4]

# ENDPOINTS FOR EXERCISE TESTING, OTHER KINDS OF EXERCISE, AND ACTIVITIES

Regardless of the type of exercise or activity a patient is doing, the physical therapist should be well aware of indications for stopping exercise (Table 9-4).[11] These signs and symptoms may indicate that the various body systems—ie, orthopedic, cardiovascular and/or respiratory systems—are not meeting the demands of the exercise and thus, possible injury is imminent. Another important reason to stop exercise is when monitoring equipment is malfunctioning especially if the monitoring is essential to ensure that exercise is carried out safely.

6-MINUTE WALK TEST REPORT

Lap counter _____

Patient Name: _____ Patient ID# _____

Walk # _____ Tech ID: _____ Date: _____

Gender: M F Age: _____ Race: _____ Height: ____ ft ___ in ____ meters

Weight: _____ lbs, _____ kg    Blood Pressure: _____ / _____

Medications taken before the test (dose and time): _____

Supplemental oxygen during the test: No  Yes, flow _____ L/min, type _____

|  | Baseline | End of Test |
|---|---|---|
| Time | ___:____ | ___:____ |
| Heart Rate | _____ | _____ |
| Dyspnea | _____ | _____ |
| Leg Fatigue | _____ | _____ |
| General Fatigue | _____ | _____ |
| $SpO_2$ | _____ % | _____ % |

Stopped or paused before 6 minutes? No  Yes, reason: _____

Other symptoms at end of exercise: angina  dizziness  hip, leg, or calf pain

Number of laps: _____ (x 60 meters) + final partial lap: _____ meters =

Total distance walked in 6 minutes: _____ meters

Predicted distance: _____ meters   Percent predicted: _____ %

Therapist comments:


Interpretation (including comparison with a preintervention 6MWT):



From:

**Figure 9-4.** Six-minute walk test report. For further details on how to perform a valid, reliable six-minute walk test, please see ATS.[4]

Table 9-4

*Absolute and Relative Indications for Stopping Exercise and Activities*

*Absolute Indications*

*General Signs and Symptoms*
- Severe chest pain suggestive of angina or increasing anginal pain
- Severe dyspnea
- Dizziness or faintness
- Marked apprehension, mental confusion
- Lack of coordination or ataxia
- Sudden onset of pallor and sweating
- Onset of cyanosis
- Patient's unwillingness to continue

*EKG Signs*
- Numerous changes indicative of myocardial instability and inability to cope with exercise stress including serious arrhythmias, high-grade ventricular arrhythmias, or atrial arrhythmias that are symptomatic

*Blood Pressure Signs*
- Any fall in systolic pressure below the resting value
- A fall of more than 20 mmHg in systolic pressure occurring after the normal exercise rise or BP persistently below baseline despite an increase in workload
- Systolic blood pressure in excess of 300 mmHg or diastolic pressure in excess of 140 mmHg

*Oxygen Saturation*
- Varies dependent on center—usually between 85% and 89%. An absolute cut-off is to stop exercising when the $SaO_2$ falls below 85%. Consult with physician

*Technical Difficulties*
- Monitoring $SpO_2$
- Monitoring BP
- Monitoring EKG

*Relative Indications*

- Fatigue, shortness of breath, wheezing, leg cramps, or claudication
- General appearance
- Increasing joint or muscle pain
- EKG changes: ST or QRS changes such as excessive ST displacement; extreme junctional depression or marked axis shift; serious arrhythmias including supraventricular tachycardias; development of bundle branch block that cannot be distinguished from ventricular tachycardia

Adapted from Fletcher GF, Froelicher VF, Hartley LH, Haskell WL, Pollock ML. Exercise standards. A statement for health professionals from the American Heart Association. *Circulation.* 1995:91(2):580-615 and Jones NL, Campbell M. *Clinical Exercise Testing.* Philadelphia, Pa: WB Saunders; 1982.

# REFERENCES

1. Gappmaier E. "220-age?"—Prescribing exercise based on heart rate in the clinic. *Cardiopulmonary Physical Therapy.* 2002;13(2):11-12.

2. Olivier FL. Suggested guidelines for the use of exercise with adults in acute care settings. *Physiotherapy Canada.* 1998;152:127-136.

3. Swain DP, Leutholz BC. *Exercise Prescription. A Case Study Approach to the ACSM Guidelines.* Champaign, IL: Human Kinetics. 2002;3-4.

4. American Thoracic Society. ATS statement: guidelines for the six-minute walk test. *Am J Respir Crit Care Med.* 2002;166:111-117.

5. Noonan V, Dean E. Submaximal exercise testing: clinical application and interpretation. *Phys Ther.* 2000;80:782-807.

6. Froelicher VF, Myers J, Follansbee WP, Labovitz AJ. *Exercise and the Heart.* St. Louis: Mosby; 1993.

7. Fletcher GF, Froelicher VF, Hartley LH, Haskell WL, Pollock ML. Exercise standards. A statement for health professionals from the American Heart Association. *Circulation.* 1995:91(2):580-615.

8. Gallagher CG. Exercise limitation and clinical exercise testing in chronic obstructive pulmonary disease. *Clin Chest Med.* 1994;15(2):305-306.

9. Wasserman K, Zhang YY, Riley MS. Ventilation during exercise in chronic heart failure. *Basic Res Cardiol.* 1996;91(S1):1-11.

10. Chua TP, Ponikowski P, Harrington D, et al. Clinical correlates and prognostic significance of the ventilatory response to exercise in chronic heart failure. *J Am Coll Cardiol.* 1996;29:1585-1590.

11. Jones NL, Campbell M. *Clinical Exercise Testing.* Philadelphia, Pa: WB Saunders; 1982.

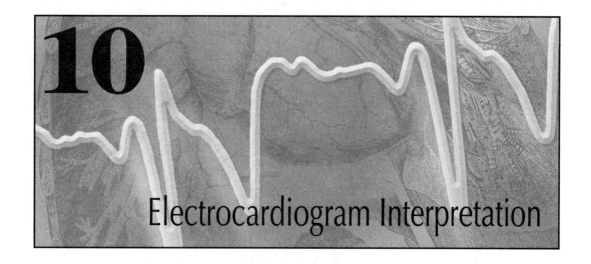

# 10

# Electrocardiogram Interpretation

## OBJECTIVES

At the end of this chapter, the reader should be able to:

1  Describe the electrical conduction system of the heart
2. Describe different recording leads
3. Interpret a 3-lead EKG tracing

The electrocardiogram (EKG) provides information about the electrical conduction system of the heart and provides essential information to help the therapist determine whether the myocardium is coping with the stress of exercise. The basic principles that underlie the EKG are easy to understand; however, interpretation of the EKG tracings recorded from various leads and recognizing the variations of all the arrhythmias is relatively complex. This chapter will provide a basic foundation that will facilitate interpretation of data presented in the case studies. The therapist is referred to several texts that will provide more detailed information on EKG interpretation.[1-3]

## ELECTRICAL CONDUCTION OF THE HEART AND COMPONENTS OF THE EKG

The electrical conduction system of the heart (Figure 10-1) consists of
- The sinoatrial (SA) node
- The atrioventricular (AV) node
- The bundle of His
- The left bundle branch (LBB) which has 2 divisions
- The right bundle branch (RBB)
- The Purkinje network of fibers

The conduction system provides a coordinated pathway for electrical conduction to travel through the heart. Arrhythmias can develop when one of the pacemakers fails to fire or fires too frequently, if one of the pathways is blocked, or if an extra focus fires an abnormal impulse also known as an ectopic beat.

The EKG is a recording of the electrical flow of current through the myocardium. When current flows toward a positive electrode, an upward deflection will be recorded, whereas when the current flows away from the positive electrode, a downward deflection occurs. The normal EKG (Figure 10-2) consists of the following components:
- The P wave, which reflects atrial depolarization
- The P-R interval, which reflects the time for conduction from the SA node to the ventricles
- The QRS complex, which reflects the depolarization of the ventricles
- The S-T segment, which represents the time when the entire myocardium is depolarized

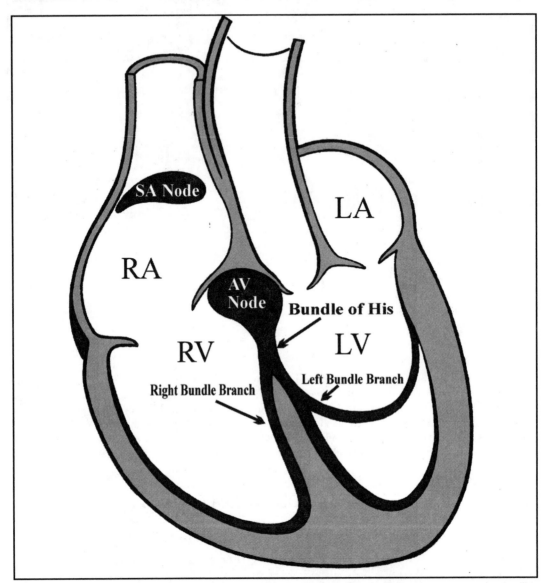

**Figure 10-1.** Electrical conduction system. The normal excitation impulse is generated in the SA node. These rhythmic impulses are immediately conducted to the surrounding atrial muscle. The impulse is delayed at the AV node and then is transmitted through the rapidly conducting bundle of His, and LBBs and RBBs to the ventricles.

- The *T wave*, which reflects ventricular repolarization
- The *R-R interval*, which is the time from one beat to the next

## RECORDING LEADS OF ELECTROCARDIOGRAM

The EKG is recorded from various electrodes placed in lead positions on the chest wall. The most common lead positions are the standard limb leads (I, II, and III), the augmented limb leads (aVR, aVL, and aVF), and the precordial leads (V1, V2, V3, V4, V5, and V6) . The 12-lead EKG reflects the electrical conduction of the heart recorded from different angles. By viewing the electrical conduction from different angles, one can discern abnormalities more specifically because some leads are especially reflective of certain heart structures. An analogy to the advantages of a 12-lead EKG versus a single lead is to ask yourself how you would inspect your car after being

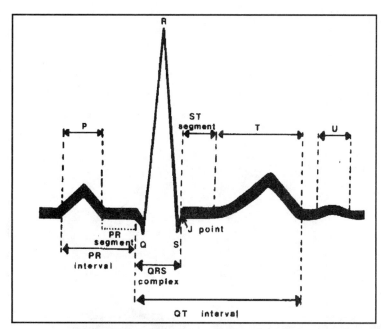

**Figure 10-2.** Components of EKG. (Reprinted with permission from: Underhill SL, Wood SL, Sivarajan ES, Halpanny CJ. *Cardiac nursing.* Philadelphia: JB Lippincott; 1983: 204.)

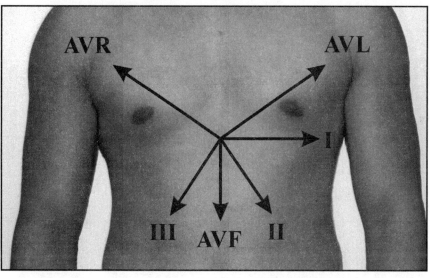

**Figure 10-3.** Vector direction of electrical recording of limb leads.

involved in a collision. It is unlikely that you would only look at your damaged car from the front. Most likely you would inspect it from the back, the front, and the sides; kneel down and look underneath; and even put the car on a hoist to examine the undercarriage more fully. Similarly, one can only ascertain a comprehensive view of whether the myocardium is conducting electrically activity normally, if it is recorded from a number of angles.

The standard and augmented limb leads view the heart in the frontal plane (Figure 10-3) whereas the precordial leads view the heart in a horizontal or transverse plane. A 12-lead EKG is able to show:

- Whether the electrical conduction is traveling via the normal conduction pathway and if part of that pathway is malfunctioning or blocked
- Whether the EKG axis is the normal direction or deviated (known as right or left axial deviation), which can happen when the heart is not positioned normally or if it is hypertrophied
- Specific signs of significant abnormalities in particular leads—eg, Q wave myocardial infarction

A normal 12-lead EKG is shown in Figures 10-4 and 10-5. Note that the R waves in lead I and II are positive because the electrical conduction is primarily going toward the lead-I and -II recording electrodes. In contrast, the R wave in lead aVR is very small and most of the QRS wave is negative because the electrical con-

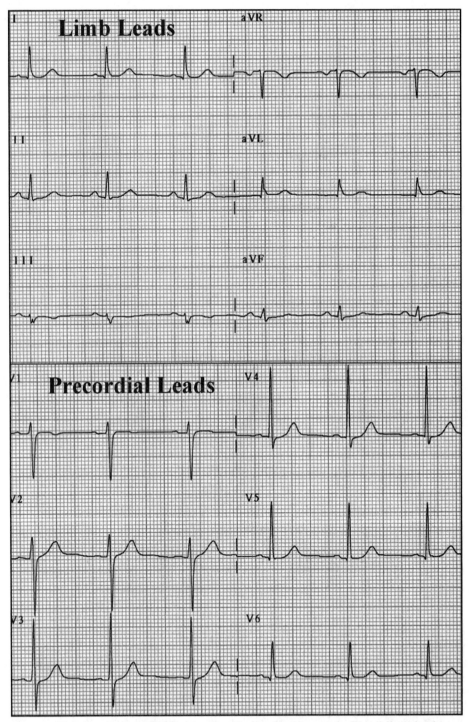

**Figure 10-4.** Twelve-lead EKG recording from a healthy adult. The 6 limb leads are shown in the upper half and the 6 precordial leads are shown in the lower half.

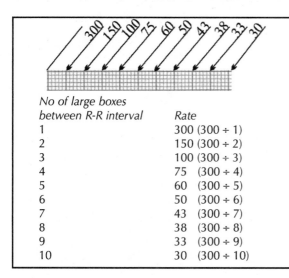

**Figure 10-5.** Determination of EKG rates. Heart rates are the shown for the intervals between the first R wave when lined up at the far left, and the second R wave aligned with the corresponding major square. See table for calculation of EKG rates according to the distance between the R-R interval of 2 beats.

| No of large boxes between R-R interval | Rate |
|---|---|
| 1 | 300 (300 ÷ 1) |
| 2 | 150 (300 ÷ 2) |
| 3 | 100 (300 ÷ 3) |
| 4 | 75 (300 ÷ 4) |
| 5 | 60 (300 ÷ 5) |
| 6 | 50 (300 ÷ 6) |
| 7 | 43 (300 ÷ 7) |
| 8 | 38 (300 ÷ 8) |
| 9 | 33 (300 ÷ 9) |
| 10 | 30 (300 ÷ 10) |

duction is going away from the aVR recording electrode. Further, the R wave normally increases in amplitude from lead V1 to lead V4 or V5 because the precordial leads provide a reflection from the thinner right ventricle to the thicker left ventricle.

A single set of leads is often used during exercise testing, especially when a stable cardiac or noncardiac patient is being assessed because the detailed electrical conduction information from a 12-lead EKG is not warranted. In this situation, often the limb lead II or V5 is used because it reflects the electrical activity of the left ventricle (which pumps blood to the systemic circulation and is highly stressed during exercise). Although a single lead EKG will not provide a 3-dimensional perspective of electrical conduction through the myocardium, it will show:

- The heart rate and the regularity of its rhythm
- Whether conduction is slowed
- Whether extra foci in the myocardium (outside of the normal conduction system) are firing ectopic beats
- Presence of ischemia in some parts of the myocardium

# APPROACH

Steps for interpreting an EKG are to examine the:

1. *Rate:* This refers to both the atrial and ventricular firing rates. See Figure 10-5 for depiction of rates. Do the atrial and ventricular firing rates match and is the rate within the normal range of 60 to 100 beats per minute (bpm)? A bradycardia is a rate slower than 60 bpm and a tachycardia is a rate higher than 100 beats per minute. If the normal conduction pathway is blocked or abnormally slow, the atrial and ventricular rates may not match.

2. *Rhythm:* Is it regular, irregular, regularly-irregular or irregularly-irregular? An irregular rhythm can arise from ectopic beats from the atria or ventricles, and slowing or blockage of the conduction pathway (see Table 10-1 for different conditions).

3. *Conduction and configuration of the waves:* Is the time for various intervals of the EKG within the normal conduction times? Are the components wider or narrower than expected? Are some of the components more peaked, notched, or M-shaped? Are the various components in the EKG pointing in the appropriate direction and is the ST segment isoelectric? Are some of the beats indicative of ectopic beats? The different components of the EKG may have slower time intervals if they are ectopic beats and if there is slowing of the conduction pathway (see Table 10-1 for different abnormalities).

4. *Axis:* Are the various components in the EKG pointing in the appropriate direction in the different 12-lead recordings? Evaluation of this aspect involves interpretation of the 12-lead EKG that will not be detailed further in this chapter.

5. *Diagnosis*

Table 10-1 lists and provides an overview of a number of EKG abnormalities.

Table 10-1

## EKG Abnormalities

| Abnormality | Configuration | Rate/Rhythm | Description |
|---|---|---|---|
| **SINUS** | | | |
| Sinus bradycardia | Normal | <60/min in adults | Electrical conduction follows the normal pathway but the rate (although regular) is lower than the lower normal limit. |
| Sinus tachycardia | Normal | 100 to 160/min in adults | Electrical conduction follows the normal pathway but the rate (although regular) is higher than the upper normal limit. |
| Sinus arrhythmia | Normal | Variable | Similar to sinus rhythm except the PP and RR intervals are irregular because the SA node is discharging at irregular intervals. |
| **REGULAR—ATRIAL OR JUNCTIONAL** | | | |
| Atrial tachycardia | P waves can be abnormal shape or inverted. | 140 to 250/min (atrial rate) | Impulses arise from an atrial pacemaker besides the SA node. At high rates not all P waves are followed by QRS waves. A 2:1 AV block can occur. |
| Atrial flutter | A "saw-tooth" appearance known as F or flutter waves reflect atrial conduction. | 240 to 340/min (atrial rate) | Impulses arise from an atrial pacemaker besides the SA node. At high rates not all P waves are followed by QRS waves. An AV block can occur which might be regular or variable. |
| Junctional tachycardia | P waves can be negative in LII lead and have variable intervals relative to QRS complexes. | 140 to 220/min | Impulses arise from the AV junctional pacemaker and travel upward to the atria and downward to the ventricles. |
| Supraventricular tachycardia | P waves are variable in shape and have variable intervals relative to QRS complexes. | 150 to 250/min | Impulses arise from the supraventricular pacemaker (above the bundle of His) and travel upward to the atria and downward to the ventricles. |
| **IRREGULAR—ATRIAL OR JUNCTIONAL** | | | |
| Premature atrial contraction (PAC) | The P wave is different shape but QRS is similar. The shape of the P wave is more abnormal when the irritable focus is further away from the SA node. | RR interval between the atrial premature beat and the previous normal beat is shorter than normal. | Arise from one or more extra "irritable" foci in the atria. |
| Atrial fibrillation | No recognizable P waves but irregular undulating baseline represents atrial fibrillatory waves. | Atrial rate of 300 to 600/min irregularly, irregular | Multifocal atrial pacemakers fire but only some are conducted to the ventricles. |

## Table 10-1 continued

## *EKG Abnormalities*

| Abnormality | Configuration | Rate/Rhythm | Description |
|---|---|---|---|
| First-degree AV block | Prolongation of PR interval greater than 0.12 sec. | Occasionally slower than 60/min | Impulses undergo normal conduction until the AV junction where conduction is slowed. |
| Second-degree AV block-Mobitz Type I (Wencke-bach) | Progressive pro-longation of the PR interval until a beat is missed. QRS complexes may be normal or wid-ened and bizarre. | P waves will have regular rate. P:QRS ratio can be 3:2, 4:3 or 5:4 or variable | Normal conduction occurs until the AV node. The conduction is progressively slowed until a ventricular contraction is missed. |
| Second-degree AV block - Mobitz Type II | An abrupt dropped QRS complex without prior PR lengthening. PR interval normal or prolonged but usually constant. QRS complexes are usually widened and bizarre. | P waves will have regular rate. P:QRS ratio can be 3:1, 4:1, or 5:1 or vari-able | Normal conduction occurs until the AV node. The conduction is intermittently blocked. |
| Idioventricular rhythm third-degree AV block | QRS complexes are widened and can be bizarre shape. | P waves are at higher rate. QRS complexes are at rate of 20 to 40 | No relationship between the atrial and ventricle contraction rates. Impulses undergo normal conduction until the AV junction where conduction is blocked. Ventricles are activated by pacemaker foci below the common bundle branch. |
| *REGULAR—VENTRICULAR* | | | |
| Ventricular tachycardia | P waves may not be observed or may be superimposed on QRS complexes. QRS complexes may be normal or slightly widened. | 100 to 250/min | Due to rapid discharge of ectopic ven-tricular foci. |
| Bundle branch block | QRS complexes are M-shaped, notched, or slurred. | | Impulses travel normally through the conduction pathways and then are blocked in the right bundle branch (RBB) or left bundle branch (LBB). |
| *REGULAR-IRREGULAR—VENTRICULAR* | | | |
| Unifocal PVC | Normal sinus rhythm intersperse with broad bizarre QRS configura-tions. | The pause after a PVC is usually compensatory—ie, the distance between the normal beat, PVC and the next normal beat is 2 RR intervals. | Arise from one "irritable" focus in the ventricles. Normal sinus rhythm inter-sperse with broad QRS configurations. Only one ventricular ectopic focus is fir-ing these extra beats, the broad QRS shapes are similar. Sometimes these PVCs can occur at regular intervals—ie, *bigeminy* is when every second beat is a PVC and *trigeminy* is when every third beat is a PVC. Unifocal PVCs do not have any clinical implications if infrequent. More frequent occurrence will result in symptoms of decreased cardiac output. |

Table 10-1 continued

## *EKG Abnormalities*

| Abnormality | Configuration | Rate/Rhythm | Description |
|---|---|---|---|
| *IRREGULAR—VENTRICULAR* | | | |
| Multifocal premature ventricular contractions | Bizarre QRS complexes that are variable in shape. | The pauses after multifocal PVCs may not be compensatory. | Arise from 2 or more extra "irritable" foci in the ventricles. Normal sinus rhythm interspersed with broad QRS configurations. If more than 1 ventricular ectopic focus is firing these extra beats, the broad QRS shapes are different. Because multifocal PVC are combined with the sinus rhythm, the rhythm is usually irregular. |
| Ventricular flutter | P waves may not be observed. QRS complex is often broad and bizarre in shape. | 250 to 350/min | Ventricular flutter is often a transient rhythm observed between ventricular tachycardia and ventricular fibrillation. |
| Ventricular fibrillation | Variable rapid fluctuation of EKG tracing. No recognizable EKG components. | | Occurs due to rapid irregular, uncoordinated and ineffective twitch-like contractions of the ventricles. Can be fatal but is reversible by defibrillation and cardiopulmonary resuscitation. |
| *ISCHEMIA/INFARCT* | | | |
| Acute myocardial infarction | T waves peak (become tall and narrow), ST segment changes, Q waves. | | After a myocardial infarct, some of the tissue becomes injured reversibly or irreversibly and no longer conducts electrical activity. An acute myocardial infarction can show changes in ST segments, T waves, and may or may not have Q waves. After weeks or months, the ST changes can disappear. After weeks to months, only the Q wave changes may be apparent if the myocardial infarct showed Q wave changes initially. |
| Angina | ST segment depression. | | ST depression can occur transiently during angina and usually returns to baseline after the angina attack has passed. If it hasn't returned to baseline, a non Q wave MI has occurred. |

# BIBLIOGRAPHY

Beasley BM. *Understanding 12-Lead EKGs: A Practical Approach*. Upper Saddle River, NJ: Prentice-Hall; 2001.

Dubin D. *Rapid Interpretation of EKGs—An Interactive Course*. 6th ed. Tampa, Fla: Cover Pub; 2000.

Stein E. *Rapid Analysis of Electrocardiograms: A Self-Study Program*. Philadelphia: Lippincott Williams & Wilkins; 2000.

Thaler MS. *The Only EKG Book You'll Ever Need*. 3rd ed. Philadelphia: Lippincott Williams & Wilkins; 1999.

Underhill SL, Wood SL, Sivarajan ES, Halpanny CJ. *Cardiac Nursing*. Philadelphia; JB Lippincott; 1983.

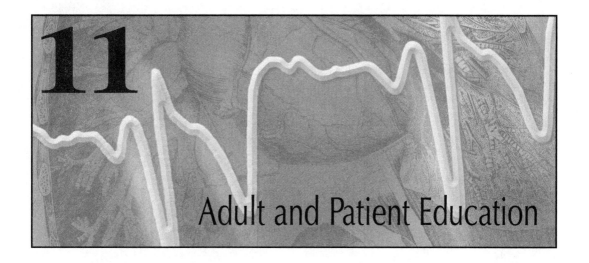

# Adult and Patient Education

## OBJECTIVES

At the end of this chapter, the reader should be able to:
1. Describe the main aspects of learning theories and models as they apply to patient education including:
   - Malcolm Knowles' Model of Adult Learning
   - Prochaska's Theory of Change
   - PRECEDE Model
   - Self-efficacy Theory
2. Describe 4 different learning styles
3. Describe the major steps for effective teaching
4. List obstacles and challenges that can be encountered during patient education

## BRIEF DESCRIPTION

Patient education can be provided on a variety of topic areas related to the person's respiratory and/or cardiovascular conditions—both in the acute and outpatient care settings. The patient education process requires not only effective teaching but also consideration of the many factors that optimize patient learning. This education often relates to self-management, lifestyle or behavioral changes, and life-long adherence to strategies to promote health.

## RATIONALE

Increased awareness of one's conditions and strategies to self-manage can promote health, minimize the impact of disease, improve quality of life, decrease emergency visits, and decrease hospital care. The ability to provide effective patient education requires thoughtful evaluation of the patient's needs and readiness, careful planning, and effective teaching to optimize learning and behavioral changes by the patient.

## EVIDENCE

*Grade B* for cardiac and pulmonary rehabilitation patient education.

## WHICH GROUPS OF INDIVIDUALS?

- Patient preoperatively and postoperatively especially for major surgeries such as upper abdominal, thoracic, cardiac, and transplant surgeries

- People with cardiovascular disease such as myocardial infarction, valvular disease, and peripheral vascular disease
- People with chronic lung disease such as COPD, interstitial lung disease, bronchiectasis, and asthma
- Less formalized and more customized for people with cystic fibrosis. Because of their early diagnosis, these individuals are often very aware of their condition

# LEARNING THEORIES

Learning theories and models provide a guideline or framework that can describe how patients learn, and illustrate obstacles or challenges to learning and behavioral changes. They do not provide specific instruction of how to deliver patient education but provide a deeper context to develop effective teaching tools and to develop evaluative measures to diagnose obstacles and challenges.

## Malcolm Knowles' Model of Adult Learning[1]

Malcolm Knowles identified some key characteristics of adult learners. Some of these features are:
1. Adults *need to know* why they need to learn the information being presented. Their learning is problem or life centered rather than topic centered
2. Adults need to be perceived and treated as independent individuals *who manage their own lives*
3. Adults can share *experiences* to enrich the learning resource material
4. Adults are *ready to learn* when the reason to learn matches the necessity to meet their identified personal challenge(s). They are motivated by factors that might improve their situation internally—ie, feeling better or externally by improving their work or living situation

## Prochaska's Theory of Change—Transtheoretical Model[2]

The primary feature of this theory is that it outlines a series of stages that most patients go through when they attempt to initiate and carry out behavioral changes. These stages are:
1. *Precontemplation*—when the person has no intention of initiating a behavioral change, which may be due to lack of awareness and information, or lack of readiness
2. *Contemplation*—when the person is carefully considering the possibility of initiating a change
3. *Preparation*—when the person has a clear intent of initiating a behavioral change in the near or immediate future
4. *Action*—when the person is actively making changes in his or her behavior
5. *Maintenance*—when the behavior is sustained or a relapse is prevented. This stage can last several months to years
6. *Termination*—when the person does not revert back to old behavioral problems. This last stage does not apply to all behavioral changes

When considering patient education on a topic that requires a major lifestyle change such as smoking cessation or initiating an exercise program, the therapist needs to evaluate what stage the patient is in so he or she can tailor the education session accordingly.

## PRECEDE Model[3]

The PRECEDE model (Preceding, Reinforcing, Enabling Causes in Educational Diagnosis and Evaluation) provides another context to examine factors that might facilitate, obstruct or reinforce the success of a patient education program. These factors can be related to the patient, society, culture, and the environment. The PRECEDE model outlines 3 main categories of factors to examine while implementing a patient education program:
1. *Predisposing factors*—relate to the beliefs, attitudes, values, and knowledge that the patient has about his or her condition. The therapist must find out and evaluate these beliefs in order to build on them or to correct misconceptions. For example, if the patient believes that exercise will cause a heart attack, this belief needs to be discussed before the therapist can outline the benefits and steps of carrying out an exercise program. If there are cultural norms that need to be adhered to, the therapist needs a full understanding of these norms so that the exercise program can be initiated within the context of these norms.

2. *Enabling factors*—are factors that enable someone to successfully carry out an activity when he or she believes he or she should be doing the behavior but are not able to do so at the present time. This involves identifying aspects that will allow the patient to master the skills required and to identify resources (home support, financial, community) that are required to carry out the task. While identifying these factors, the therapist should try to facilitate the patient in determining the solutions rather than the therapist simply providing the "easy" answer to the patient.

3. *Reinforcing factors*—are factors that reinforce the changed behavior. These can include support and encouragement by family, friends, and health care providers. As the new behavior continues, a very important reinforcer is that the patient feels better; however, the patient needs to be apprised of the timing between the behavior change and feeling better. For example, some medications act almost immediately, whereas the benefits of exercise may take a minimum of 10 days to 2 weeks. If the patient is not aware of the length of time for the benefit to occur, they may discount the potential merit from the therapy and discontinue the new behavior.

## *Self-Efficacy Theory*[3,4]

The main premise of this theory is that the patient's belief or lack of belief is a major determinant of his or her motivation and ability to carry out the task. Further, their self-efficacy can be enhanced by mastering a technique, modeling behavior after a patient who has overcome a similar problem, improving understanding of symptoms, and being persuaded (which is usually more successful if the steps are small). All 4 of these approaches can be used to facilitate behavioral changes in pulmonary and cardiac rehabilitation programs.

# LEARNING STYLES[5,6]

Everyone learns in different ways. A better understanding of learning styles will facilitate the development of more effective patient education tools and approaches. In a group setting, one cannot individualize the session to meet one person's style, however, by using a number of approaches, the therapist is likely to optimize learning for most participants. Different types of learning styles include:

1. *Diverging*—People with this style often learn by observing from different points of view. They may enjoy group sessions when a number of ideas are generated such as a brainstorming session.

2. *Assimilating*—People with this style can examine a wide range of information and integrate it into a concise, logical form. They are often less people oriented and more interested in abstract ideas and concepts.

3. *Converging*—People with this style are directed toward finding practical applications for theories and ideas.

4. *Accommodating*—People with this style primarily learn from active hands-on experimentation.

Other details of these learning styles are provided in Table 11-1. When planning your patient education session, consider these different learning styles and understand that your presentation and teaching approach may be more appealing to certain individuals more so than others regardless of the content of your session.

# OBSTACLES IN PATIENT EDUCATION

- Anxiety and depression
- Fatigue, pain, dyspnea
- Lack of literacy—more than 40% of Americans and Canadians have poor literacy skills or can only deal with material that is simple and clearly laid out (Level 1 or 2) when using information from brochures or instruction manuals.[7,8]
- Culture and ethnicity
- Competing priorities and habits—eg, work schedule, home demands from young children
- Diminished cognition especially if hypoxemia is present
- Loss of sight or hearing
- Lack of support and resources—eg, financial, transportation to health clinic, community resources, home support

Table 11-1

## Learning Styles

| Learner's Style | Teacher's Style | Learning Strategies | Teaching Methods |
|---|---|---|---|
| *Diverger* Concrete/reflexive learner. Likes to discover the "why" of a situation | Motivator | Searching for information Evaluating current information | Information presented in a detailed, systematic, reasoned manner: specific lectures, hands-on exploration |
| *Assimilator* Abstract conceptualization/ reflective observers Likes to answer "What is there to know?" | Expert or resource person | Predicting outcomes Inferring causes | Information presented in a highly organized format: lectures followed by demonstration, presentations, laboratories |
| *Converger* Abstract conceptualization/ active experimenters Likes to understand "how" things work | Coach | Testing theories Designing experiments | Information: applied and useful interactive instruction, case studies, workbooks, computer-assisted learning |
| *Accommodator* Concrete experience/ experimenter likes to ask "What if?" and "Why not?" | Tasks' assigner and supervisor | Trying different solutions Independent learning | Information unstructured: experimentations, active learner's participation |

Reprinted with permission from Nault D, Dagenais J, Perreault V, Borycki E. Patient education. In: Bourbeau J, Nault D, Borycki E, eds. *Comprehensive Management of Chronic Obstructive Pulmonary Disease.* Hamilton, ON: BC Dekker Inc; 2002; 301-318.

# KEY STEPS IN EFFECTIVE TEACHING

Regardless of whether a therapist is providing education to a patient, work colleague, or student, the content of the lesson should have some major components.

1. *Use well-established patient education resources*—There are many resources of patient education readily available from well-established rehabilitation or outpatient programs, hospital departments, and local and national agencies such as the lung and heart associations (see Web sites at the end of this chapter). Rather than "reinventing the wheel" for patient education content, the therapist is encouraged to access these resource materials so that one can focus more time on developing his or her teaching approaches.

2. *Motivate learners with a "hook"*—After your introduction, one needs to clearly explain the relevance of what you are about to teach in order to *motivate* the learner. Think of this as the *hook*. This needs to be short and catchy; the therapist needs to have the patient's attention and motivation to learn, otherwise the rest of the learning session is wasted.

3. *Assess the needs of the learner*—The hook is followed by a *needs assessment*. Identification of what the patient needs to learn rather than having a preset agenda will optimize the patient's benefit from the

exchange of information. The instructor needs to identify the individual's readiness, willingness, and abilities to learn health education. This will include consideration of their physical and emotional condition in addition to their baseline level of knowledge. A needs assessment will help determine priorities and barriers to learning.

4. *Organize the session with clear objectives*—The *objectives* of the lesson plan needs to be clearly stated in a patient-focused format. These objectives should be defined and refined by both the therapist and learner.

5. *Involve patients with participatory learning*—The body of the lesson should primarily consist of *participatory learning*. This will ensure that the patient remains actively engaged in the learning experience and also provides feedback regarding how the lesson content is being received. Depending on the patient's comments, the therapist can shift the lesson to a slightly different direction, simplify content or expand on a particular topic.

6. *Close the lesson with a post-test*—The last part of the lesson is a post-test when the patient is asked about content of the lesson. This provides important reinforcement of the main points of the lesson as well as providing more feedback regarding the comprehension of the material.

## STRATEGIES FOR DIAGNOSING OBSTACLES

In order to determine whether the patient understands and is implementing patient education material, the therapist should:

- Ask questions
- Review a typical day
- Review the treatment plan and ask for a demonstration

## REFERENCES

1. Knowles M. *The Adult Learner—A Neglected Species*. 4th ed. Houston: Gulf Publishing Company; 1990.
2. Prochaska JO, Redding CA, Evers KE. The transtheoretical model and stages of change. In: Glantz K, Lewis K, Rimer B, eds. *Health Behavior and Health Education: Theory, Research and Practice*. 2nd ed. San Francisco, Calif: Jossey-Bass; 1997;60-84.
3. Goeppinger J, Lorig K. What we know about what works: one rationale, two models, three theories. In: Lorig K, ed. *Patient Education: A Practical Approach*. 2nd ed. Thousand Oaks, Calif: Sage Publications; 1996;195-226.
4. Bandura A. *Social Learning Theory*. Englewoods Cliffs, NJ: Prentice Hall; 1977.
5. Kolb DA. *Learning Style Inventory*. Version 3. Boston, Mass: Experience Based learning Systems, Inc. Hay/McBer Training Resources Group; 1999.
6. Nault D, Dagenais J, Perreault V, Borycki E. Patient education. In: Bourbeau J, Nault D, Borycki E, eds. *Comprehensive Management of Chronic Obstructive Pulmonary Disease*. Hamilton, ON: BC Dekker Inc; 2002;301-318.
7. Doak CC. *Teaching Patients With Low Literacy Skills*. Philadelphia: Lippincott; 1996.
8. Statistics Canada. Literacy in the information age: final report of the international adult literacy survey. Cat. No. 89-571-XPE. Available at: www.statcan.ca. Accessed April 1, 2004.

## WEB SITES FOR PATIENT EDUCATION RESOURCES AND CONTENT

### *Heart Information*

- www.heartandstroke.ca     The Canadian Heart and Stroke Foundation
- www.americanheart.org     The American Heart Association
- www.aacvpr.org     The American Association of Cardiovascular and Pulmonary Rehabilitation

## Lung Information

- www.lung.ca                    The Canadian Lung Association
- www.lungusa.org                The American Lung Association

## Cigarette Smoking

- www.medbroadcast.com/health_topics/smoking/index.shtml?costs_of_smoking.html
  The med broadcast smoking cessation page

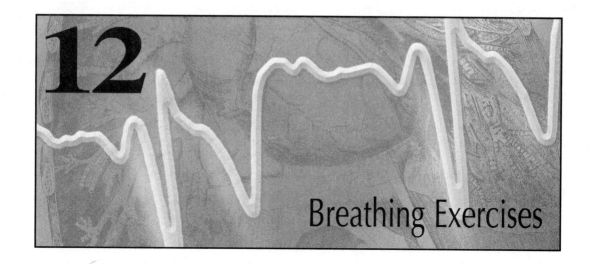

# Breathing Exercises

## OBJECTIVES

Upon completion of this chapter, the therapist should be able to:
1. Describe the therapeutic rationale for different breathing exercise techniques
2. Describe the level of evidence to support different breathing exercise techniques
3. Effectively prescribe and instruct breathing exercises for acute medical and surgical patients and those with chronic respiratory disease

## BRIEF DESCRIPTION

Breathing exercises can be used to optimize gas exchange, promote lung expansion, minimize atelectasis, decrease dyspnea, and promote secretion removal. This chapter will focus on 2 major types of breathing exercises:
1. Those used to promote lung expansion and minimize atelectasis. These techniques include deep breathing, deep breathing with breath stacking, deep breathing with inspiratory hold, and incentive spirometry.
2. Those used to reduce dyspnea and to promote lung expansion or minimize atelectasis in individuals with moderate to severe chronic respiratory disease. These include breathing control and pursed lip-breathing techniques.

## RATIONALE—FACTORS THAT AFFECT VENTILATION

### Time Constants

A time constant is the product of the compliance and resistance of an alveolar unit. In healthy individuals, the time constants of the 3 million alveolar units in the lungs are relatively uniform. In lung disease, the alveoli may become more or less compliant (less or more stiff) and the small airways leading to these alveoli can develop increased resistance. Those alveolar units with increased resistance will take longer to fill. Those alveoli that are stiffer will take a greater inspiratory effort to fill.

### Inspiratory Flow Rate

Slower deeper breaths allow regions with long time constants to fill more. This is thought to be a major reason why breathing control and pursed lip breathing techniques result in improved gas exchange; however, the evidence supporting this postulate is speculative. It has been shown that slow inspiration (<0.2 L/s) from FRC will fill lower lung regions and a faster inspiration will fill upper lung regions in subjects with healthy lungs.[1] Slow deep inspiration with an inspiratory hold also tends to produce a more uniform distribution of ventilation with a minimal gradient between the apices and bases when compared to rapid inspiration.

### *Voluntarily Altering Regional Ventilation—Can We Instruct Patients to Ventilate a Specific Lung Region?*

In the 1970's, unilateral breathing techniques by applying pressure with either a hand or a towel over 1 side in order to facilitate regional lung expansion were considered to be viable treatment options[2,3]; however, Martin et al[4] showed that instruction to enhance or restrict unilateral breathing had no effect on rate of ventilation, perfusion, nor oxygen uptake. Subsequent research has shown that healthy people are able to direct inspiration to upper or lower lung regions upon instruction.[5-7] Whether this technique may be of benefit in patients has not yet been shown.

### *Gravity and Closing Volume*

Both gravity and closing volume have profound effects on regional ventilation. See Chapter 13 for more details.

## EVIDENCE

*Grade B*—Evidence from small, randomized trials support the use of breathing exercises and incentive spirometry[8,9] to promote lung expansion postoperatively.[10] A similar level of evidence supports the use of breathing control/pursed lip techniques but not diaphragmatic breathing in people with chronic respiratory disease.[11-13]

## BREATHING EXERCISES OR MOBILIZATION ONLY IN ACUTE CARE PATIENTS

The answer to that question is to do both. After upper abdominal surgery, patients who did deep breathing exercises had significantly larger increases in tidal volume whereas ambulation alone did not result in a significant increase.[14] Of likely greater benefit, the therapist should instruct patients to breathe deeply while ambulating.

## INDICATIONS FOR BREATHING EXERCISES IN PATIENTS WITH NO CHRONIC LUNG DISEASE

- Postoperatively especially in high-risk individuals:
  - Elderly
  - Smokers
  - Obese
  - Compounding medical conditions—eg, immunosuppressed, neuromuscular dysfunction
- Postoperatively especially in those following *high-risk surgeries:*
  - Thoracic or upper abdominal surgery
  - Long duration of general anesthetic and surgery
- Clinical signs of atelectasis or lung infection:
  - Elevated temperature
  - Chest x-ray signs consistent with atelectasis or lung infection
  - Abnormal physical and auscultatory signs consistent with atelectasis or lung infection
  - Hypoxemia

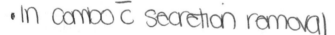
• In combo c̄ secretion removal

# INDICATIONS FOR INCENTIVE SPIROMETRY

Same indications as those shown previously *and:*
- Those who are *high-risk* cases, including patients with *restricted mobility*
- The use of incentive spirometry in patients with sickle cell anemia was shown to decrease pulmonary complication rate[8]
- Routine use of incentive spirometer in conjunction with respiratory physical therapy is questionable[15]
- *Contraindicated* in patients with moderate to severe COPD and acute asthma who have an increased respiratory rate and hyperinflation. In these patients, if the incentive spirometer technique does not allow the patient to fully expire, it should not be used

# IS INCENTIVE SPIROMETRY
# SUPERIOR TO BREATHING EXERCISES?

Two systematic reviews[16,17] reported no advantage of the use of incentive spirometry over other treatment techniques such as deep breathing exercise, and continuous positive airway pressure. A common problem with the studies selected by these reviews was small sample sizes, resulting in a lack of statistical power to identify a significant difference if a difference existed. In other words, with the small sample sizes used in these studies, only treatments with very large effect size could have been identified. In addition, it is difficult to control other confounding factors such as deep breathing, coughing, and ambulation in clinical studies, which will likely affect the effectiveness of incentive spirometry.

Two recent randomized control trials that reported beneficial effects with the use of incentive spirometer were not included in the 2 systematic reviews. Bellet et al[8] compared incentive spirometry to no incentive spirometry in patients with sickle cell diseases. The incidence of pulmonary complications was significantly lower in the incentive spirometry group—1/19 in spirometry group versus 8/19 in the nonspirometry group. This study showed an important decrease in complication rate for those patients who used incentive spirometry. Whether this benefit will be shown in other patient groups needs to be tested. Weiner et al[9] compared the use of incentive spirometry and inspiratory muscle training on pulmonary function after lung resection. They reported improvement in pulmonary function 2 weeks before surgery and 3 months after surgery between the treatment and nontreatment groups. However, it is not known whether incentive spirometry or inspiratory muscle training alone was more beneficial.

# INDICATIONS FOR BREATHING EXERCISES
# IN PATIENTS WITH CHRONIC RESPIRATORY DISEASE

Pursed lip breathing exercises have primarily been shown to be effective in patients with chronic obstructive respiratory diseases but may also benefit those with other chronic respiratory problems. These techniques can be used for in- and outpatients with chronic respiratory disease based on the following criteria:
- Clinically significant dyspnea at rest or with activities and exercise
- Atelectasis
- Pneumonia
- As an adjunct for relaxation techniques
- As an adjunct for secretion removal techniques

**Figure 12-1.** Volumetric type incentive spirometer. Voldyne, Sherwood Medical, St. Louis, Mo.

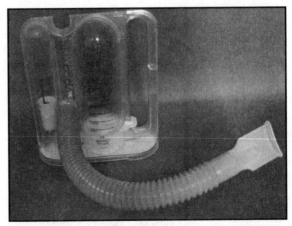

**Figure 12-2.** Flow rate type incentive spirometer. Portex incentive spirometer, Sims Portex Inc, Fort Myers, Fla.

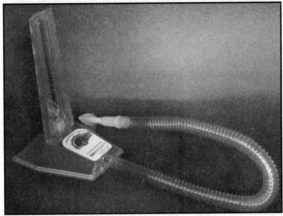

*Don't forget analgesics + bronchodilators*

## Breathing Exercises   Side lying & high sitting preferred

For all breathing exercises, position patient in an upright position when possible.

1. *Those to promote basal lung expansion and minimize atelectasis*—use when patient has <u>no chronic obstructive pulmonary disease</u>

   - Assesses the inspiratory effort of the patient and position the patient accordingly.
   - Frequent position change and deep breathing in different positions are encouraged.
   - Deep breathing exercises with slow sustained inspiration:
     o Emphasize diaphragmatic and lateral costal expansion. Place hands over lower lateral aspects of chest wall.
     o Emphasize minimal upper chest movement.
   - Deep breathing exercises with maximum end-inspiratory hold.
     o Same as above—deep breathing exercises with <u>slow</u> sustained inspiration—except inspiration is to a full vital capacity with an end inspiratory hold for 3 to 5 seconds to maximize alveolar expansion.
   - Deep breathing exercises using incentive spirometer.
     o There are 2 main types of incentive spirometers commercially available: flow and volume. Volumetric incentive spirometers (Figure 12-1) are theoretically better because they provide the appropriate feedback for a slow sustained inspiration and volume. In contrast a flow incentive spirometer (Figure 12-2, Figure 12-3) will have the marker reach the appropriate level with a quick or sustained deep breath so long as a sufficient flow is achieved. Slow sustained inspirations are much more effective to promote lung expansion rather than fast inspirations.

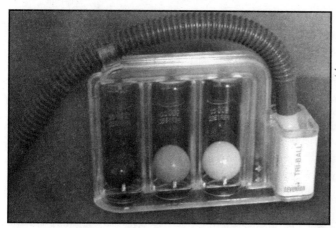

**Figure 12-3.** Flow rate type incentive spirometer. Tri Ball, Leventon, Barcelona, Spain.

*\* Don't take O₂ mask off if on >40%*
*-35-40% - use caution*
*- monitor sats*

Table 12-1

## Instructions in the Use of Incentive Spirometer

1. Position patient in an upright sitting position. The incentive spirometer has to be positioned upright for it to show accurate volumes and flows.
2. Instruct the patient to:
   - Exhale to functional residual capacity.
   - Put the mouthpiece in his or her mouth and inhale slowly.

### Using the Flow Meter Type

- Inhale so that the ball stays at the top for as long as possible or so that all the balls stay up in the air.
- For those units that offer different flow rates, the therapist can change the flow rate to provide different levels of challenge. However, the higher flow rate settings are frequently misused to achieve a large inhalation.

### Using the Volumetric Type

- Inhale within an "ideal" flow rate by keeping the flow indicator within the prescribed range while at the same time inhaling as deeply as possible.

### Additional Considerations for Incentive Spirometry

- Select an incentive spirometer that measures inspiratory volume and provides feedback on inspiratory flow rate.
- Monitor the use and compliance of its use. Patients should use the incentive spirometer at least 10 times every 1 to 2 hours during their waking hours.
- Monitor the patient's effort when using the incentive spirometer.
- Obtain the maximum inspiratory volume before surgery when possible and use it as the target volume after surgery.
- Allow the patients to be familiar with the incentive spirometer by having them practice with the device at home prior to surgery.

o Instructions for the use of different incentive spirometers are provided in Table 12-1.
o Clear and precise instructions need to be provided to patients. Frequently, patients have complained that their incentive spirometer does not work because they have blown into the device! Allowing the patient to practice incentive spirometry before surgery may facilitate patient learning.

- Deep breathing exercises with breath stacking:
  - Avoid forced exhalation below FRC because breathing may be below closing volume (see Chapter 13 for more explanation). Breath stacking is a series of deep breaths building on top of the previous one without expiration until a maximum volume tolerated by the patient is reached.[18] Each inspiration consists of a few seconds of a brief inspiratory hold. It is often used when a large breath is too painful.    → slows down expiration

2. *Breathing control/pursed lip breathing*—is primarily used to promote relaxation and reduce dyspnea in patients who have <u>significant chronic obstructive pulmonary disease</u> (dyspnea and hyperinflation). These techniques can also be used by other patients who are dyspneic such as those with restrictive lung disease. The patient is instructed to :

- Breathe in through the nose and out through his or her mouth
- Gently expire and not to force expiration at all. Often expiration through pursed lips is promoted.
- Expire 2 to 3 times longer than inspiration
- Do not focus on the use of diaphragm. Many patients with COPD have a partially or totally flattened diaphragm; thus, they cannot use their diaphragm to any extent. Patients should not be criticized for not being able to do diaphragmatic/abdominal breathing.[19,20] Rather, they should be asked to fill air into the abdominal regions as much as possible.
- Promote optimal use of accessories by ensuring the shoulder girdle is relaxed. The therapist may instruct the patient to be positioned with arms supported in order to facilitate accessory muscle use (See Chapter 13 for positioning).

Pursed lip breathing can improve oxygenation in some COPD patients[13,21] and those with other respiratory disorders. The deleterious effects of breathing exercises, however, need to be considered when prescribing them to patients. In COPD, diaphragmatic breathing has been associated with decreased mechanical efficiency, a tendency for increased dyspnea[12,19,20] and a decrease in respiratory drive in some patients[11] when compared to their natural breathing pattern.

Because of the potential for deleterious effects from breathing exercises, the therapist should monitor $SpO_2$, dyspnea, and chest wall motion while the patient is performing pursed lip breathing, especially in those individuals with moderate to severe COPD associated with marked hyperinflation and/or poor arterial blood gases. Any instruction in modifying breathing pattern should not be associated with deterioration in $SpO_2$, increased dyspnea, and asynchronous chest wall motion.

## Coordination of Breathing Exercises With Other Treatments

It is essential to coordinate physical therapy treatment with administration of medication in 2 cases:
- Pain medication in postoperative patients or those with significant chest trauma[22-24]
- Bronchodilator medication in those with COPD, asthma, or other conditions that result in bronchoconstriction

## Other Considerations

- *Positioning in bed.* If the patient has to rest in bed, side lying is best to preserve the FRC. Slumped sitting and supine tend to decrease the FRC. However, studies have been shown that sitting in the upright position and standing will increase the FRC and the vital capacity (VC). Avoid or minimize the period of bed rest. A rotation bed (see Chapter 13) or frequent position change might be beneficial for those patients requiring prolonged immobilization in bed.
- *Mobilization* used in conjunction with breathing exercises will often promote better lung expansion than breathing exercises alone. See Chapter 14 for more details about mobilization.
- *Secretion removal.* When the patient is congested and unable to expectorate by deep breathing and positioning alone, manual techniques should be used concurrently with deep breathing and must finish with deep breathing exercises to ensure full expansion of the treated area.

# REFERENCES

1. Bake B, Wood L, Murphy B, et al. Effect of inspiratory flow rate on regional distribution of inspired gas. *J Appl Physiol.* 1974;37:8-17.

2. Gaskell DV, Webber DA. *The Brompton Hospital Guide to Chest Physiotherapy.* 2nd ed. Oxford: Blackwell Scientific Publications; 1973.

3. Cash J. Introduction to the treatment of medical chest conditions. In: Downie P, ed. *Cash's Textbook of Chest, Heart, and Vascular Disorders for Physiotherapist.* 1st ed. London: Faber and Faber; 1979.

4. Martin CJ, Ripley H, Reynolds J, Best F. The distribution of ventilation. *Chest.* 1976;69:174-178.

5. Lloyd JJ, James JM, Shields RA, et al. The influence of inhalation technique on Technegas particle deposition and image appearance in normal volunteers. *Eur J Nucl Med.* 1994;21:394-8.

6. Roussos CS, Fixley M, Genest J, et al. Voluntary factors influencing the distribution of inspired gas. *Am Review Respir Dis.* 1977;116:457-467.

7. Tucker B, Jenkins S, Cheong D, et al. Effect of unilateral breathing exercises on regional lung ventilation. *Nucl Med Commun.* 1999;20:815-821.

8. Bellet PS, Kalinyak KA, Shukla R, et al. Incentive spirometry to prevent acute pulmonary complications in sickle cell diseases. *N Eng J Med.* 1995;333:699-703.

9. Weiner P, Man A, Weiner M, et al. The effect of incentive spirometry and inspiratory muscle training on pulmonary function after lung resection. *J Thorac Cardiovasc Surg.* 1997;113:552-557.

10. Brooks D, Crow J, Kelsey CJ, Lacy JB, Parsons J, Solway S. A clinical practice guideline on perioperative cardiorespiratory physiotherapy. *Physiotherapy Canada.* 2001;Winter:9-25.

11. Sackner MA, Gonzales HF, Jenouri G, Rodrigez M. Effects of abdominal and thoracic breathing on breathing pattern components in normal subjects and in patients with chronic obstructive pulmonary disease. *Am Rev Respir Dis.* 1984;130:584-587.

12. Cahalin LP, Braga M, Matsuo Y, Hernandez ED. Efficacy of diaphragmatic breathing in persons with chronic obstructive pulmonary disease: a review of the literature. *J Cardiopulm Rehab.* 2002;22:7-21.

13. Dechman G, Wilson CR. Evidence underlying cardiopulmonary physical therapy in stable COPD. *Cardiopulmonary Physical Therapy.* 2002;13(2):20-22.

14. Orfanos P, Ellis E, Johnston C. Effects of deep breathing exercise and ambulation on pattern of ventilation in post-operative patients. *Aust J Physiother.* 1999;45:173-182.

15. Crowe JM, Bradley CA. The effectiveness of incentive spirometry with physical therapy for high-risk patients after coronary artery bypass surgery. *Phys Ther.* 1997;77:260-268.

16. Overend TJ, Anderson CM, Lucy SD, et al. The effect of incentive spirometry on postoperative pulmonary complications. A systematic review. *Chest.* 2001;120:971-978.

17. Thomas JA, McIntosh JM. Are incentive spirometry, intermittent positive pressure breathing, and deep breathing exercises effective in the prevention of postoperative pulmonary complications after upper abdominal surgery? A systematic overview and meta-analysis. *Phys Ther.* 1994;74:3-16.

18. Baker WL, Virnita JL, Marini LL. Breath-stacking increases the depth and duration of chest expansion by incentive spirometry. *Am Rev Respir Dis.* 1990;141:343-346.

19. Gosselink RA, Wagenaar RC, Rijswijk H, et al. Diaphragmatic breathing reduces efficiency of breathing in patients with COPD. *Am J Respir Crit Care Med.* 1995;151:1136-1142.

20. Vitacca M, Clini E, Bianchi L, et al. Acute effects of deep diaphragmatic breathing in COPD patients with chronic respiratory insufficiency. *Eur Respir J.* 1998;11:408-415.

21. Tiep BL, Byrns M, Kao D, et al. Pursed lips breathing training using ear oximetry. *Chest.* 1986;90:218-221.

22. Dureuil B, Viires N, Caantineau JP, et al. Diaphragmatic contractility after upper abdominal surgery. *J Appl Physiol.* 1986;61:1775-1780.

23. Ford GT, Whitelaw WA, Rosenal TW, et al. Diaphragm function and upper abdominal surgery in humans. *Am Rev Respir Dis.* 1983;127:431-436.

24. Vassilakopoulos T, Mastora Z, Paraskevi P, et al. Contribution of pain to inspiratory muscle dysfunction after upper abdominal surgery. A randomized controlled trial. *Am J Respir Crit Care Med.* 2000;161:1372-1375.

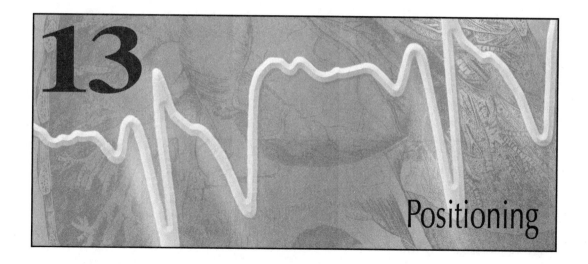

# OBJECTIVES

Upon completion of this chapter, the therapist should be able to:

1. Describe the effects of positioning on the cardiovascular and respiratory systems
2. Describe the therapeutic rationale for different positions
3. Describe the level of evidence to support the therapeutic use of different positions
4. Prescribe appropriate positions for acute medical and surgical patients and for those with chronic respiratory disease

# BRIEF DESCRIPTION

Physiotherapists prescribe the therapeutic use of different body positions in a variety of patient groups with cardiovascular and respiratory problems. Positioning can be used to:

- Optimize relaxation
- Provide pain relief
- Improve ventilation, ventilation-perfusion matching, and gas exchange
- Minimize dyspnea
- Minimize the work of breathing—ie, promote efficient diaphragm and accessory muscle function
- Promote airway clearance (described in Chapter 15)

<u>Common Clinical Issue</u>

In healthy subjects during tidal breathing, the apex (upper most or nondependent region) has larger alveolar volumes than in the bases (lower most or dependent region) of the lung. During deep inspiration, the base (dependent region) of the lung has the most ventilation. Where is the most common site of atelectasis in surgical patients? Why? How do you position these patients to improve ventilation and gas exchange?

You should be able to answer these questions by the middle of this chapter.

**Figure 13-1.** Distribution of ventilation at FRC and low lung volumes. At FRC (top panel), the alveoli at the top of the lung become stiffer sooner and fill less whereas the alveoli at the bottom remain compliant and fill with more volume during a normal breath. The key point about this concept is that it applies to healthy individuals with no pathology. Many patients postoperatively are breathing at lower lung volumes (bottom panel) so that a normal tidal breath results in minimal or no volume change in the alveoli at the bases, whereas volume change of apical alveoli are greater.

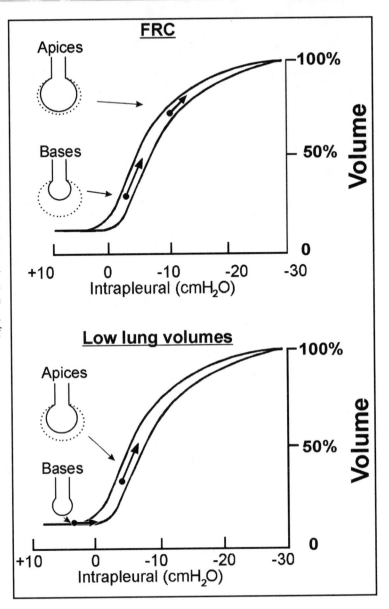

# RATIONALE FOR POSITIONING TO PROMOTE OPTIMAL GAS EXCHANGE AND VENTILATION

## Gravity and the Pleural Pressure Gradient

Clinical Note
The lowermost lung regions may not inflate well in individuals postoperatively. Be sure to position atelectatic regions upper most or promote frequent position change.

Gravity results in a vertical pleural pressure gradient that causes the alveoli at the top of the lung to have a larger resting volume and the alveoli at the bottom of the lung to have a smaller resting volume at FRC (end of expiration). Thus, in healthy people, the alveoli at the top of the lung become stiffer *sooner* and fill less whereas the alveoli at the bottom remain compliant and fill with more volume during a normal breath (Figure 13-1). The key point about this concept is that *it applies to healthy individuals with no pathology* and to those not experiencing postoperative changes in their lungs. Many patients with acute respiratory conditions—such as those postoperatively—are breathing at lower lung volumes so that a normal tidal breath results in minimal volume change in the alveoli at the bases (see Figure 13-1). The lung bases are on the lower asymtotic region of "pressure-volume" curve and a smaller inspiratory effort due to incisional pain may not be sufficient to inflate the alveoli in the bases.

### Closing Volume

Closing volume is the lung volume that dependent airways close. In young healthy adults, closing volume occurs well below FRC or even below RV (for young adults in their early 20's or younger). In healthy elderly adults and smokers, closing volume may occur close to or above FRC. General anesthetic and the sequelae that follow postoperatively result in a decrease in FRC such that closing volume may occur above FRC in younger adults and this is further accentuated in smokers and older adults. In other words, the small airways in the lower lung regions may close during a normal tidal breath resulting in no ventilation of some alveoli—and much less efficient ventilation overall.

> A higher closing volume in the elderly is considered to be one reason why these individuals have a lower arterial oxygen partial pressure even when healthy.

### Cardiovascular and Pulmonary Effects of Positioning

The upright position can improve pulmonary function but can have negative hemodynamic effect, whereas the supine or head-down position tends to have the opposite impacts (Table 13-1). Other issues to consider in some patients are the effects of different positions on the diaphragm, accessory inspiratory and expiratory muscle use. Table 13-1 outlines the usual responses of healthy people to different positions. These factors should be considered and weighed carefully when selecting the most advantageous positions because patients can have many pathologies such that they respond in an atypical manner. After positioning, the therapist needs to carefully monitor the therapeutic impact of each position in every patient.

### Cardiopulmonary Effects of Positioning Based on Clinical Trials

In recent years, there have been many clinical trials on positioning in different medical conditions. Most of the trials are based on pre- and post-repeated measures designs with small sample sizes. The results of some of these studies are summarized in Appendices A and B.

Less has been published regarding the benefit of relaxation positions. Bracing the arms and the lean-forward position has been shown to improve the function of the inspiratory muscles in healthy people and those with COPD.[1-3]

# POSITIONING FOR ACUTE
# MEDICAL AND SURGICAL PATIENTS

### Evidence: B

For details of evidence, see Summary section and Appendix A.

### Which groups?

- All patients who are allowed to be mobilized or mobility status is "activity as tolerated" (AAT). Some patients, however, might require other physical therapy interventions in addition to specific positioning.

Note:

- Among patients that are allowed to be mobilized, only some of the more unstable patients are sensitive to position change.

- In these patients, the change in oxygenation between positions is usually minimal. One common exception is the use of prone position in patients with acute lung insufficiency.

Table 13-1

## Cardiovascular and Pulmonary Effects of Different Positions

### Upright

- Increases FRC
- Increases FVC
- Decreases closing volume
- Increases chest wall anterior-posterior diameter
- Decreases venous return and cardiac output
- Increases pooling of secretions in the bases of the lung
- Better basal expansion with large inspiration (except when breathing at low lung volumes or during positive pressure mechanical ventilation)
- Decreases curvature of diaphragm at end-expiration—especially in those patients with weak abdominals

### Supine

- Decreases chest wall AP diameter
- Reduces FRC
- Pooling of secretions to the posterior (dependent) lung zone
- Increases central blood volume
- Increases airway closure
- Increases curvature of diaphragm at end-expiration—especially in those with weak abdominals

### Head Down

- Further increases central blood volume more so than supine
- Promotes basal expansion
- Increases curvature of diaphragm at end-expiration but imposes a greater load to inspire against Can increase dyspnea

### Side-Lying

- Increases chest wall AP diameter of the dependent region
- Increases ventilation to the dependent region but decreases tidal volume and FRC
- Theoretically speaking, positioning the good lung lowermost should improve oxygenation

### Prone

- Improves oxygenation in patients with ARDS or acute lung injury

### Arms-Supported

- Can facilitate accessory muscle contraction
- Decreases dyspnea

### Sitting With Lean Forward, Arms Supported on Knees

- Improves diaphragm contraction and efficiency
- Facilitates accessory muscle contraction
- Decreases dyspnea

## *Side to Side, Upright and Supine Positioning*

General guidelines for positioning:
- Use pillows to ensure comfort
- Ensure patient is safely positioned in bed
- Use bed rails appropriately
- Ensure proper body alignments when positioning patients
- Keep patient's joints in neutral or relaxed positions
- Use pressure-reducing materials such as dressings or mattresses for patients who are susceptible to pressure sores
- Frequently change position to patient's tolerance

## *When Changing Position*

- Encourage "log" rolling
- Ask patient to participate when changing position as much as possible
- Incorporate leg circulation exercises especially when getting the patient upright from the horizontal position
- When getting the patient upright from the horizontal position, raise the head of the bed gradually to the upright position to avoid postural hypotension
- Ensure all lines are not kinked or stretched during and after the position change
- Evaluate cardiovascular and pulmonary responses to the new position

# PRONE POSITIONING FOR ACUTE MEDICAL PATIENTS

## *Evidence: B*

For details of evidence, see Summary section and Appendix B.

The prone position can positively impact gas exchange.[4-13] Considerations for positioning patients in prone are outlined below.

### Which Groups of Individuals?

- Early acute respiratory distress syndrome (ARDS)
- Pulmonary edema
- Acute lung insufficiency as defined by a $PaO_2$/$F_iO_2$ ratio <300. In other words the $PaO_2$ is very low relative to the $F_iO_2$

### Contraindications for Prone Position

- Unstable spinal injury with or without trauma (ie, patients with severe spinal problems and neurological signs, rheumatoid arthritis, ankylosing spondylitis, or fractures)
- Unstable cardiac arrhythmias that might require defibrillation or chest compressions
- Hemodynamic instability
- Cerebral hypertension unresponsive to therapy
- Active intra-abdominal processes
- Facial trauma, burns, open chest, or abdominal wounds

### Precautions for Prone Position

- Tracheotomy tube, chest tube(s), and central lines

### Turning From Supine to Side Lying and Then to Prone Lying

1. Preparation prior to turning the patient:
   - Position patient in supine. Ensure patient is sedated and medical condition is optimized before turning
   - Stop tube feeding at least ½ hour before turn

- Temporarily disconnect nonessential monitoring devices, drainage tubing, and intravenous lines Position the remaining tubings and related equipment towards the foot or head of the bed
- Remove limb-supporting cushions
- Record all vital signs before turning
- Patient does not have to be disconnected from the ventilator for the turn
- If patient is on paralytic agents, be sure to support and do not pull on limbs, as they will be prone to dislocation
- Depending on the size of the patient, a minimum of 4 people is recommended for the turn

2. Steps to take during the turn:
    - Slide patient on his or her back toward the side of the bed (away from the ventilator)
    - Position the arm (on the side that the patient is turning towards) very close to the body and roll the patient onto that side
    - Ensure all lines, wires, catheters, and ventilator tubings have ample room to move and remain patent
    - Roll the patient to prone with 2 pillows under the upper chest. This should provide adequate clearance for the endotracheal tube and help keep the patient's head in a neutral position (ie, lying face down with pillow on the forehead)
    - Support forehead and face with foam or cushion. The anaesthesiology department might have a special cushion for prone ventilation
    - Every 2 hours, alternate head position with the head turned toward the ventilator or resting face down on the "cut out donut"
    - Put one pillow underneath the pelvis. Put one pillow underneath the anterior aspect of the ankle for comfort
    - Check to ensure that there is no pressure on the eyes and ears. Pressure should be on the forehead and/or cheeks
    - Check to ensure that the abdomen is pressure-free
    - Monitor all vital signs after turning
    - Elevate the head of the bed slightly so that the head is higher than the right atrium to promote venous return yet not too high to compromise neck and back alignment

## When the Patient is in Prone

- Avoid pressure on the eyes and ears; excessive arching of the low back; excessive pressure to forehead, chin, and nipples; and putting arm(s) overhead for prolonged periods of time[14]
- Allow proper alignment of the limbs. Alternate head position every 2 hours (face down or face toward the ventilator)
- Expect some facial edema. The head of the bed can be elevated (reverse Trendelenberg position) to decrease facial swelling and to decrease the risk of aspiration from a previous feeding
- Enteral feeding intolerance and aspiration have been reported in some patients[15,16]
- Consider nasal duodenal feedings and a dietary consult
- Antiembolic stockings for legs are recommended
- Monitor vital signs routinely

## Duration in Prone Lying

- Prone positioning for 2 to 20 hours in 1 session has been reported in the literature
- Two to 10 hours are suggested. The duration should be determined on a case-by-case basis
- Patients that respond positively to prone but deteriorate in supine should be kept in the prone position longer and more often (eg, 10 hours prone, 2 hours supine)
- If initial prone positioning does not show any improvement, periodic attempts should still be made to reassess their response

## End Points

- Patient has improved oxygenation ($PaO_2/FiO_2$ >300) in supine or rotation
- No response or improvement in prone position
- Patient has a negative response such as an arrhythmia with hemodynamic instability, skin breakdown, or eye damage

## Possible Mechanisms by Which the Prone Position Improves Oxygenation[4,8,9,11,12]

- Prone position produced more uniform pleural pressures between dorsal and ventral lung regions promoting more even distribution of tidal volume by recruiting dorsal lung regions but perfusion in the dorsal and ventral lung region did not differ between the supine or prone positions. In other words, gravity does not have a major influence on distribution of ventilation and perfusion in supine and prone position. As a result, the ventilation-perfusion distribution in the dorsal lung region is more uniform in the prone position.
- Prone positioning could prevent ventilator-associated lung injury by preventing repeated opening and closing of small airways or the excessive stress at margins between aerated and atelectatic dorsal lung units.
- Chest wall compliance tends to decrease in the prone position.
- In the prone position, the anterior chest wall may be constricted between the bed surface and the weight of the body above it. This might result in some redistribution of tidal volume to dorsal lung units close to the diaphragm.

# CONTINUOUS ROTATION FOR ACUTE MEDICAL PATIENTS

## Evidence: B

For details of evidence, see Summary section and Appendix A.

Special rotating beds are used to improve gas exchange, hemodynamic function, airway clearance and resolution of atelectasis.

## Which Groups?

- Mechanically ventilated patients similar to those selected for prone lying

## Steps for Continuous Rotation

- Obtain baseline measures of cardiopulmonary functions and other clinical measures of interest.
- Set patients up to maximum tolerable angles of rotations. In time, the aim is to increase the angle of rotation to the maximum allowable by the bed (which depends on the make of the bed).
- Determine the time that the patient should stay in 1 position. The range is usually between 2 to 30 minutes. The goal is to minimize the time in 1 position and to simulate continuous rotation.

# RELAXATION POSITIONS

## Evidence: B for COPD Patients

There is a lack of evidence to use these positions in other patient groups. The lean-forward sitting position has been shown to reduce dyspnea in COPD patients[3] and bracing arms increased the sustained maximal ventilation in healthy people.[2] Bracing arms during walking on a wheeled walker reduced dyspnea in COPD patients[17]; however, bracing arms during walking is different than a similar standing position while at rest.

Different relaxation positions can be instructed to people with chronic respiratory disease to decrease dyspnea and to facilitate rest. Five different positions are often instructed (Figure 13-2) that could be adopted by patients when trying to sleep (Figure 13-2 A and B), when resting where chairs are available (Figure 13-2 B and C), and when they are outside walking (Figure 13-2 D and E).

**Figure 13-2.** Relaxation positions. Five different relaxation positions are often instructed (A) when the person is sleeping, (B & C) when the person is resting where chairs are available, and (D & E) when patients are outdoors or indoors walking when a chair is unavailable.

C = ↓ diaphragm EMG

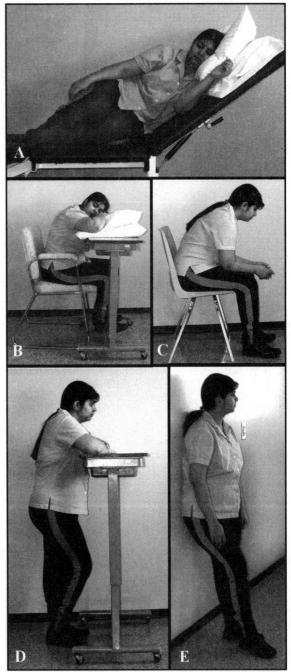

## Which Groups?

- Those patients with clinically significant dyspnea
- To facilitate relaxation in those patients with excessive accessory muscle use

## Steps for Relaxation Positions

- In most positions, the upper body is supported. Be sure that the trunk is straight in all positions.

- Support with adequate pillows for positions A and B in Figure 13-2.
- Have patient perform breathing control and pursed lip breathing (See Chapter 12 for details) while in relaxation positions.
- Ensure head is supported and/or turned to side in B and C in Figure 13-2. Do not have patients bury their head in a pillow. This could make them feel more dyspneic.
- Keep in mind that all positions do not work for all patients. Select positions based on patients' needs and comfort, then modify accordingly.

# SUMMARY OF THE CARDIOVASCULAR AND PULMONARY EFFECTS OF POSITIONING BASED ON CLINICAL TRIALS

1. With unilateral lung disease, the "good lung down" is not always beneficial. Furthermore, none of the studies published thus far (Appendix A) support the theory of "good lung down." Close monitoring is needed to select the best position for patients.

2. The upright position may be beneficial in nonventilated patients with mild to moderate disease, postoperative patients, and the elderly. However, in some conditions[18-20] (liver cirrhosis with portal hypertension, in patent foramen ovale) the supine position can be more beneficial. Stable COPD patients may show little change in lung volumes or desaturation from sitting, to horizontal, to 25-degree head-down position.[21] Therefore, it is important to select positions on a case-by-case basis and to consider all the effects of each position that can optimize comfort and minimize dyspnea.

3. In ventilated patients, the supine position increases the risk of aspiration of gastric contents and nosocomial pneumonia.[22,23] However, the upright position decreases oxygenation especially in patients with ARDS or acute lung injury.[5-7,11-13]

4. The rotating bed maybe beneficial in early acute respiratory distress syndrome (ARDS) or atelectatic patients (Appendix A)

5. In ARDS patients, the prone position has been shown to improve oxygenation (Appendix B)

6. Choosing the most beneficial position is not always very straightforward. Determine ahead of time what you want to accomplish (eg, comfort, improved gas exchange, normalize HR and BP), position accordingly, and always monitor the impact of the position on the patient.

# REFERENCES

1. Prandi E, Couture J, Bellemare F. In normal subjects bracing impairs the function of the inspiratory muscles. *European Respiratory Journal.* 1999;13:1078-1085.
2. Banzett RF, Topulos GP, Leith DE, Nations CS. Bracing arms increases the capacity for sustained hyperpnea. *Am Rev Respir Dis.* 1988;138:106-109.
3. Druz WS, Sharp JT. Electrical and mechanical activity of the diaphragm accompanying body position in severe chronic obstructive pulmonary disease. *Am Rev Respir Dis.* 1982;125:275-280.
4. Brower RG, Ware LB, Berthiaume Y, et al. Treatment of ARDS. *Chest.* 2001;120:1347-1367.
5. Curley MAQ. Prone positioning of patients with adult respiratory distress syndrome: a systematic review. *Am J Crit Care.* 1999;8:397-405.
6. Dries DJ. Prone position in acute lung injury. *J Trauma.* 1998;45:849-852.
7. Force TR, Saul JD, Lewis M, et al. Adult respiratory distress syndrome. Patient position and motion strategies. *Resp Care Clin N Am.* 1998;4:665-677.
8. Jones AT, Hansell DM, Evans TW. Pulmonary perfusion in supine and prone positions: an electron-beam computed tomography study. *J Appl Physiol.* 2001;90:1342-1348.
9. Lamm WJ, Graham MM, Albert RK. Mechanism by which the prone position improves oxygenation in acute lung injury. *Am J Respir Crit Care Med.* 1994; 50:184-193.
10. Messerole E, Peine P, Wittkopp S, et al. The pragmatics of prone positioning. *Am J Respir Crit Care Med.* 2002;165:1359-1363.

11. Mure M, Domino KB, Lindahl SG, et al. Regional ventilation-perfusion distribution is more uniform in the prone position. *J Appl Physiol.* 2000;88:1076-1083.

12. Pelosi P, Tubiolo D, Mascheroni D, et al. Effects of the prone position on respiratory mechanics and gas exchange during acute lung injury. *Am J Respir Crit Care Med.* 1988;157;387-393.

13. Tobin A, Kelly. Prone ventilation—it's time. *Anesth Int Care.* 1999;27:194-201.

14. Willems MC, Voets AJ, Welten RJ. Two unusual complications of prone dependency in severe ARDS. *Intensive Care Med.* 1998;24:276-277.

15. Albert RK. The prone position in acute respiratory distress syndrome: where we are, and where do we go from here. *Crit Care Med.* 1997;25:1453-1454.

16. Blanch L, Mancebo J, Perez M, et al. Short-term effects of prone position in critically ill patients with acute respiratory distress syndrome. *Intensive Care Med.* 199723:1033-1039.

17. Solway S, Brooks D, Lau L, Goldstein R. The short-term effect of a rollator on functional exercise capacity among individuals with severe COPD. *Chest.* 2002; 122(1):56-65.

18. Robin ED, Harmann PD, Horn BR, et al. Platypnea related to orthodeoxia caused by true vascular shunts. *N Eng J Med.* 1976;294:941.

19. Robin ED, Laman ML, Goris ML, et al. A shunt is (not) a shunt is (not) a shunt. *Am Rev Respir Dis.* 1977;115:553-557.

20. Smeenk FW, Postmus PE. Interatrial right-to-left shunting developing after pulmonary resection in the absence of elevated right-sided heart pressures: review of the literature. *Chest.* 1993;103:528-531.

21. Marini JJ, Tyler ML, Hudson LD, et al. Influence of head-dependent positions on lung volume and oxygen saturation in chronic air-flow obstruction. *Am Rev Respir Dis.* 1984;129:101-105.

22. Drakulovic MB, Torres A, Bauer TT, et al. Supine position as a risk factor for nosocomial pneumonia in mechanically ventilated patients: a randomised trial. *Lancet.* 1999;354:1851-1858.

23. Torres A, Serra-Batlles J, Ros E, et al. Pulmonary aspiration of gastric contents in patients receiving mechanical ventilation: the effect of body position. *Ann Intern Med.* 1992;116:540-543.

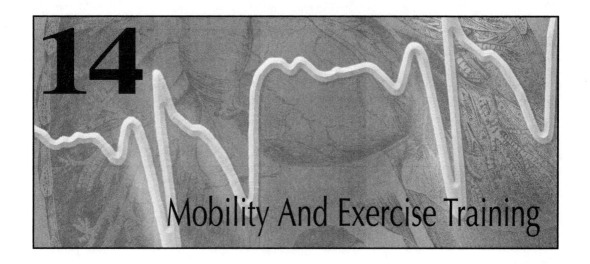

# Mobility And Exercise Training

## OBJECTIVES

At the end of this chapter, the reader should be able to describe:
1. The rationale, indications, and contraindications for mobilization and exercise training
2. The key steps to consider when mobilizing patients in the acute care setting
3. Major components of an exercise training program that should be considered when designing a training program for different patients

## BRIEF DESCRIPTION

One of the most effective treatments the physical therapist can prescribe is an effective exercise program. In the acute care setting, this is often termed mobilization, whereas in the outpatient setting it is referred to as exercise prescription and training. The extremely low exercise tolerance and complexity of health conditions in some patients can preclude the use of training regimens designed for healthy individuals or cardiovascular patients; however, many of the basic training principles apply.

## RATIONALE

Immobility can negatively impact a number of body systems (Table 14-1). Increasing mobility and exercise can have many positive impacts on the body (Table 14-2). Because many of the hospital patients are very ill and can have multiple comorbidities, the therapist has to be more cautious when prescribing exercise to this type of patient than to those in the outpatient clinic. Regardless of the setting and complexities of the patient's conditions, the effects of prolonged bed rest, and inactivity are more detrimental than earlier ambulation or short-term bed rest.[1]

## EVIDENCE

- A—for healthy people,[2] those with coronary artery disease,[3] and those with COPD[4-8]
- C—The evidence is less well defined for individuals in the acute care setting although the effects of immobilization and bed rest are well described

### Indications—Which Patients?

- The physical therapist should endeavor to implement and progress an effective exercise program for all patients, except with those with extremely unstable medical conditions.
- Bed rest is often prescribed for acute back pain, spontaneous premature labor, unstable hemodynamic or cardiovascular status, severe respiratory failure, and acute infectious hepatitis or after medical procedures

Table 14-1

# Physiological Changes and Functional
## Consequences of Immobilization and Reduced Activity

*Cardiovascular System*
- Decreased total blood and plasma volume
- Decreased red blood cell mass and hemoglobin concentration
- Increased basal HR
- Decreased transverse diameter of the heart
- Decreased maximum oxygen uptake and fitness level
- Decreased vascular reflexes and responsiveness of blood vessels in lower extremities to constrict leading to postural hypotension fainting, dizziness
- Deep vein thrombosis and increased risk for pulmonary embolus

*Respiratory System*
- Decreased arterial level of oxygen
- Decreased lung volumes
- Changes in blood flow and ventilation distribution in lungs
- Closure of small airways in dependent regions of lungs leading to lung collapse
- Pooling of secretions increasing potential for infection
- Increased aspiration of food and gastric contents

*Metabolic System*
- Increased calcium excretion leading to increased risk of kidney and ureteral stones
- Increased nitrogen excretion
- Decreased resistance to infection
- Increased diuresis
- Increased blood lipids related to heart disease

*Skeletal Muscle*
- Decreased enzymatic activity and muscle bulk due to increased catabolism and decreased synthesis leading to decreased strength and endurance
- Muscle length can shorten if immobilized at shortened length

*Tendons, Ligaments, and Bones*
- Decreased bone density leading to decreased strength
- Decreased cross-sectional diameter of ligaments and tendons leading to decreased strength
- Joint contracture
- Increased incidence of injury from minor trauma

*Central Nervous System*
- Slowing of EEG activity
- Decreased reaction time and mental functioning
- Emotional and behavioral changes such as increased anxiety and depression
- Decreased psychomotor performance
- Disorientation
- Regression to childlike behavior
- Changes in sleep patterns

*Gastrointestinal System*
- Difficulty in eating and swallowing
- Poor digestion
- Constipation

*Skin*
- Skin breakdown

Table 14-2

## Cardiovascular, Respiratory, Skeletal Muscle, and Bone Mass Adaptations to Aerobic Training[9,10]

| System/Factor | | Rest | Submaximal Exercise | Maximal Exercise |
|---|---|---|---|---|
| Measures of work performance | Oxygen consumption (VO$_2$) | — | — | ↑ |
| | Workload/rate - Work capacity | | | ↑ |
| Heart | HR | ↓ | ↓ | — |
| | Stroke volume | ↑ | ↑ | ↑ |
| | Cardiac output | — | — | ↑ |
| | Heart mass | | ↑ | |
| Blood | Blood and plasma volume | | ↑ | |
| | Red cell mass | | — | |
| Distribution of blood flow | Blood flow to exercising muscle | ↓ | — | ↑ |
| | Coronary blood flow | ↓ | ↓ | ↑ |
| | Brain blood flow | — | — | — |
| | Splanchnic blood flow | — | — | — |
| | Skin blood flow | — | — | — |
| Ventilation - amount of air in and out of lungs | Ventilation (VE) | — | — | ↑ |
| | Respiratory rate | — | ↓ | ↑ |
| | Tidal volume (TV) | — | — | — |
| Lung volume | Vital capacity | | — | |
| | Blood lactate | — | ↓ | ↑ |
| **also affected by other acidoses | Blood pH | — | ↓ | ↑ |
| Skeletal muscle | Anaerobic enzymes in muscle— eg, phosphofructokinase (PFK) | | — | |
| | Myoglobin | | ↑ | |
| | Oxidative enzymes | | ↑ | |
| | Amount of mitochondria | | ↑ | |
| | Muscle capillarization | | ↑ | |
| | Oxygen extraction | | ↑ | |
| | Fat mobilization and oxidation | | ↑ | |
| | Muscle glycogen | | ↑ | |
| Fiber type size | Type I | | ↑ | |
| | Type II | | — | |
| Neuromuscular recruitment and transmission | | | ↑ | |
| Muscle strength | | | ↑ | |
| Muscle endurance | | | ↑ | |
| Bone | Bone mineral density | | ↑ | |
| | Urinary calcium excretion | | ↓ | |

Abbreviations: ↓: decreases; ↑: increases; —: does not change

Note: For some factors, the change occurs after training regardless of whether it's measured during rest, submaximal exercise or maximal exercise. For these factors, the 3 columns for rest, submaximal, and maximal exercise were merged.

such as lumbar puncture, spinal anesthetic, radiography, and cardiac catheterization; however, ambulation and bed exercises should be promoted as early as possible.

# CONTRAINDICATIONS, PRECAUTIONS, AND SCREENING FOR EXERCISE RISK

- Tables 9-1 and 9-2 of Chapter 9 outline contraindications and precautions for exercise with an emphasis on conditions often seen in acute care settings. Patients should be carefully screened for the conditions in these tables when determining the type and progression of mobilization.
- For outpatients, a detailed chart is often unavailable. When requisite information is unavailable in the chart or referral letter, the patient should be cleared for those conditions outlined in the screening questions determined by ACSM as described in Table 9-3.

## Pretraining Evaluation

- The patient should be optimally managed medically.
- The patient should be properly nourished. If not, exercise should be mild and progression should be slow.
- Pretraining evaluation is essential to screen for underlying medical conditions as well as determining whether any adjuncts or medications are essential for safe exercise such as walking aids, weight bearing status, bronchodilators, nitroglycerin, oxygen.

## The Art of Bed to Chair Transfer of Frail or Newly Postoperative Patients in Acute Care Setting—Steps to Take to Perform a Bed to Chair Transfer

- Lower extremity range of motion exercises—especially in postoperative patients to stimulate circulation and venous return—should be performed prior to mobilization
- Change patient position gradually from horizontal to upright position in bed. Patients who are on prolonged bed rest, on new hypertensive medication, have cardiovascular problems, on strong sedatives or narcotics are prone to postural hypotension
- Follow proper postural mechanics. Log rolling and get patient up from high sitting in bed may be useful
- Avoid tension to incision, lines, wires, and tubings. If patient has a chest tube, disconnecting chest tube from wall suction and utilizing water seal only might decrease the duration of air leak
- Sit patient at the edge of the bed first and if it is well tolerated, proceed to chair
- Early ambulation should be performed whenever patient's condition permits

## The Art of Mobilization in the Acute Care Setting—Steps to Take to Prepare for and Mobilize Patients

### Step 1: Who Are We Dealing With?

- What is the functional status before hospital admission?
- Relevant past medical history
- What impact does the acute illness have on patient mobility (eg, weakness from bed rest, incision, trauma, and pain)?
- Medication effects (eg, beta blocker effects on exercise heart rate, effects of analgesia on BP, and balance)
- Others obstacles (eg, drainage, intravenous, and oxygen tubings)

### Step 2: Mobilize or Not?

- Weigh the benefit: risk ratio for mobilizing your patient.

### Step 3: How Much Can the Patient Do?

- Be prepared. Set up chairs along the way. Provide appropriate walking aids, use of a transfer belt, and if required, alert nursing staff before hand. Use proper body mechanics during transfer and allow gradual change from lying to upright position. Encourage circulation exercises—ie, foot and ankle, knee flexion/extension before and during transfer.

- Obtain baseline vital signs before activity.

## Step 4: When to Quit While You Are Still Ahead

- Have objective endpoints such as limits of BP, HR, oxygen saturation, and level of exertion predetermined before mobilization. Other indicators for stopping exercise are listed in Chapter 9, Table 9-4.
- Look patient in the face and eyes. Watch for signs of fatigue, pain, diaphoresis, and intolerance during activity. Frequently ask patient how he/she feels.

## Step 5: Quitting Time Yet?

- Look at patient's exercise responses.

## Step 6: Monitor and Progress

- Determine the limiting factor of the mobilization.
- Think of objective outcome measures that you can use to monitor progress—eg, ease of transfer, sitting duration, walking distance, HR, respiratory rate, oxygen saturation, Borg scales, and pain scales.
- After mobilization, monitor patient until vital signs have returned to pre-activity level.

## *Exercise Prescription and Training of Outpatients*

The main focus of this section will be to provide general over-riding principles for exercise training outpatients. The benefits of exercise training are well defined for individuals in cardiac and pulmonary rehabilitation. However, the length of this text does not allow for further details to be outlined here. The reader is encouraged to read other references[4,11-14] for further details of cardiac and pulmonary rehabilitation and exercise training of other conditions.

All programs should be based on basic training principles: overload, specificity of training, individual differences, and reversibility. An *overload* needs to be applied to bring about a training response. Varying frequency, duration, intensity, or a combination of these factors can alter the overload. Due to the *specificity* of training, maximal benefit will occur when the training techniques are similar to the functional outcomes desired. It is obvious that training programs are optimized when they are planned to meet the *individual's* needs and capacities. The *reversibility* principle states that detraining will occur when a person is immobilized or decreases his or her activity level.

### Supervision

More success has been shown when the training program is supervised. This provides feedback to the patient and an opportunity to modify the program as the needs of the patient change. Supervision by the physiotherapist should be quite frequent initially and then usually tapers as the patient becomes more proficient in the exercise program. Successful programs have been conducted in hospitals, in outpatient departments, or at home.

### Monitoring

HR and BP should be monitored before, during, and after the supervised exercise training sessions. Monitoring the electrocardiogram is important in new patients to exclude arrhythmias and in those patients with cardiovascular disease. Monitoring of oxygen saturation is usually essential for all individuals with chronic respiratory disease and will facilitate assessment of the need for oxygen therapy. Similarly, the respiratory rate may also be a suitable guide for exercise intensity.

### Components of the Training Program

All programs should include a *warm-up*, a performance of an aerobic activity at a *specific training intensity*, and a *cool-down* period. Adequate warm-up and cool-down not only ensure optimal performance but are safer and less stressful to the cardiovascular system. Further, a warm-up of approximately 15 minutes at 60% of maximum oxygen consumption about 30 minutes before exercise can reduce exercise-induced asthma (EIA) and an adequate cool-down can also minimize EIA. In those patients who are less able, thoracic, upper extremity, and lower extremity mobility exercises can be used for the warm-up and cool-down rather than walking or using a modality at a lower intensity.

## Modalities

Modalities include walking, running, rowing, using a stairmaster, stationary bicycling, stair climbing, or a combination of these. The specificity of training and ease of access to exercise facilities should be considered in selecting the most appropriate modality or activity for endurance training. Availability of equipment and climate are also important factors to consider. In most cases, combinations of walking and unsupported arm exercise are the most desirable training modalities for older people with chronic respiratory disease. Younger people with cystic fibrosis or post MI can often select exercises that are similar to those performed by healthy individuals. Because many activities are performed with the upper extremities, a comprehensive exercise program should incorporate strength and endurance training of both the upper and lower extremities. Respiratory muscle training may be indicated in those individuals who have weak respiratory muscles and in those who are more dyspneic.

## Training Intensity

Details of exercise testing are provided in Chapter 9. All patients entering a rehabilitation program should be exercise tested to screen for their physiologic, subjective, and untoward responses to exercise. Advantages of exercise testing are that monitoring can be done more carefully, and supervised more closely than the higher patient: therapist ratio during treatment sessions. Baseline training intensity is based on:

- The patient's condition(s)
- Assessment findings including his or her response to the exercise test
- The limits of an exercise intensity that is within the training-safety zone as described in Chapter 9 are:
  o The minimum intensity to provide an effective training program
  o The maximum intensity that should not be exceeded to ensure safe training

Depending on the specific population, other parameters for exercise prescription may be considered including:
- Calculation of the HR reserve
- Calculation of a MET level
- An exercise intensity that elicits a comfortable level of dyspnea. Often the sing-talk-gasp test is an easy guideline for some patients. The exercise should be strenuous enough that they don't have enough breath to sing but can talk comfortably.

A more cautious exercise prescription should be formulated in the elderly, those with multiple conditions, and those who are uncomfortable or anxious about an exercise training program. Further details about exercise prescription for pulmonary patients are provided by Cooper,[13] and for cardiac patients are provided by Brannon.[12]

Age-predicted heart rate is not usually useful for prescription of exercise in many groups of patients because the heart rate of patients with chronic respiratory disease is elevated with respect to oxygen consumption compared with the heart rate-oxygen consumption relationship in the healthy individual. Further, the 95% confidence interval is a 40- to 60-BPM variation.[15] Once a person is exercise tested, however, monitoring heart rate can be useful in detecting those patients who experience exercise-induced arrhythmias or determining the upper limit to safely exclude myocardial ischemia or other untoward effects.

*Progression of training intensity* should consider the training-safety zone. Exercise needs to be progressed to maintain an intensity stimulus as training adaptations occur. This well-known training principle is often ignored clinically. Endurance exercise can be progressed by increasing duration, intensity, and frequency. Progression of training intensity should be very slow in most patients. Slow progression is essential for some individuals because an apparently trivial progression may be a substantial training load in the very debilitated. Further, some patients with chronic conditions have a very limited capacity for training adaptations because of the contributing factors of their condition, nutrition, and medications.

Do not increase more than one of three variables—duration, intensity, and frequency—each week and only a small increase should be prescribed (not more than 5% of 1 parameter per week). Exercise training is a lifelong commitment so progression can be very slow to avoid injury yet still be effective because the person has the rest of his or her life to reach the desired training intensity.

*Range of Training Intensities.* The range of training intensity can be very low for people with COPD (Table 14-3) and some cardiac myopathies. For other individuals with conditions like asthma, cystic fibrosis, and post MI the training intensity can be above or may be in the normal training range for healthy people of similar ages.

> When weighing the pros and cons of a higher versus lower training intensity, it is important to remember that *high intensity will show more physiologic improvement but is riskier and some patients don't like it.*

Table 14-3

### Range of Training Intensities for People With COPD and Interstitial Lung Disease

| Modality | Warm-Up Workload | Training Workload |
|---|---|---|
| Cycle ergometer | Free wheeling at 50 rev/min 0 kiloponds (kp) at 50 rev/min 0 kilopond meters (kpm) | 0.5 to 1.0 kp 150 to 300 kpm 25 to 50 watts (1 watt = 6.1 kpm) |
| Arm ergometer | Free wheeling or unsupported arm exercises. Usually 30-40 rev/min | 5 to 10 watts |
| Treadmill | Slowest speed (~1.0 mph) and flat grade | Usually 1 to 2 mph and flat—10 % grade |

Abbreviations: rev/min:revolutions per minute

## Frequency of Training

Frequency should be performed 3 to 5 times per week. Less frequent training may produce no training effect, whereas more frequent training may not allow sufficient time for recovery.

## Duration of Training Session

The training session may initially have to be very short. A good rule of thumb is that any duration greater than what the patient is doing will elicit a training response—ie, 2 or 3 minutes of walking is better than absolute bed rest. A very short training duration or an interval program might be necessary for those patients with a very low exercise tolerance. An interval-training program consists of higher-intensity training workloads interspersed with low-intensity workloads or periods of rest. Ideally, the target duration should gradually increase to a period of 25 to 30 minutes of aerobic exercise. Interval training can minimize EIA in some individuals.

## Length of Training Program

Exercise training is a life-long commitment. The effects of training are totally reversible once training discontinues. Lifestyle changes are more likely to occur with a longer supervised component and assisting the client with the transition into community-based programs.

# SUMMARY OF THE EFFECTS OF MOBILIZATION AND TRAINING

In summary, mobilization and exercise training are beneficial to patients but do have associated risks. The avoidance of exercise and inactivity has more detrimental effects. High-risk patients should be monitored using both subjective and objective outcome measures. Starting intensities should be low and progression should be slow. The exercise program should be varied to encompass endurance, strength, and flexibility as well as training of all muscle groups used in the patient's daily activities. Exercise training is a life-long commitment for the benefits to be sustained.

# REFERENCES

1. Allen C, Glasziou P, Del Mar C. Bed rest: a potentially harmful treatment needing more careful evaluation. *Lancet.* 1999;354:1229-1233.
2. Franklin BA, Roitman JL. Cardiorespiratory adaptations to exercise. *ACSM's Resource Manual for Guidelines for Exercise Testing and Prescription.* 3rd ed. Philadelphia: Lippincott, Williams & Wilkins: 1998;156-163.

3. Wenger NK, Froelicher ES, Smith LK, Ades PA, Berra K, Blumenthal JA. Cardiac rehabilitation as secondary prevention. Clinical practice guideline. *Quick Reference Guide for Clinicians*. No. 17. Rockville, MC: Agency for Health Care Policy and Research and National Heart, Lung and Blood Institute. AHCPR Pub. No. 96-0673. October 1995.

4. AACVPR. *Guidelines for Pulmonary Rehabilitation Programs*. 2nd ed. Champaign, IL, Human Kinetics, 1998.

5. ACCP/AACVPR Pulmonary Rehabilitation Guidelines Panel. Pulmonary Rehabilitation. Joint ACCP/AACVPR evidence-based guidelines. *Chest*. 1997;112:1363-1396.

6. Celli B. Is pulmonary rehabilitation an effective treatment for chronic obstructive pulmonary disease? Yes. *Am J Respir Crit Care Med*. 1997;155:781-783.

7. Chavannes N, Vollenbeerg JJ, van Schayck CP, Wouters EF. Effects of physical activity in mild to moderate COPD: a systematic review. *Br J General Practice*. 2002;52(480):574-578.

8. Lacasse Y, Guyatt GH, Goldstein RS. The components of a respiratory rehabilitation program. A systematic overview. *Chest*. 1997;1111:1077-1088.

9. Brooks GA, Fahey TD, White TP, Baldwin KM. *Exercise Physiology, Human Bioenergetics and its Applications*. Mountain View, Calif: Mayfield Publishing Company. 2000;319,332.

10. McArdle WD, Katch FI, Katch VL. *Exercise Physiology: Energy, Nutrition, and Human Performance*. 5th ed. Philadelphia: Lippincott, Williams & Wilkins; 2001.

11. ACSM's Resources for Clinical Exercise Physiology: Musculoskeletal, Neuromuscular, Neoplastic, Immunologic, and Hematologic Conditions. Baltimore: Lippincott Williams and Wilkins; 2002.

12. Brannon FJ. *Cardiopulmonary Rehabilitation: Basic Theory and Application*. Philadelphia: FA Davis; 1993.

13. Cooper CB. Exercise in chronic pulmonary disease: aerobic exercise prescription. *Med Sci Spo Exerc*. 2001; 33(7) Suppl:S671-S679.

14. Chapters 21-23. *ACSM's Resource Manual for Guidelines for Exercise Testing and Prescription*. 4th ed. Baltimore: Lippincott Williams and Wilkins; 2001:191-208.

15. Gappmaier E. "220-age?"—Prescribing exercise based on heart rate in the clinic. *Cardiopulmonary Physical Therapy*. 2002;13(2):11-12.

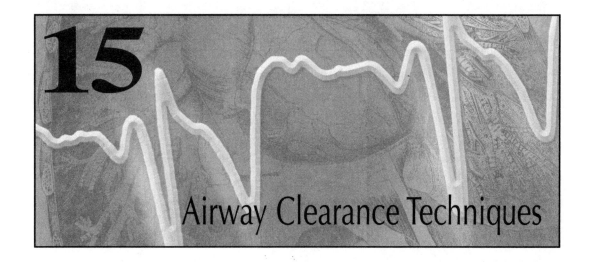

# Airway Clearance Techniques

## OBJECTIVES

Upon completion of this chapter, the reader should be able to:
1. Describe factors that affect mucociliary clearance
2. Describe various airway clearance techniques
3. Describe the level of evidence to support different airway clearance techniques
4. Effectively prescribe and instruct airway clearance techniques for patients with mucus congestion

This chapter describes anatomical and physiological factors affecting airway clearance; airway clearance techniques; clinical trials on airway clearance; their relative effects; and the level of evidence of these techniques on secretion removal. Basic airway clearance techniques include thoracic expansion exercises, huffing, coughing and breathing control exercises. Manual techniques such as percussion, vibrations, and postural drainage are used less often nowadays. Other newer airway clearance techniques such as the flutter device, autogenic drainage, and the positive expiratory pressure mask are gaining popularity.

## FACTORS THAT AFFECT MUCOCILIARY CLEARANCE

The respiratory mucous membrane consists of goblet cells, mucus, and serous glands and cilia (Table 15-1). Their functions are to entrap foreign particles and the mucus is moved toward the nasopharynx to be disposed of by swallowing and/or expectoration. Mucociliary clearance is an important lung defense mechanism; unfortunately, inhaled irritants such as cigarette smoke, air pollutants, and disease can damage this mechanism.[1] Mucociliary clearance also decreases with age and sleep but is stimulated by exercise. When exposed to irritants, the mucus secretion is increased to protect the airways.

Mucus is viscoelastic material (an equal combination of solid like—eg, spring and liquid like responses). Many factors affect mucus flow (Table 15-2). Vigorous agitation destroys its biorheologic structure, making it less viscous, which is known as reversible shear-thinning, or thixotrophic. In general, purulent sputum samples (eg, from patients with chronic bronchitis) tend to have a higher viscosity and elasticity than nonpurulent sputum, and hence less mucociliary transportability.[1] When using chronic bronchitis as the reference point, asthma subjects have higher sputum viscosity while cystic fibrosis or bronchiectasis subjects have lower sputum viscosity. Some viral infections and diseases, such as COPD and especially asthma, reduce mucociliary clearance rates.

## CLINICAL IMPLICATIONS OF FACTORS THAT AFFECT MUCUS

- Mucus flow is slower near openings, branchings, and junctions of airways
- Increased roughness of airway surfaces increases the frictional resistance and decreases flow

Table 15-1

## The Mucociliary Clearance System

### The Ciliary System

- The cilia extend down the pharynx, larynx, trachea, bronchi, and bronchioles.
- Below the small bronchi (about 11 generation of bronchioles), the epithelium is lacking cilia.
- The contact between the cilia and mucus is facilitated by tiny claw-like appendages seen at the tips of the cilia.
- Each ciliated epithelial cell contains about 275 cilia.
- Cilia beat in an asymmetric pattern, with a fast, forward stroke, during which the cilia are stiff and outstretched, and a slower return stroke, during which the cilia are flexed.
- Each cilium beats slightly out of phase with its neighbor, producing a wave-like motion.
- The cilia beat frequency is between 11 and 15 beats per second.

### The Mucus System

- Mucus lines the airways from the nasal opening to the terminal bronchioles.
- Alveolar macrophages, lymphocytes and polymorphonuclear leukocytes are important in defending the distal airways against foreign particles.
- The lower layer or periciliary layer contains nonviscid serous fluid that lines the airway epithelium where the cilia beat.
- The upper layer or the mucus layer contains viscoelastic material and is propelled by the cilia.
- The optimal depth of the periciliary layer is approximately the length of an outstretched cilium.
- In contrast, the depth of mucus layer has very little influence on ciliary beats.

Table 15-2

## Factors That Affect Mucus Flow

### Physical Properties of Mucus (Rheology)

- Viscosity is defined as the quality of being adherent. Viscosity in the lung consists of the sticking together of mucus molecules or the adhering of mucus to the wall of the airways. When mucus viscosity doubles, the mucus flow will be at least decreased by a half.
- Elasticity is the ability of a substance to return to its resting shape following the cessation of a distortional force. Liquid with high elasticity has a lower flow rate.
- Surface tension is the force exerted by molecules moving away from the surface and toward the center of a liquid. Low surface tension is related to increased flow. For example, an increase in temperature would decrease surface tension and increase flow.
- Water content helps to liquefy mucus and increase flow.

### Physical Characteristics of Airways

- Flow rate increases with an increase in diameter. In small airways, the adhesion is higher because the area of mucus in contact with the airway is proportionally higher than in large airways. Layered mucus depositions, solid mucus plugs, bronchospasm, and edema can reduce the size of the airway.
- Mucus flow is decreased in longer airways. When airways are disrupted or obstructed, mucus has to flow through alternate routes resulting in slower flow rates.

### Gravity

- Airflow and gravity are important at mucus depths greater than 20 μm. This depth is far greater than the length of cilia in subsegmental bronchi, which is 3.6 μm. For a size comparison, the aerosol particulate diameter from a nebulizer is also about 3.5 μm.

**Figure 15-1A.** Postural drainage positions. (Reprinted from *Principles and Practice of Cardiopulmonary Physical Therapy*. 3rd ed., Frownfelter D, Dean E, 340-341, Copyright [1996], with permission from Elsevier.)

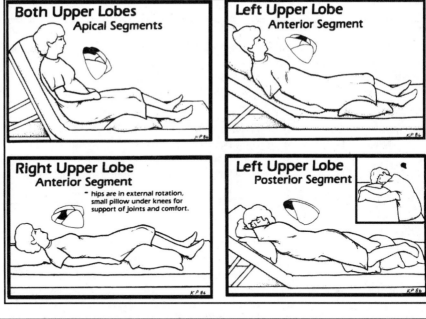

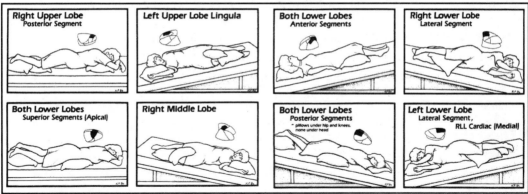

**Figure 15-1B.** Postural drainage positions. (Reprinted from *Principles and Practice of Cardiopulmonary Physical Therapy*. 3rd ed., Frownfelter D, Dean E, 340-341, Copyright [1996], with permission from Elsevier.)

- There is an optimal viscosity/elasticity ratio. Mucus that has decreased viscosity, elasticity, and surface tension but increased water content is less tenacious and easier to expectorate. Therefore, medications such as bronchodilators, drugs that alter the viscosity or elasticity of the mucus, and nebulizers can be used to increase mucus flow.
- Decreased ciliary beat frequency and alteration of the periciliary fluid depth can decrease mucociliary clearance rate.
- Gravity (15- to 25-degree head-down position) increases mucociliary clearance especially in diseased populations.

# HOW TO PERFORM AIRWAY CLEARANCE TECHNIQUES

## Postural Drainage

Postural drainage (PD) has been shown to increase mucociliary clearance in patients by means of measuring sputum collection dry weight, volume, or radionuclide particles clearance rate. The classic postural drainage positions are designed to drain individual segments of the lungs (Figure 15-1 and Table 15-3). However the

Table 15-3

## Tracheal Bronchial Tree and Drainage Positions

| Lung (Lobe and Segment) | Direction of Branching (Proximal to Distal) | Postural Tipping Requirement (Degrees From Horizontal) |
|---|---|---|
| *Right upper lobe* | | |
| Apical | Ascends vertically | Sitting |
| Posterior | Runs posteriorly and in a horizontal direction | Not required |
| Anterior | Runs anteriorly and horizontally | Not required |
| *Right middle lobe* | Descends downward and anterolaterally | 15-degree head-down position |
| *Right lower lobe* | | |
| Apical | Runs horizontally and posteriorly | Not required |
| Medial | Downward and medially | 30-degree head-down position |
| Anterior | Downward and anteriorly | 30-degree head-down position |
| Posterior | Descends posteriorly | 30-degree head-down position |
| Lateral | Descends laterally | 30-degree head-down position |
| *Left upper lobe* | | |
| Anterior | Ascends at 45 degrees anteriorly | Lean backward sitting |
| Apical | Ascends vertically and posteriorly | Lean forward sitting |
| Lingular | Descends anterolaterally like the right middle lobe | 15-degree head down position |
| *Left lower lobe* | | |
| Apical | Runs posteriorly in a horizontal direction | Not required |
| Anteromedial | Descends anteriorly | 30-degree head-down position |
| Posterior | Descends posteriorly | 30-degree head-down position |
| Lateral | Descends laterally | 30-degree head-down position |

head-down positions produce lower peak expiratory flow and pressure.[2] Thus, to maximize the strength of expiratory maneuvers during treatments, patients should be asked to adapt to a more upright position when coughing or huffing during the PD. For patients with mucus congestion who are not able to cough or mobilize (eg, paralyzed or heavily sedated patients in intensive care unit), PD can be an important component of airway clearance techniques.

## Evidence: C

For details about evidence, see Appendices C and D, the Summary section, and Figure 15-2.

## Steps for Postural Drainage Technique

The usual recommendation is 2 to 10 minutes per position for a total treatment time of 30 to 40 minutes. The mucociliary clearance rate is about 5 to 15 mm/min in the nasopharynx in normal subjects and much lower in the small airways with thick mucus. It will take more than 10 minutes for foreign particles to get from the alveoli or the lower airways to the nasopharynx.

The classical postural drainage positions are usually modified in the clinical setting:

- To meet the needs and tolerance of the patient
- Due to nonspecific diagnoses or diffuse involvements of lung segments
- Due to the therapist's work load and time management

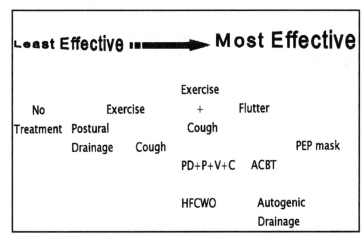

**Figure 15-2.** The relative effectiveness of secretion removal techniques. Abbreviations: ACBT: active cycle of breathing techniques; HFCWO: high frequency chest wall oscillation; PEP: positive expiratory pressure; PD+P+V+C: postural drainage, percussion, vibrations, and cough.

## Cough and Huff

Cough is stronger when the patient is in an upright position.[2] After a deep inspiration to total lung capacity, a cough is initiated by an active sudden contraction of expiratory muscles against a closed glottis. There is a sudden, sharp rise in pleural pressure that can cause dynamic airway compression especially in subjects with decreased elastic recoil of the lung. During a cough, the near-explosive expulsion of air from the lung imparts very high shearing forces to the mucus lining the upper airways. Exposed to high shear stress, the mucus flows easily forward because of lowered effective viscosity. After the cough with the cessation of the shear force, the mucus does not flow back into the lung because its effective viscosity is higher again.

Cough alone is only effective in clearing the central lung regions (ie, up to the sixth generation of airways). Coughing can also produce a milking action on peripheral airways thus facilitating mucus clearance. In patients with an ineffective cough and artificial airways, manual hyperinflations with a resuscitation bag are sometimes used.

### Evidence: B

For details about evidence, see Appendices C and D, the Summary section, and see Figure 15-2.

### Steps for Manual Hyperinflation

- Six cycles of inflation and then suctioning
- Inflation involves a slow squeeze of the resuscitation bag followed by a pause
- The rate of bagging usually coincides with the patient's respiratory rate
- Additional oxygen may be needed if the oxygenation is at the lower limit of the normal range

### Steps for Huffing

A huff is a modified cough and it is reported to clear mucus from the seventh generation of bronchi and beyond. The rate of expiratory flow varies with the degree of airflow obstruction and disease and is specific to the individual. Crackles would be heard if excess secretions were present and coughing might be required to clear the mucus from the large airways. The patient is instructed to:

- Open the mouth to an O-shape and to keep the back of the throat (glottis) open
- To perform a forced expiration from mid-to-low lung volume in order to move the more peripheral secretions or a forced expiration from high-to-mid lung volume in order to move the more proximal secretions.
- Contract the chest wall muscles and abdomen simultaneously during this forced expiratory maneuver. The sound is like a sigh, but forced
- Often the patient is instructed using the analogy of "pretend you are holding a ping-pong ball in your mouth and then to blow it out with a forced breath."

## Manual Percussion and Vibrations

The aim of this technique is to remove mucus from the airways. Manual percussion is performed with cupped hand onto the designated portion of the chest (Table 15-4). The technique does not need to be very forceful to be effective. This can be done using a single- or double-handed technique. It is widely believed in the clinical

Table 15-4

## *Manual Percussion and Vibrations*

### Manual Percussion Technique

1. Clap the "congested" area.
2. "Fast" clapping is 240 cycles/min and has sufficient magnitude to produce quivering of the voice.
3. "Slow" (6 to 12 cycles/minutes) one-handed percussion is clapping the chest wall once at the beginning of a relaxed expiration following a maximal inspiration.
4. "Fast" or "slow" clapping should coincide with slow deep breathing exercises and should last between 30 to 60 seconds.
5. This is followed by 2 to 3 huffs or coughs.
6. The patient should perform breathing control exercises until oxygen saturation is adequate and breathing has stabilized.

### Indications for Percussion, Vibrations, and Postural Drainage

- Excessive secretion retention—history of excessive secretion is usually defined as 25 ml a day or more—eg, many patients with bronchiectasis, select patients with chronic bronchitis, or lung abscess.
- Aspiration of fluid into lungs—eg, post cardiac arrest, swallowing dysfunction, etc.
- Clinical signs of mucus retention such as rattly sounds on auscultation or palpation, congested cough, etc.
- Suspicion of secretion retention on other clinical bases (eg, in comatose or uncooperative patients, acute on chronic infection, etc.).

### Contraindications, Limitations, and Adverse Effects

- Oxygen desaturation. Percussion and vibrations in addition to postural drainage can cause severe hypoxemia in critically ill patients. Postural drainage on its own has a lower incidence of oxygen desaturation than percussion and vibrations. Patients with the least secretions to remove tend to have the most desaturation.
- Bronchospasm. High frequency and intense percussion is known to induce bronchospasm in asthmatics. Single-handed slow percussion is usually advocated. Use of bronchodilators prior to treatment may help to minimize this effect.
- Fractured ribs. Fragile patients with advanced COPD and other chronic disease can be on corticosteroids and may be osteoporotic. The hyperinflated rib cage also becomes very rigid. Elderly women tend to have decalcification of bones.
- Bruising. Patients on anti-coagulation medication or those who have coagulopathy.
- Patient intolerance. Pain and discomfort is associated with overly aggressive treatment. Some patients who are more sensitive are post-thoracotomy patients, and those with open wounds or chest tubes.
- Cardiovascular consequences. In acute cerebral vascular accident patients, some brain surgery, unstable cardiovascular patients, and uncontrolled seizures.
- Recent bright red hemoptysis.
- Recent pacemaker insertion.
- Pulmonary embolism.
- Increased intracranial pressure.
- Tube feeds need to be stopped at least ½ hour prior to treatment to minimize risk of aspiration.

Table 15-5

### Recommendations by Professional Societies Regarding Chest Physiotherapy and the Clearance of Airway Secretions in the Management of Acute Exacerbations of COPD

| Professional Society | Recommendations |
| --- | --- |
| American College of Chest Physicians and American College of Physicians—American Society of Internal Medicine[3-6] | Not recommended |
| European Respiratory Society[7] | Recommended: coughing to clear sputum: physiotherapy at home |
| American Thoracic Society[8] | Recommended for hospitalized patients with >25 ml of sputum/day |
| Global initiatives for chronic obstructive lung disease[9] | Manual or mechanical chest percussion and postural drainage possibly beneficial for patients with lobar atelectasis or >25 ml of sputum/day; facilitating sputum clearance by stimulating coughing |

field that slow single-handed percussion induces a lower incidence of bronchospasm. The aim of percussion is to loosen up mucus plugs and increase mucociliary clearance (perhaps by applying external shear force or decreasing viscosity of the mucus). It is also known in the literature as the "ketchup bottle" method. Manual vibrations can be applied to the areas that are percussed such as on the peripheral chest wall or progressively applied more centrally toward the large airways. Sometimes it is only applied to the chest wall closer to the central airways.

Classical or modified postural drainage positions are usually used with these manual techniques. Both manual percussion and vibration techniques can be used alone or in combination.

The essential prerequisite for these types of "chest physiotherapy" techniques is a volume of secretions large enough to be jarred loose by percussion or vibrations and carried to the pharynx by gravity and coughing. In other words, the bottle must contain some ketchup before it can be emptied.

### Precautions

- Manual vibrations are applied at the onset of expiration and usually become more vigorous at the end of expiration. Properly carried out manual vibrations likely decreases lung volume to below FRC.
- In patients on a ventilator, positioning patients to alternate side lying and chest percussion can increase oxygen demand and cardiovascular responses (HR, BP, etc.). The increased oxygen demand is thought to be related to muscular activity and is suppressed by vecuronium (muscle relaxant). However, the increase in cardiovascular response is thought to be a stress-like response by enhanced sympathetic output and is not suppressed by vecuronium.[10]

### Evidence on the Use of Manual Percussion and Vibrations: B

For details about evidence, see Appendices C and D, the Summary section, and see Figure 15-2.

In the last decade, 3 out of 4 international professional societies have recommended manual percussion and vibrations to patients with acute exacerbations of COPD producing greater than 25 ml of sputum/day (Table 15-5). The American College of Chest Physicians (ACCP) and American College of Physicians—American Society of Internal Medicine[3-6] however, did not recommend chest physiotherapy. The rationale for this last recommendation was seriously flawed. For details, see Appendix C for a critique of the above guideline.

## Mechanical Vibration

The mechanical vibrator was popularized in the 1980's and is one of the most frequently used techniques. In some instances, mechanical vibration replaces percussion and manual vibrations.[11]

**Evidence: C**

For details about evidence, see Appendices C and D, the Summary section, and see Figure 15-2.

## Steps for Mechanical Vibrations

The vibrator is firmly applied against the chest wall over the affected area. The vibrator is moved around usually at 15- to 30-second intervals to the adjacent areas in order to cover the whole affected region. Usually 5- to 10-minute treatments are applied to each affected region. The aim is to improve mucociliary clearance and ventilation especially in acutely ill patients when postural drainage and manual percussion and vibrations cannot be tolerated.

## Potential Therapeutic Effects of Mechanical Vibrations

- Improves ventilation of lung units with poor ventilation
- Promotes muscle relaxation in chest wall, therefore altering chest wall mechanics
- Improves intrapulmonary mixing by transmission of vibration to lung tissue leading to improved diffusion and gas exchange
- Alters physical properties of sputum (perhaps by decreasing effective viscosity)
- Dislodges mucus plugs
- Enhances ciliary beat frequency

## Active Cycle of Breathing Techniques

Active cycle of breathing techniques (ACBT) utilizes cycles of breathing exercise, forced expiration, and relaxed breathing. ACBT is thought to have the effect of shearing mucus from the small airways and progressively mobilizing it to the upper airway. When the secretions reach the upper airways, a cough or huff is used to expectorate the mucus. The ACBT can be done without using postural drainage positions and may be better tolerated by some patients.[12]

**Evidence: B**

For details about evidence, see Appendices C and D, the Summary section, and see Figure 15-2.

## Steps for ACBT

- Position the patient in an upright or PD position
- Instruct the patient to:
  - o Perform breathing control exercises for about 1 minute
  - o Perform thoracic expansion exercises or deep breathing exercises for about 30 seconds. This involves slow sustained inspirations from FRC to TLC
  - o To huff or cough 2 to 3 times
  - o Perform breathing control exercises for 1 to 2 minutes before repeating the cycle. Effective breathing control involves gentle breathing using the lower chest at normal tidal volumes and at a natural rate with unforced expiration.
- The cycles continue to the tolerance of the patient or until the mucus congestion is clear. A minimum of 3 to 4 cycles, however, is recommended.

# NEW AIRWAY CLEARANCE TECHNIQUES

## Flutter

The flutter is an easy-to-use physiotherapy device based on oscillations of a steel ball during expiration through a pipe-type device. During exhalation, the steel ball vibrates, producing a variable positive expiratory pressure up to 20 cm $H_2O$ and an oscillating intratracheal pressure wave frequency of 6 to 20 Hz.

**Evidence: B**

For details about evidence, see Appendices C and D, the Summary section, and see Figure 15-2.

Brief instructions on use the flutter device (more detailed instructions are included in the package insert with the device). The patient is instructed to:

- Seal his or her lips around the mouthpiece
- Inhale deeply through the nose 10 to 15 times and hold each breath for 2 to 3 seconds

- Exhale deeply into the flutter device
- Tilt the flutter up or down until maximal vibration is felt throughout the chest wall
- Once the secretions are loosened to more proximal lung regions, use the huffing technique to remove secretions
- Treatment time is at least 15 minutes once or twice a day

## Positive Expiratory Pressure Mask

Positive Expiratory Pressure (PEP) consists of a mask and a 1-way valve resistor for expiration. A manometer is used to help select the resistor that provides a steady PEP of 10 to 20 cm $H_2O$ during mid expiration.

### Evidence: B

For details about evidence, see Appendices C and D, the Summary section, and see Figure 15-2.

### Brief Instructions on the Use of the PEP Mask

More detailed instructions are included in the package insert with the device. The patient is instructed to:
- Breathe for about 15 breaths at normal tidal volumes and a slightly forced expiration through the mask
- Huff off the mask 2 to 3 times and/or cough to remove mucus
- To perform a breathing control phase for 1 to 2 minutes in order to relax
- To perform a minimum of 6 sequences or a 20-minute session, once or twice a day

## Autogenic Drainage

AD is a breathing technique performed at different lung volumes and with different tidal volumes to assist in secretion removal.

### Evidence: B

For details about evidence, see Appendices C and D, the Summary section, and see Figure 15-2.

### Brief Overview of Steps for Autogenic Drainage

This technique is fairly complicated for the therapist to learn how to instruct and for the patient to learn how to do. It is highly recommended that a course be taken on the AD before instructing it to patients. The different components of AD include:
- Phase I: Peripheral loosening of mucus—After a deep inspiration, the patient inhales to mid-tidal volume and exhales to just below functional residual capacity. The peripheral airways are compressed and secretions are mobilized upward away from the peripheral lung field.
- Phase II: Collection of mucus in large airways—Breathing exercises are done at mid lung volumes (using a larger inspiration and less emptying than phase I during expiration).
- Phase III: Transport of mucus from the large airways to the mouth—Progressively larger inspirations are used with expiration to the functional residual capacity. A small burst of very gentle coughs is used to help expectorate the mucus.

## High Frequency Chest Wall Oscillation

High frequency chest wall oscillation (HFCWO) consists of a chest vest that is connected to a piston pump that compresses and decompresses the chest wall at 6 to 19 Hz. The treatment usually involves chest wall compressions for 4 to 5 minutes followed by deep breathing exercises and huffing techniques. The cycle of treatment usually takes 20 to 30 minutes to complete.

### Evidence: B

For details about evidence, see Appendices C and D, the Summary section, and see Figure 15-2.

## Clinical Trials on Secretion Removal Techniques

Evidence on airway clearance techniques is based on a reviews of clinical trials related to these techniques which are summarized in Appendix C, Clinical Trials on Secretion Removal Techniques, and Appendix D, Clinical Trials of Exercise Programs and Secretion Removal in Patients With Cystic Fibrosis.

# SUMMARY

The relative effectiveness of secretion removal techniques when applied to patients with copious secretions is controversial. In order to provide the reader with some guidance in the relative effectiveness of different tech-

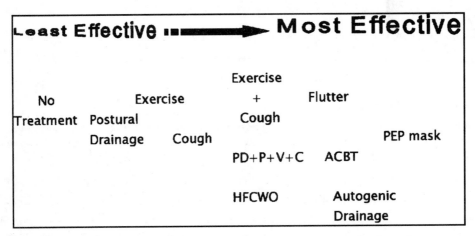

niques, the above figure (also shown as Figure 15-2 on page 109) is an attempt by the authors to rate some of the common techniques. Large variations in response to treatment and individual preferences do exist; clinicians should base their choice of treatment on patients' responses and other related outcome measures.

## REFERENCES

1. Wilson R, Cole PJ. The effect of bacterial products on ciliary function. *Am Rev Resp Dis.* 1998:138:S49-S53.
2. Badr C, Elkins MR, Ellis ER. The effect of body position on maximal expiratory pressure and flow. *Aust J Physiother.* 2002;48:95-102.
3. Bach PB, Brown C, Gelfand SE, McCrory DC. Management of exacerbations of chronic obstructive pulmonary disease: a summary and appraisal of published evidence. *Ann Intern Med.* 2001;134:600-620.
4. McCrory DC, Brown C, Gelfand SE, Bach PB. Management of exacerbations of COPD: a summary and appraisal of the published evidence. *Chest.* 2001;119:1190-1209.
5. Snow V, Lascher S, Mottur-Pilson C, et al. The evidence base for management of acute exacerbations of COPD: clinical practice guideline, part 1. *Chest.* 2001;119:1185-1189.
6. Snow V, Lascher S, Mottur-Pilson C, et al. Evidence base for management of acute exacerbations of chronic obstructive pulmonary disease. *Ann Intern Med.* 2001;134:595-599.
7. Siafakas NM, Vermeire P, Pride NB, et al. Optimal assessment and management of chronic obstructive pulmonary disease (COPD). *Eur Respir J.* 1995;8:1398-1420.
8. American Thoracic Society. Standards for the diagnosis and care of patients with chronic obstructive pulmonary disease. *Am J Respir Crit Care Med.* 1995;152:S77-S121.
9. Pauwels RA, Buist AS, Calverley PMA, Jenkins CR, Hurd SS. Global strategy for the diagnosis, management, and prevention of chronic obstructive pulmonary disease: NHLBI/WHO Global Initiative for Chronic Obstructive Lung Disease (GOLD) Workshop summary. *Am J Respir Crit Care Med.* 2001;163:1256-1276.
10. Horiuchi K, Jordan D, Cohen D, et al. Insights into the increased oxygen demand during chest physiotherapy. *Crit Care Med.* 1997;25:1347-1351.
11. Thomas J, Dehueck A, Kleiner M, et al. To vibrate or not to vibrate: usefulness of the mechanical vibrator for clearing bronchial secretions. *Physiotherapy Canada.* 1995;47:120-125.
12. Cecins NM, Jenkins SC, Pengelley J, et al. The active cycle of breathing techniques—to tip or not to tip? *Respir Med.* 1999;93:660-665.

## BIBLIOGRAPHY

Bates D. *Respiratory Function in Disease.* 3rd ed. Philadelphia: WB Saunders Company; 1989.

Stoller JK. Acute exacerbations of chronic obstructive pulmonary disease. *N Eng J Med.* 2002;346:988-994.

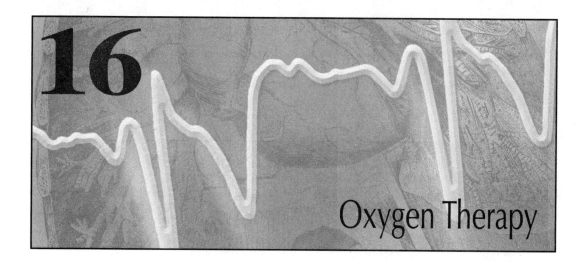

Oxygen Therapy

## OBJECTIVES

At the end of this chapter, the therapist should be able to describe:
1. The diagnostic requirements for home oxygen use
2. The implications of oxygen administration during exercise and at rest
3. The dangers, potential problems, and contraindications associated with oxygen administration
4. Different oxygen delivery systems

## BRIEF DESCRIPTION

Oxygen can be stored in liquid or compressed gas form and delivered from wall ports or from cylinders and small portable units for therapeutic use. Oxygen therapy can improve oxygen delivery to tissues in people with respiratory and cardiac disorders. There are a number of dangers associated with the administration of oxygen—both in terms of untoward effects in patients and the handling of the oxygen delivery systems.

## EVIDENCE: A

Long-term oxygen therapy administered for 12 or 24 hours in COPD patients with hypoxemia decreased mortality, reduced hematocrit, and ameliorated the increase in pulmonary vascular resistance and pulmonary arterial pressure found in the control group.[1,2]

## INDICATIONS FOR OXYGEN IN ACUTE CARE SETTING

- *Hypoxemia*, which can be defined as a $PaO_2$ of less than 80 mmHg or $SaO_2$ less than 90%; the absolute $PaO_2$ or $SaO_2$ may vary dependent on the patient, the nature of the condition being treated, other conditions, age, etc.
- *To decrease the work of breathing.*
- *To decrease myocardial work.* This may be done to target a specific organ in order to prevent ischemic damage and pain.

## PRIMARY CRITERIA FOR HOME OXYGEN

- Resting $PaO_2$ less than 55 mmHg at rest on room air
- Resting $PaO_2$ of less than 56 to 60 mmHg with polycythemia or cor pulmonale as shown by:
  o Edema, p pulmonale, pulmonary artery hypertension, polycythemia

- Can be prescribed for COPD patients with resting normoxia ($SaO_2$ > 88%) who transiently desaturate during exercise if the patient shows a significant improvement in dyspnea and exercise performance with oxygen. Its widespread use for this group is not recommended because some patients who transiently desaturate during exercise neither improve exercise performance nor reduce dyspnea with supplemental oxygen.[3-5]
- Can be prescribed for nocturnal sleep desaturation in sleep apnea, chronic respiratory failure, and some patients who have considerable transient nocturnal sleep desaturation—ie, greater than 30% of the time at a $SpO_2$ of less than 88%.
- Ischemic heart disease is rarely an indication for oxygen therapy. Hypoxemia needs to be documented in refractory cardiac failure for prescription of long-term oxygen therapy.
- Note: Criteria for home oxygen paid for by third-party payers can vary so it is important that physical therapists facilitate the administrative arrangements for home oxygen for those patients requiring extra assistance.

# DANGERS, PROBLEMS, AND CONTRAINDICATIONS FOR OXYGEN

1. *Diminishing Hypoxic Drive*—People who are chronically hypercapnic (elevated arterial $PaCO_2$) with COPD have some equilibration of their arterial pH. Increased $CO_2$ levels stimulate breathing in healthy people, whereas this stimulus is blunted in people with chronic hypercapnia or a chronic respiratory acidosis; thus, these individuals are more dependent on their hypoxic drive to breathe. In a small percentage of people with a chronic respiratory acidosis, administering high concentrations of oxygen will remove their hypoxic drive to breathe; they will hypoventilate and go into respiratory failure. Therefore, in people with chronic respiratory disease, the aim is to use the lowest concentration of oxygen that will provide a sufficient oxygenation, which is often 2 L/min.

2. *Absorption Atelectasis*—About 80% of the gas in the alveoli is nitrogen. If high concentrations of oxygen are administered, the nitrogen is displaced. When the oxygen diffuses across the alveolar-capillary membrane into the blood stream, the nitrogen is no longer present to distend the alveoli contributing to their collapse and atelectasis.

3. *Oxygen Toxicity*—High levels of oxygen administration for 24 hours usually results in some lung damage because of oxygen radical production. Oxygen radical production occurs because of incomplete reduction of oxygen to water. Oxygen radicals are very reactive molecules that can damage membranes, proteins, and many cell structures in the lungs.

4. *Retrolental Fibroplasia*—occurs in premature infants if maintained on high levels of $O_2$ because this leads to retinal vasoconstriction that causes fibrosis behind the ocular lens and blindness.

5. *Pulmonary vasodilation*—High inspired oxygen may be contraindicated in some cardiac lesions when an elevated pulmonary vascular resistance is required.

# OXYGEN DELIVERY SYSTEMS

Different types of oxygen delivery systems are summarized in Table 16-1. Physical therapists are not usually involved in the adjustment, supplying, or fitting of these systems to patients. It is essential that physical therapists are aware of the oxygen therapy prescription for their patients and regularly check to ensure that patients are receiving their oxygen as prescribed.

Table 16-1

## Oxygen Delivery Systems

| Delivery System | Flow Rate | FiO$_2$* | Comment |
|---|---|---|---|
| Nasal prongs | 1 to 6 L/min | 0.24 to 0.44 | Most common delivery system. |
| Simple mask | 6 to 10 L/min | 0.25 to 0.50 | Second most common delivery system. |
| Partial rebreathing | 10 to 15 L/min | 0.40 to 0.60 | Oxygen flow should always be supplied to mask. Maintain the reservoir bag at least one-third to one-half full on inspiration. |
| Non-rebreathing mask | | ~0.60 to 0.80 | One valve is placed between the bag and mask to prevent exhaled air from returning to the bag. There should be a minimum flow of 10 L/min. The delivered FiO$_2$ of this system is 60% to 80%. |
| Aerosol or venturi face mask with and without star wars | 7 to 15 L/min | 0.25 to 0.50 | Air entrainment nebulizer blends the FiO$_2$ with humidity. The "star wars" refers to has large bore tubing reservoirs attached to the mask |
| Face tent | | | Used for patients with poor tolerance of nasal prongs or facemask. |
| Trach mask | | | Used to deliver humidity and oxygen. |
| T-piece | | variable | Can be used for weaning and when very precise control of the FiO2 is required. |

*Note that the FiO$_2$ is the abbreviation for the fractional concentration of inspired oxygen. It is a measure of the proportion of inspired oxygen. For example, an FiO$_2$ of 21% or 0.21 means that 21% of the inspired air is oxygen. The precise FiO$_2$ delivered via a particular delivery system depends on the breathing pattern and the fit of the mask on the patient.

# REFERENCES

1. Medical Research Council Working Party. Long-term domiciliary oxygen therapy in chronic hypoxic cor pulmonale complicating chronic bronchitis and emphysema. *Lancet.* 1981;1:681-6.

2. Nocturnal Oxygen Therapy Trial (NOTT) Group. Continuous or nocturnal oxygen therapy in hypoxemia chronic obstruct lung disease; a clinical trial. *Ann Intern Med.* 1980;93:391-8.

3. Ishimine A, Saito H, Nishimura M, Nakano T, Miyamoto K, Kawakami Y. Effect of supplemental oxygen on exercise performance in patients with chronic obstructive pulmonary disease and an arterial oxygen tension over 60 Torr. *Nihon Kyobu Shikkan Gakkai Zasshi.* 1995;33:510-519.

4. Jolly EC, Di B, Aguirre VL, Luna CM, Berensztein S, Gene RJ. Effects of supplemental oxygen during activity in patients with advanced COPD without severe resting hypoxemia. *Chest.* 2001;120:437-443.

5. Matsuzawa Y, Kubo K, Fujimoto K, et al. Acute effects of oxygen on dyspnea and exercise tolerance in patients with pulmonary emphysema with only mild exercise-induced oxyhemoglobin desaturation. *Nihon Kokyuki Gakkai Zasshi.* 2000;38:831-835.

# BIBLIOGRAPHY

Kallstrom TJ. AARC clinical practice guideline: oxygen therapy for adults in the acute care facility—2002 revision and update. *Respiratory Care.* 2002;47:717-720.

Stubbing D, Beaupre A, Vaughan R. Long-term oxygen treatment. In: Bourbeau J, Nault D, Borycki E, eds. *Comprehensive Management of Chronic Obstructive Pulmonary Disease.* Hamilton, BC Decker; 2002;109-130.

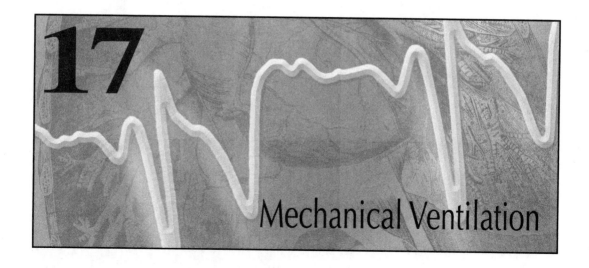

# OBJECTIVES

At the end of this session, the student should be able to describe:
1. The indications and rationale for using mechanical ventilation
2. The different modes of mechanical ventilation
3. The different ventilatory parameters of mechanical ventilation

Patients with severe hypercapnia or those with severe hypoxemia despite high flow oxygen therapy can require mechanical ventilation to sustain life. This chapter defines and describes different types and modes of mechanical ventilation commonly used in the clinical setting.

# INVASIVE MECHANICAL VENTILATION

## Overview

Positive pressure ventilators (Figure 17-1) expand the lungs by increasing the pulmonary pressure resulting in an increase in the transpulmonary pressure. The ventilator's pressure, volume, flow, and time are the main variables determining ventilation delivered to the patient. Two common modes of delivering mechanical ventilation are pressure-limited or volume-limited ventilation. Inspiration is usually set but can also be triggered by the patient. During the inspiratory phase, the ventilator pumps the air into the lungs until a predetermined pressure or volume limit is reached. Once the limit is reached, it signals the end of the inspiratory phase and passive expiration begins. The ventilator is connected to the patient by an oral or nasal endotracheal (ET) tube (Figure 17-2) or a tracheostomy tube (Figure 17-3). In-line suction catheters, used to clear secretions, are commonly used and connected to the ET or tracheostomy tube.

## Common Conditions Where Mechanical Ventilation is Indicated[1]

- 66% of patients have acute lung injury (adult respiratory distress syndrome,[2] heart failure, pneumonia, sepsis, complications post-surgery, and trauma)
- 15% of patients have decreased level of consciousness
- 13% of patients have acute exacerbations of COPD
- 5% of patients have neuromuscular disorders

## Rationale for Using Mechanical Ventilation

- To decrease the work of breathing
- To maintain normal oxygenation
- To maintain normal levels of ventilation and acid-base balance[3-6]

**Figure 17-1.** Positive pressure mechanical ventilator. (A) connector to endotracheal or tracheostomy tube.

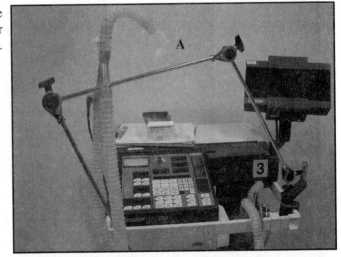

**Figure 17-2.** Endotracheal tube with an in-line suction catheter. (A) oral endotracheal tube. (B) connector to ventilator and in-line suction catheter. (C) in-line suction connector. (D) instillation port. (E) suction on-off switch. (F) suction catheter covered in a plastic aseptic barrier.

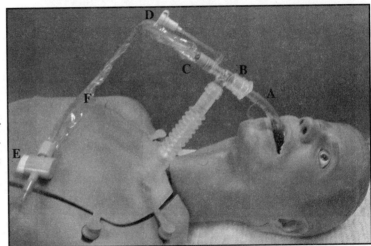

**Figure 17-3.** Front view of tracheostomy tubes with collar (right) and without collar (left). The inflatable cuff (A) is used to prevent leakage between the trachea and tracheostomy tube of air from the lungs and aspiration of fluid into the lungs. Note the relatively short length of the tracheostomy tube.

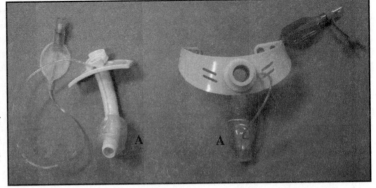

## Table 17-1

### *Potential Adverse Effects of Positive Mechanical Ventilation*

*Hemodynamic Effects*

- Decreased venous return
- Decreased cardiac output
- Decreased renal perfusion
- Decreased blood pressure

*Pulmonary Effects*

- Increased ventilation/perfusion ratio and dead space/tidal volume ratio
- Air trapping
- Barotrauma can cause
  - o Release of proinflammatory cytokines, which can lead to multi-system failure
  - o Pneumothorax, subcutaneous emphysema
- Increased work of breathing and respiratory distress (eg, narrow diameter ET tube, discomfort associated with mechanical ventilation, incoordination with ventilator)
- Respiratory muscle weakness
- Infection—nocosomial or aspiration pneumonia

*Other Effects*

- Increased use of narcotics or sedative agents
- Use of other invasive measures (eg, arterial lines, feeding tube)
- Increased intracranial pressure
- Decreased mobility

## Table 17-2

### *Features of Common Ventilation Modes*

| Mode | Mandatory Breath | Assisted Breath | Spontaneous Breath |
|---|---|---|---|
| Controlled mandatory ventilation (CMV) | Yes | | |
| Assisted control ventilation (ACV) | Yes | Yes | |
| Intermittent mandatory ventilation (IMV) | Yes | | Yes |
| Synchronized intermittent mandatory ventilation (SIMV) | Yes | Yes | Yes |

The increase in the pulmonary pressure during positive pressure ventilation could potentially have adverse effects on the patient (Table 17-1). Hence efforts are made to minimize or limit the amount of positive pressure the patient receives during mechanical ventilation.

## Ventilatory Modes Frequently Used With Positive Pressure Ventilation

- In pressure-controlled ventilation, the inspiration phase ends when a set peak pressure limit is reached. The tidal volume can therefore vary between breaths. In volume-controlled ventilation, the inspiration phase ends when a set volume or a set peak pressure limit (as a safety feature) is reached. The tidal volume is therefore controlled. Pressure-controlled or volume-controlled ventilation can be used with the following modes of ventilation. The common modes of mechanical ventilation are outlined below and in Table 17-2.

- CMV—Ventilation is completely controlled by the ventilator
- ACV—Patients may breathe above the mandatory rate with ventilator-assisted breaths at the mandatory tidal volume
- IMV—Patients may breathe above the mandatory rate with spontaneous breaths
- SIMV—Assisted controlled ventilation and allows spontaneous breaths in between ventilator-assisted breaths

## Supportive Modes Frequently Used With Mechanical Ventilation

- Pressure support ventilation (PSV)
  - o Because the patient has to breath through the ET tubing, which is much smaller in diameter than the normal upper airways, the work of breathing is much higher. PSV is used to decrease the airway resistance and make breathing easier for the patient.
  - o PSV delivers a preset inspiratory pressure to assist spontaneous breathing. It can be used to ventilate or wean patients off the ventilator. However, pressure support (PS) is frequently used to provide ventilatory support. For a set PS, the patient determines the rate, volume and breath-by-breath inspiratory time. It is frequently used to help decrease the work of breathing imposed by the ET tube and ventilator. Pressure support can also be added during volume-controlled ventilation.
- Continuous positive airway pressure ventilation (CPAP)
  - o CPAP provides continuous positive airway pressure during both the inspiratory and expiratory phases. During CPAP, the patient is breathing spontaneously and has to generate all the inspiratory effort. CPAP is frequently used to wean patients off the ventilator.

## Ventilatory Parameters

- RR
  - o 12 to 20 breaths per minute for normal lungs.
  - o A high RR tends to increase the probability of air trapping especially in patients with chronic obstructive pulmonary disease. However, high RR can be required for patients with acute lung injury.
- $V_T$
  - o 10 to 15 ml/kg of body weight for normal lungs.
  - o A higher $V_T$ tends to optimize the $V_T$ and dead space ventilation ratio but at the expense of an increased risk of barotrauma.
  - o A lower $V_T$ is recommended in patients with restrictive lung disease or acute lung injury. Allowing permissive hypercapnia while using a lower $V_T$, causes less lung damage and has been shown to increase survival in patients with adult respiratory distress syndrome.
  - o Serial arterial blood gas analyses are used to adjust the RR and $V_T$ settings to an acceptable pH.
- Inspiratory flow pattern
  - o The inspiratory time: expiratory time ($T_i : T_E$) ratio is usually maintained at greater than 1:2.
  - o In general, a prolonged $T_i$ allows for more even distribution of ventilation amongst alveoli but at the expense of a shortened $T_E$, which can increase air trapping in patients with obstructive lung diseases.
  - o An inverse $T_i$ and $T_E$ ratio is occasionally used in patients with ARDS.
- Inspiratory waveforms
  - o Usually square or decelerating waves are used because they deliver more rapid initial flows and improve gas exchange.
- Trigger sensitivity
  - o It is the effort that the patient has to exert in order to trigger ventilatory support in the assisted mode. The sensitivity is usually set at a pressure of –1 to –2 cm of $H_2O$.
- Peak inspiratory flow rate
  - o The peak inspiratory flow rate is usually set at 60 to 90 L/min or a $T_i$ of 0.8 to 1.2 seconds in patients with spontaneous breathing. Increased peak inspiratory flow rates will shorten the $T_i$ and lengthen the $T_E;$ however, this can cause an increase in the RR in some patients.

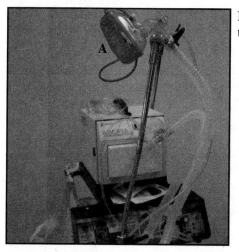

**Figure 17-4.** Nasal mask (A) connected to a bilevel continuous positive airway pressure ventilator.

- Oxygenation
    - A high fraction of inspired oxygen ($FiO_2$) and positive end expiratory pressure (PEEP) are used to maintain adequate oxygenation. Both of these parameters, however, can have adverse effects. A high $FiO_2$ can induce oxygen toxicity and cause reabsorption atelectasis. High PEEP can impede venous return, decrease cardiac output, decrease systemic blood pressure, and increase the risk of overdistending alveoli.

# NONINVASIVE MECHANICAL VENTILATION

## Indications and Common Conditions for Using Noninvasive Positive Pressure Ventilation

- Signs of respiratory failure as defined by:
    - $PaCO_2$ > 50 mmHg and $PaO_2/FiO_2$ < 200
    - Moderate to severe dyspnea with RR > 24/min or paradoxical breathing
- Common conditions that noninvasive positive pressure ventilation (NPPV) is used in the event of respiratory failure are: restrictive chest wall disease, sleep apnea, neuromuscular disorders, COPD, and acute pulmonary edema.
- Patients need upper airway control and an intact cough to be suitable for NPPV, otherwise intubation and positive pressure invasive mechanical ventilation will be used.

## Negative Pressure Ventilation

Negative pressure ventilation (NPV) expands the lungs by pulling out the chest wall. Each of the NPV devices provides an airtight enclosure around the thorax. The negative pressure applied to the chest wall mimics normal ventilation during which the inspiratory muscles pull out the chest wall. Examples of NPV are iron lungs, body wrap, or cuirass ventilators. NPVs are bulky and restrictive, and patients are usually kept in the supine position. Patients frequently complain of back and shoulder pain and pressure sores. With the refinement of NPPV, NPV use has become more rare.

## Abdominal Displacement Ventilator

Examples of abdominal displacement ventilators are rocking beds and pneumobelts. These devices are relatively ineffective and are of limited use.

## Noninvasive Positive Pressure Ventilation

An oronasal mask or nasal mask (Figure 17-4) is used to interface the patient with the positive pressure ventilator. Mouthpieces with lip seals are also available especially for use with neuromuscular patients. The oronasal mask covers the nose and mouth, which prevents air leakage through the mouth. It is frequently used in acute patients. Some patients complain of claustrophobia. Other concerns are increased risk of asphyxiation and aspiration in some patients. The use of a nasal mask permits talking and eating. It is popular with chronic and more experienced patients.

## Ventilator Modes Frequently Used With Noninvasive Positive Pressure Ventilation

Ventilators frequently use a bilevel of continuous positive airway pressure (BiPAP) that provide positive airway pressure during inspiration (IPAP) and expiration (EPAP). Patients with spontaneous breathing needing some ventilatory support are prime candidates for the use of BiPAP ventilation (see Figure 17-4). People with sleep apnea often benefit from the use of CPAP or BiPAP for nocturnal ventilation.[7-10] For the more disabled patients, assisted control or full ventilation in either volume- or pressure-controlled ventilation are available.

# REFERENCES

1. Tobins MJ. Advances in mechanical ventilation. *N Eng J Med.* 2001;344:1986-1996.

2. Brower RG, Ware LB, Berthiaume Y, et al. Treatment of ARDS. *Chest.* 2001;120:1347-1367.

3. Dries DJ. Permissive hypercapnia. *J Trauma.* 1995;39:984-989.

4. Hickling KG, Joyce C. Permissive hypercapnia in ARDS and its effect on tissue oxygenation. *Acta Anaesthesiol Scand Suppl.* 1995;107:201-208.

5. Mutlu GM, Factor P, Schwartz DE, Sznajder JI. Severe status asthmaticus: management with permissive hypercapnia and inhalation anesthesia. *Crit Care Med.* 2002;30:477-480.

6. Pfeiffer B, Hachenberg T, Wendt M, Marshall B. Mechanical ventilation with permissive hypercapnia increases intrapulmonary shunt in septic and nonseptic patients with acute respiratory distress syndrome. *Crit Care Med.* 2002;30:285-289.

7. Kohnlein T, Welte T, Tan LB, et al. Central sleep apnoea syndrome in patients with chronic heart disease: a critical review of the current literature. *Thorax.* 2002;57:547-554.

8. Claman DM, Piper A, Sanders MH, et al. Nocturnal noninvasive positive pressure ventilatory assistance. *Chest.* 1996;110:1581-1588.

9. International Consensus Conferences in Intensive Care Medicine: noninvasive positive pressure ventilation in acute respiratory failure. *Am J Respir Crit Care Med.* 2001;163:283-291.

10. Mehta S, Hill NS. Non-invasive ventilation. *Am J Resp Crit Care Med.* 2001;163:540-577.

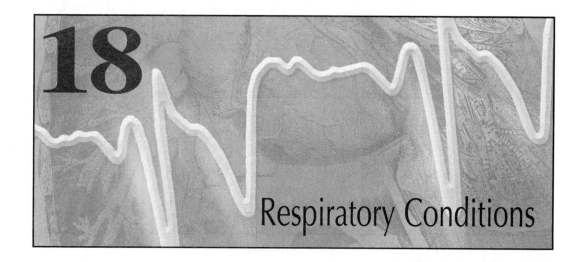

# OBJECTIVES

Upon completion of this chapter, the reader should be able to:

1. Describe the definition, etiology, pathophysiology, presentation, and medical and physical therapy management of the acute respiratory conditions including: pneumonia, atelectasis, chest trauma, ARDS, respiratory failure, pulmonary infarct, lung abscess, pleural effusion, and pulmonary edema

2. Describe the definition, epidemiology, etiology, pathophysiology, clinical presentation, medical management, and physical therapy management of the chronic respiratory conditions including: restrictive lung disease, restrictive chest wall disorders, COPD, asthma, bronchiectasis, cystic fibrosis, and lung cancer

3. Describe changes in the respiratory system or pathology that can compound the deleterious impact of respiratory conditions including changes that occur in the elderly, smoking, and obesity

4. Describe the pathophysiology that is reversible by physical therapy and other health professionals in these respiratory disorders

5. Outline the medical management and physical therapy interventions that can be provided for different respiratory disorders

*Note: In this section, an outline of problems and possible physical therapy interventions are provided to facilitate the reader in making the connection between preceding content and various respiratory conditions. Evidence to support these treatments is provided in the previous chapters. Further, treatment plans in this chapter are suggested guidelines only; the optimal treatment plan for each patient needs to be individualized to his or her specific needs.*

# PNEUMONIA

## *Definition*

Pneumonia is inflammation of the substance of the lung.

## *Epidemiology*

The leading cause of death from infection and the sixth most common cause of death overall in Canada is influenza and pneumonia. It is the second most common cause of hospital-acquired infection second to urinary tract infection.

## *Etiology*

An etiological agent can be found in 70% of patients. Possible causes include:

1. *Aspiration* of contaminated oropharyngeal contents. 70% of normal individuals aspirate oropharyngeal contents during deep sleep; this occurs much more frequently in patients with swallowing difficulties and ventilated patients.[1-3]

Table 18-1

### Risk Factors That Will Lead to Readmission
### or Increase Mortality in Pneumonia Patients[4]

#### Risk Factors That Are Present on the Day of Hospital Discharge

- Temperature above 37.8° C or 100°F
- Heart rate above 100 BPM
- Respirations of more than 24/minute
- Systolic BP below 90 mmHg
- Oxygen saturation below 90%
- Inability to maintain oral intake
- Abnormal mental status

Overall 32.8% of pneumonia patients were not able to return to their preadmission activity level within 30 days of discharge from hospital.[4]

- The supine body position increases the risk of aspiration pneumonia in mechanically ventilated patients.[1]
- Mechanically ventilated patients have a lower incidence (8% versus 39% respectively) of ventilator-associated pneumonia when treated with chest physical therapy (modified postural drainage, vibration and suction) than those treated with sham physical therapy (positioning from side to side and suction).[5]
- Continuous subglottic suctioning may prevent aspiration pneumonia in mechanically ventilated patients.[2,3]
- Swallowing dysfunction including silent aspiration happens in more than 50% of patients intubated for longer than 48 hours. Neck muscle strengthening might improve patient swallowing in patients with swallowing problems.[6,7]

2. *Inhalation* of airborne infectious agents such as bacteria, viruses, microplasma, and fungi
3. *Hematogenous* occurs more often in immunosuppressed people
4. *Direct extension*—eg, trauma or chest tube

Those more prone to severe lower respiratory tract infections include: infants, the elderly, those with chronic cardiac or respiratory disease, and those who are immunosuppressed

## Pathophysiology

Pneumonias can be classified both anatomically and on the basis of etiology:

1. *Anatomical*
   - Lobar pneumonia, which is localized to the lobe of the lung
   - Bronchopneumonia, which primarily involves spread and involvement along the bronchi and bronchioles
2. *Etiological*
   - For example, streptococcal pneumonia is named after the causative organism.

## Clinical Presentation and Course

The presentation of pneumonia varies considerably depending on the etiological agent, the condition of the patient, and the time of diagnosis. Factors that worsen prognosis are listed in Table 18-1. Many pneumonias are not treated beyond the care given for general malaise, flu, and cold symptoms. In other instances, the pneumonia can result in respiratory failure and death. Signs and symptoms associated with pneumonia vary but can include: fever, chills, pleuritic pain, headache, fatigability, weight loss, generalized aches and pains, cough with or without expectoration of sputum or blood, or patchy or lobar opacity on chest x-ray.

Severe acute respiratory distress syndrome (SARS) is an atypical pneumonia of viral origin that can progress to ARDS in its end stages. See www.who.int/csr/sars/en/ for updated information on SARS.

## Medical Interventions

Medical interventions are aimed at identifying the etiologic agent and treating with the appropriate antimicrobial agent if indicated. Supportive measures of oxygen therapy, intravenous fluids, nutritional support, and mechanical ventilation may be required in more severe cases.

SARS is highly infectious especially in a hospital setting or with close personal contact. Preventing cross-contamination or spreading of infectious diseases is important. Frequent hand-washing is essential. In highly contagious diseases such as SARS, stringent isolation procedures and protective gear such as a N-95 facemask, face shield, eye goggles, double gloves, and protective clothing is required.

## Physical Therapy Interventions

Problems and possible treatments for this condition include:

1. *Poor gas exchange in affected regions*

   Possible treatments: deep breathing, positioning, ensure patient is using oxygen if prescribed.

2. *Pain, due to coughing or pleuritis*

   Possible treatments: relaxation, supported cough.

3. *Retained secretions can be present. Need to assess carefully.*

   Possible treatments: airway clearance techniques such as coughing, huffing, and active cycle breathing techniques, increase mobility to tolerance as soon as able.

4. *Decreased mobility*

   Possible treatments: bed exercises; gradually increase mobility to patient tolerance and as their condition permits; position upright as soon as possible.

5. *Exercise to improve swallowing in patients with dysphagia[6,7]*

   A suprahyoid muscle strengthening exercise program is effective in restoring oral feeding in some patients with swallowing difficulties due to abnormal upper esophageal sphincter opening. The patient should be instructed in the supine position to:

   • Perform 3 sustained head raisings for 1 minute and follow by a 1-minute rest period
   • Perform 30 consecutive repetitions of head raising

   The head should be raised high and forward enough that the patient could see his or her toes without lifting the shoulders off the bed.

What aspects of pneumonia are reversible by physical therapy?

# ATELECTASIS

## Definition

Atelectasis is collapse of lung tissue. This can have a patchy, segmental, or lobar distribution.

## Etiology & Pathophysiology

Atelectasis can be due to:

1. Blockage of a bronchus or bronchiole (the distal lung will collapse)
2. Compression from a pneumothorax, a pleural effusion, or other space-occupying lesions
3. Postanesthetic—due to the effects of anesthesia and prolonged recumbency during surgery resulting in hypoventilation, decreased sighing, and other pathophysiologic effects of surgery. Physical therapists often see patients with atelectasis due to anesthetic and postanesthetic effects.

## Clinical Presentation and Course

The clinical presentation can vary depending on the extent and distribution of the atelectasis, the cause of atelectasis, and other patient characteristics. Some atelectasis is clinically insignificant in patients. The primary presentation of atelectasis that needs to be managed is poor gas exchange including low $PaO_2$ and $SpO_2$ levels. Other signs are a fever and increased opacity apparent on the chest x-ray with signs consistent with volume loss (see Chapter 6 for further details of possible chest x-ray changes).

## Medical Interventions

Medical interventions are directed toward identifying and treating the underlying cause. Bronchoscopy can clear an obstructed airway. Supportive measures of oxygen therapy, intravenous fluids, nutritional support, and mechanical ventilation may be required in more severe cases.

## Physical Therapy Interventions

Problems and possible treatments for this condition include:

1. *Poor gas exchange in affected regions*

   Possible treatments: deep breathing with inspiratory hold, positioning, ensure patient is using oxygen if prescribed

2. *Pain, if atelectasis is due to surgery or trauma*

   Possible treatments: coordinate treatment with pain medication if indicated; educate patient regarding pain medications; support painful area with pillows; and positioning during deep breathing and coughing

3. *Decreased mobility*

   Possible treatments: bed exercises; gradually increase mobility to patient tolerance and as his or her condition permits; position upright as soon as possible

4. *Retained secretions can be present. Need to assess carefully.*

   Possible treatments: airway clearance techniques such as coughing, huffing, active cycle breathing techniques, increase mobility to tolerance as soon as able

What aspects of atelectasis are reversible by physical therapy?

# CHEST TRAUMA

## Definition

Blunt and penetrating trauma to the chest can injure the bony skeleton; rupture the diaphragm, the lungs, and the airways; contuse or lacerate the heart; and rupture major vessels.

## Etiology & Pathophysiology

The leading cause of blunt trauma is motor vehicles accidents followed by falls usually in the home. Penetrating wounds to the chest are usually caused by shooting or stab wounds. Blunt trauma often affects several structures whereas a penetrating wound can be more specific. A number of structures can be injured.

- *Rib fractures*—may not be treated if the fractured rib does not damage underlying tissue or result in significant pain. Complications arise with multiple fractures and when the underlying lung or blood vessels are damaged. Complications include atelectasis, pneumothorax, and hemothorax. Most rib fractures result in a 10% to 20% decrease in lung volume due to a pneumothorax but pneumothoraces can be larger.

- *Fractured sternum* may result in minimal problems or if a flail segment occurs, then internal fixation is necessary.

- *Flail chest* occurs in the case of multiple fractures of ribs and/or sternum when bony connections of the ribs or sternum of the fractured segment are disconnected from the rest of the rib cage. The flail segment moves in the opposite direction of the rib cage on inspiration and expiration that can result in very inefficient ventilation and impairment of gas exchange.

- *Trauma to lung and lung contusion* results in hemorrhage into the lung parenchyma that can lead to hemoptysis.

- *Damage to the major airways* including the trachea and main-stem bronchi can occur. These airways can be disconnected in blunt trauma and can be lacerated with penetrating trauma.

- *Contusions to the heart and rupture or laceration of major blood vessels*—treatment depends on the extent of damage; immediate repair may be essential if person survives.

## Clinical Presentation and Course

The presenting signs and symptoms depend on the extent of injury to the underlying structures and whether adequate oxygenation and perfusion can be maintained. Often other regions of the body are injured, which are usually the head, extremity fractures, and the abdomen.

## Medical Interventions

Medical interventions are directed toward pain control, stopping bleeding, maintaining cardiovascular stability, and maintaining adequate gas exchange.

- The amount of atelectasis is related to pain and thus *management of pain* is important to ensure that adequate ventilation and removal of secretions are maintained.
- *Surgical repair* may be necessary to repair lacerated vessels, lacerated main airways, damaged cardiac structures, or a flail sternum.
- Often there is a combination of blood and air in the pleural space that can be drained by the insertion of 1 or 2 *chest tubes* if large.
- If there is a large flail segment, flail sternum, or substantial lung injury, *mechanical ventilation* may be required.
- Cardiac instability will be managed with *pharmaceuticals* and *fluid balance*.
- Neurological and musculoskeletal problems associated with the initial injury or resultant shock will be managed accordingly.

## Physical Therapy Interventions

Problems and possible treatments focused on the cardiopulmonary system include:

1. *Poor gas exchange in affected regions*

   Possible treatments: deep breathing with inspiratory hold; positioning; ensure patient is using oxygen if prescribed

2. *Pain*

   Possible treatments: co-ordinate treatment with pain medication; patient education regarding importance of adequate pain medication; support trauma area with pillows while moving or coughing; relaxation techniques; gentle ROM exercises; can inquire about intercostal nerve blocks for pain relief

3. *Retained secretions can be present. Need to assess carefully*

   Possible treatments: airway clearance techniques, positioning, supported cough, increase mobility

4. Decreased mobility

   Possible treatments: bed exercises; gradually increase mobility to patient tolerance and as their condition permits; position upright as soon as possible. Use caution when mobilizing patient with drainage device such as a chest tubes. The chest fluid collection chamber should always be positioned lower than the chest tube insertion site.

What components of chest trauma are reversible by physical therapy?

# PLEURITIS AND PLEURAL EFFUSIONS

## Definition

Pleuritis is inflammation of the pleura and a pleural effusion is a collection of fluid between the lungs and chest wall.

## Etiology and Pathophysiology

### Causes of Dry Pleuritis or Pleurisy

- Pneumonia (bacterial or viral), tuberculosis, pulmonary infarction, connective tissue diseases, chest wall trauma, carcinoma, mesothelioma

## Causes of Pleural Exudates

- Diseases of the lungs such as bacterial pneumonia, pulmonary infarction, malignancy, tuberculosis. Other conditions can cause pleural exudates such as postmyocardial infarction syndrome, acute pancreatitis, and primary pleural tumors

## Causes of Pleural Transudates

- Congestive heart failure, pericarditis, cirrhosis, peritoneal dialysis

## Clinical Presentation and Course

The signs and symptoms can vary but can include:
- Pain with deep breathing and cough, which is worse in dry pleuritis
- Fever may or may not occur
- Dyspnea especially with a large pleural effusion
- Fluid collection can shift mediastinum to the unaffected side, decrease chest movement on affected side, and decrease vital capacity
- Over time adhesion formation can result from the organization of the exudate
- An empyema can occur if the pleural effusion becomes infected:
  o More often there is organization of exudate with formation of dense tough fibrous adhesions
  o Signs and symptoms are often an erratic temperature, dyspnea, and pain in chest

## Medical Interventions

Medical management can vary. In some cases, the pleural effusion will be observed to await resolution without intervention. If treated, the medical intervention will be directed at the underlying cause. The fluid may be drained by insertion of chest tube or needle aspiration (thoracocentesis).

## Physical Therapy Interventions

Problems and possible treatments for *pleural effusion* and other space-occupying lesions* such as *hemothorax, pneumothorax, if closed and chest tube is inserted* include:
1. *Poor gas exchange in affected regions*

   Possible treatments: deep breathing (only if chest tube is inserted in pneumothorax), positioning, especially upright positions to facilitate draining, ensure patient is using oxygen if prescribed
2. *Decreased mobility*

   Possible treatments: bed exercises; gradually increase mobility to patient tolerance and as his or her condition permits; position upright as soon as possible; assist with chest tube and collection equipment
3. *Decreased ROM of shoulder on side where chest tube is inserted*

   Possible treatments: encourage active use of shoulder while tube is in place; assess ROM when chest tube is removed

   *Similar treatment considerations might be provided for patients with a hemothorax and pneumothorax if it is closed and a chest tube is inserted.

What components of pleuritis and pleural effusions are reversible by physical therapy?

# LUNG ABSCESS

## Definition

A lung abscess is a localized inflammatory response resulting in a collection of pus around an inciting agent such as a bacteria or fungi. The localized area of pus formation can proceed to necrosis of lung tissue and sometimes liquefaction resulting in an air-fluid level surrounded by fibrosis that is apparent on chest x-ray.

## Etiology & Pathophysiology

A lung abscess can result from aspiration of a foreign body, cavitary tuberculosis, obstruction of a bronchus from a neoplasm, unresolved pneumonia, infection of an infarct, or from sepsis.

## Clinical Presentation and Course

The presentation of an abscess is usually dominated by the underlying lung disease, the size of the abscess, and the presentation of complications, if any. Often its initial presentation is on a chest x-ray. A fever and other symptoms of malaise may occur. The abscess can rupture into a bronchus resulting in its evacuation and often expectoration of purulent, foul sputum. Alternatively an empyema can result.

## Medical Interventions

Medical interventions are aimed at identifying the etiologic agent and treating the underlying cause. Supportive measures of oxygen therapy, intravenous fluids, and nutritional support may be required in more severe cases.

With extensive abscess formation, lung resection may be indicated.

## Physical Therapy Interventions

Problems and possible treatments for this condition include:

1. *Poor gas exchange in affected regions*

   Possible treatments: deep breathing exercises, positioning, ensure patient is using oxygen if prescribed.

2. *Decreased mobility*

   Possible treatments: bed exercises; gradually increase mobility to patient tolerance and as his or her condition permits; position upright as soon as possible

3. *Retained secretions, if lung abscess is communicated* (draining into airway)

   Possible treatments: airway clearance techniques such as coughing, huffing, active cycle breathing techniques, increase mobility to tolerance as soon as able

What components of lung abscess are reversible by physical therapy?

# PULMONARY EDEMA

## Definition

Pulmonary edema is the abnormal accumulation of fluid in the extravascular space, which can initially occur in the interstitium and then progress to the alveolar spaces.

## Etiology and Pathophysiology

Normally, the fluid balance in the lungs is tightly controlled; there is an outflow of fluid into the extravascular space of about 20 mL/hr in the normal lung but this is drained by the lymphatic system. Pulmonary edema can occur from high-pressure or low-pressure causes. The underlying causes can be best explained by examining the Starling equation:

$$\text{net fluid out} = K\,[\,(P_c - P_i) - k\,(\pi_c - \pi_i)\,]$$

where  $K$ is a constant
$P_c$ is the hydrostatic pressure in the capillaries
$P_i$ is the hydrostatic pressure in the interstitium
$k$ is a constant that describes the permeability of pulmonary endothelium and alveolar epithelium
$\pi_c$ is the osmotic pressure in the capillaries
$\pi_i$ is the osmotic pressure in the interstitium

Pulmonary edema occurs because of an increase in hydrostatic pressure, an imbalance of the osmotic pressure, or because of a loss of integrity of the pulmonary endothelium and alveolar epithelium. For example, in left-sided heart failure, increased hydrostatic pressure of the capillaries results in *high-pressure pulmonary edema*. Other causes of high-pressure pulmonary edema are MI, and mitral valve disease. Increased pressure within the pulmonary capillaries pushes fluid into the interstitial and alveolar spaces. Other names for high-pressure pulmonary edema are hydrostatic pulmonary edema, cardiogenic pulmonary edema and hemodynamic pulmonary edema. An example of *low pressure pulmonary edema*, also known as ARDS, is when toxins or trauma cause increased permeability of the capillary endothelium and alveolar epithelium resulting in a disruption in the balance of the osmotic pressure. This can cause flow of proteins (that are normally only in the capillaries) into the interstitium and alveolar spaces. The increased osmotic pressure and permeability allow the influx of fluid as well.

## Clinical Presentation and Course

Presentation depends on the underlying cause of the pulmonary edema and its severity. Increased airways resistance, shunting and ventilation-perfusion mismatch occurs. There is an increased work of breathing and associated dyspnea. Sputum expectorated in cardiogenic pulmonary edema can be light pink and frothy.

## Medical Interventions

In cardiogenic pulmonary edema, treatment is directed toward decreasing cardiac preload and venous return. Supplemental oxygen and mechanical ventilation may be necessary to maintain gas exchange. Medical treatment for noncardiogenic pulmonary edema, also known as ARDS, will be outlined below.

## Physical Therapy Interventions

Physical therapy is primarily aimed at preventing the deleterious effects of inactivity. Cardiogenic pulmonary edema is not amenable to any physical therapy technique and must be treated medically. Of considerable importance to the physical therapist is not to use airway clearance techniques to promote removal of cardiogenic pulmonary edema. Suctioning may be indicated, however, to maintain a patent airway in the intubated patient.

What components of pulmonary edema are reversible by physical therapy?

# ACUTE RESPIRATORY DISTRESS SYNDROME

## Definition

ARDS is acute lung injury characterized by increased permeability of the alveolar capillary membrane and severe hypoxemia. It is not a single disease but rather the term given to the clinical manifestation of the common pathway of several indirect lung injuries.

## Epidemiology

The incidence of ARDS is 1.5 to 8.4 cases per 100,000 population per year.[8]

## Etiology and Pathophysiology

Causes of ARDS include: shock, severe viral pneumonia, sepsis, aspiration, drugs, multiple leg or pelvic fractures, extensive burns, and high inspired levels of oxygen resulting in *oxygen toxicity*. Significant airway, parenchymal and interstitial disease processes occur in addition to increased water in the lung, which results in low pressure or "noncardiogenic" pulmonary edema. As the disease progresses, the rate of collagen deposition is very rapid in ARDS compared to other causes of pulmonary fibrosis.

## Clinical Presentation and Course

The pathophysiology may vary depending on the cause but the presenting signs and symptoms are nearly always identical. Patients are acutely ill, very dyspneic, often restless, and can be disoriented. Severe hypoxemia occurs that is characteristically not responsive to increasing $FiO_2$, which is indicative of pulmonary shunting. The lungs have a decreased compliance; high pressures and a high $FiO_2$ are required in an attempt to obtain adequate oxygenation.

Approximately 50% of patients with ARDS develop multisystem failure. The cause of death is not usually due to hypoxemia but rather multisystem failure and hemodynamic instability. The mortality rate is approximately 30% to 40%, which may vary in different centers.

## Medical Interventions

Medical interventions are aimed at:
- Treating the underlying cause of ARDS
- Obtaining adequate oxygenation via mechanical ventilation (often with a high PEEP)
- Maintaining adequate nutrition and electrolyte support

- Preventing complications; once mechanical ventilation has begun, complications include: barotrauma, hyperoxia damage, and infections

## *Physical Therapy Interventions*

Problems and possible treatments for this condition include:

1. *Poor gas exchange in affected region*

   Possible treatments: positioning—trial of prone position might be indicated; refer to Chapter 13 for more details

2. *Retained secretions*

   Possible treatments: airway clearance techniques if indicated—manual or mechanical vibrations, positioning

3. *Decreased mobility*

   Possible treatments: bed exercises; gradually increase mobility to patient tolerance and as his or her condition permits; position upright as soon as possible

# PATHOPHYSIOLOGY OF RESPIRATORY FAILURE

## *Definition*

Respiratory failure is the inability to maintain adequate gas exchange. The absolute $PaO_2$ and $PaCO_2$ are not as important in defining the seriousness of this condition but rather how quickly these values deteriorate.

## *Etiology and Pathophysiology*

There are 2 types of respiratory failure. *Type I* or lung failure results from a problem in the lungs such as a severe pneumonia or ARDS. Clinically, the $PaO_2$ is lower than normal but the $PaCO_2$ may be normal or even low. Type II results from a problem with the chest wall or the respiratory muscles such as central nervous system depression, inspiratory muscle fatigue, or multiple rib fractures resulting in a flail chest. Clinically, the $PaO_2$ is lower than normal and the $PaCO_2$ is elevated above the normal range. Chronic respiratory conditions can lead to a slower, more insidious onset of respiratory failure when the deterioration may take months or years to develop. For example, severe kyphoscoliosis and COPD can result in type II respiratory failure.

## *Clinical Presentation and Course*

The clinical presentation and course will depend on the underlying cause. In the more acute causes, the patient will present with increasing dyspnea and cyanosis as well as poor arterial blood gases and low $SpO_2$. Arrhythmias, headache, lightheadedness and decreased level of consciousness are associated symptoms. In chronic conditions, dyspnea may not be associated with poor arterial blood gases. Key clinical features are poor arterial blood gases, low $SpO_2$, cyanosis, and fatigue. As arterial blood gases progressively deteriorate, central nervous signs of headache, lightheadedness, and decreased level of consciousness may also be present.

## *Medical Interventions*

Medical interventions are aimed at:

- Treating the underlying cause of respiratory failure
- Obtaining adequate oxygenation via mechanical ventilation if required; in individuals with chronic respiratory failure, noninvasive mechanical ventilation is often instituted intermittently or nocturnally
- Preventing complications; if mechanical ventilation is instituted by oral or nasal intubation, complications include: barotrauma, hyperoxia damage, and infections

## *Physical Therapy Interventions*

Problems and possible treatments for this condition include:

1. *Poor gas exchange in affected regions—if Type I respiratory failure*

   Possible treatments: deep breathing, positioning, ensure patient is using oxygen if prescribed

2. *Pain, if underlying cause is chest trauma*

   Possible treatments: relaxation, ensure treatment coincides with adequate pain medication

3. *Retained secretions* can be present. Need to assess carefully

   Possible treatments: airway clearance techniques such as manual or mechanical percussion and positioning with suctioning in ventilated patients

4. *Decreased mobility*—active or passive bed exercises if mechanically ventilated. Dangle or mobilize patient out of bed as soon as possible as tolerated

5. *Inspiratory muscle fatigue*—inspiratory muscle training may be of benefit in select patients, however, one needs to proceed cautiously to avoid further fatigue and muscle injury[9]

# PATHOPHYSIOLOGY OF PULMONARY EMBOLUS AND LUNG INFARCTION

## Definition

Pulmonary emboli result from a clot dislodging from a systemic vein and lodging in the pulmonary circulation.

## Etiology and Pathophysiology

Thrombi are most often formed in the lower extremities. Risk factors include immobilization due to bed rest, prolonged travel, or fracture stabilization especially of the lower extremities. Other risk factors include aging, congestive heart failure, obesity, cancer, chronic deep venous insufficiency, trauma, oral contraceptives, and pregnancy. Once a thrombus is lodged in the pulmonary circulation, it can cause a pulmonary embolus. Edema and hemorrhage can occur in the lung parenchyma followed by atelectasis. In less than 10% of the cases, the blood flow to the lung tissue is totally infarcted and necrosis of the lung parenchyma will occur. The decrease in pulmonary cross-sectional area can increase pulmonary arterial resistance increasing the right ventricular workload and cause right-sided heart failure.

## Clinical Presentation and Course

Most patients have an acute onset of dyspnea and an increased respiratory rate. Often this is accompanied by a tachycardia and less often by pleuritic chest pain. Bloody sputum is expectorated in some cases. Factors that predispose patients to a pulmonary embolus are: recent surgery, history of previous thromboembolic event, older age, and hypoxemia. Ventilation-perfusion scan, spiral computer tomogram (CT), and pulmonary angiography are frequently used to diagnose a pulmonary embolism. The outcome is variable. Those with no shock and early treatment have a mortality rate of 8% whereas those with a large embolism leading to increases in right ventricular pressures can have a 90% mortality rate.

## Medical Interventions

The most important intervention is prevention of thrombose formation by decreasing the risk factors and prophylactic anticoagulant therapy. Heparin is the most common anticoagulant therapy used preventatively, and once a thrombose or pulmonary embolus has occurred. In selected patients, thrombolytic therapy, placement of a vena cava filter, and pulmonary embolectomy are sometimes required.

## Physical Therapy Interventions

The most important intervention is prevention of thrombose formation by promoting bed exercises and early mobilization. Anti-embolic stockings, continuous passive motion machine, and sequential compression devices are other measures used by physical therapists to prevent blood clots. Once the deep vein thrombosis and pulmonary embolus are suspected, all mobilization is halted until adequate anticoagulation is achieved.

# CHRONIC RESPIRATORY CONDITIONS

Chronic respiratory conditions are divided in 2 main categories: (1) those that result in a restricted chest wall (nonparenchymal) and/or lungs (parenchymal), and (2) those that result in obstruction of the airways.

# RESTRICTIVE CHEST WALL DISEASES

## Definition

Many different conditions such as neuromuscular disease and connective tissue disorders can reduce chest wall compliance and result in restrictive chest wall disease. This is usually followed by decreased compliance of the lungs over time.

## Etiology & Pathophysiology

The etiology can be a *neuromuscular* condition such as a spinal cord lesion, polio, Guillain-Barré, and amyotrophic lateral sclerosis. The underlying muscle weakness results in decreased respiratory muscle strength and a reduced vital capacity. The chest wall becomes progressively stiffer due to shallow breathing. Decreased expansion of lung parenchyma leads to microatelectasis that can progress to fibrosis. Reduced expiratory muscle strength and an ineffective cough can result as well.

Different *connective tissue disorders* that result in arthritis can affect the thoracic joints and reduce chest wall compliance. For example, ankylosing spondylitis and rheumatoid arthritis are chronic inflammatory conditions that affect the chest wall.

*Kyphoscoliosis*, which is often of an unknown origin (85% of the cases), is characterized by an increased anteroposterior and lateral curvature of the thoracic spine. The very rigid chest wall results in an increased work of breathing, respiratory muscle fatigue, and eventually decreased compliance of the lungs.

*Obesity* results in chest wall restriction because of the thick layer of adipose on the chest wall and also often results in restriction of the diaphragm by a large abdomen.

## Clinical Presentation and Course

The clinical presentation is varied, dependent on the underlying cause. If the inspiratory muscles are affected by paralysis or overuse resulting in fatigue, respiratory failure will ensue and mechanical ventilation will be required. In progressive conditions such as amyotrophic lateral sclerosis, death usually occurs due to respiratory failure.

## Medical Interventions

Treatment will be directed toward the underlying disease process if it is reversible. Noninvasive or invasive mechanical ventilation can be required especially during acute exacerbations.

## Physical Therapy Interventions

The physical therapy interventions are varied dependent on the underlying etiology. Breathing exercises aimed at maximizing vital capacity and inspiratory muscle endurance training might be indicated. In the case of neuromuscular weakness, facilitated cough, expiratory muscle strength training might be indicated. Other airway clearance techniques, and general strength and mobility training might be required.

What features of restrictive chest wall diseases are reversible by physical therapy?

# RESTRICTIVE LUNG DISEASES

## Definition

Restrictive lung diseases are a group of conditions that usually have an inflammatory process in the lungs followed by lung fibrosis.

## Epidemiology

Prevalence estimates for interstitial pulmonary fibrosis are 3 to 6 cases per 100,000 and incidence estimates are 9.1 cases per 100,000.[10]

## Etiology and Pathophysiology

The most common cause of lung restriction is idiopathic pulmonary fibrosis when the underlying etiologic agent is unknown. Other restrictive lung diseases can arise from a large variety of known causes, some of which are due to exposure to different agents in the occupational environment. Some examples are inhalation of mineral dusts such as silicosis, coal worker's pneumoconiosis, asbestosis, inhalation of organic dusts such as farmer's lung, and pigeon breeder's lung.

Initially, the inciting agent results in edema and infiltration of inflammatory cells into the lung interstitium. Next, there is progression to chronic inflammation and type II epithelial cells lining the alveoli proliferate to repair the damaged epithelium. Laying down of collagen resulting in "pulmonary fibrosis" follows this. In some conditions such as sarcoidosis, there is formation of granulomas, which are huge masses of epithelioid cells evolved from macrophages.

Ventilation-perfusion mismatch is the major cause of poor gas exchange followed by diffusion limitation. The increased work of breathing and corticosteroid treatment can result in respiratory muscle dysfunction.

## Clinical Presentation and Course

These patients are often cyanotic, or dyspneic and have a shallow, rapid breathing pattern. They may have a chronic unproductive cough. These patients can quickly desaturate with exertion. The mean survival is 2 to 4 years with only 30% to 50% surviving to 5 years.

## Medical Interventions

The inciting agent is removed if it can be identified. This involves avoiding offending particles or discontinuing suspected medications. Therapy is usually directed towards controlling the inflammatory process. Often the inflammatory process will respond to steroids. Other care is supportive and aimed at optimizing cardiopulmonary function including oxygen therapy, nutritional support, smoking cessation, and mechanical ventilation as the disease progresses or during exacerbations.

## Physical Therapy Interventions

Because of the many different etiologies and variable progression, research examining physical therapy interventions in this group of patients is scarce. Potential problems and treatments are outlined; however, physical therapy interventions are often based on clinical experience rather than well-established evidence-based practice:

1. *Dyspnea*

   Possible treatments: breathing control and relaxation positions, relaxation techniques

2. *Poor gas exchange and may desaturate with exercise*

   Possible treatments: Ensure patient is using oxygen properly (if prescribed), monitor $SpO_2$ during exercise, and may modify $O_2$ flow rate if prescribed; may position in order to maximize $SpO_2$

3. *Poor exercise tolerance*

   Possible treatments: ensure safe to exercise; devise exercise program which may incorporate both strength and endurance components; educate in modification of activities of daily living (ADL) and conservation of energy techniques; walk using devices which support upper body—ie, wheeled walker, shopping cart, wheelchair

4. *Increased use of accessory muscles*

   Possible treatments: neck and thoracic mobility exercises to maintain range of motion of these muscles; relaxation positions to decrease use during rest

5. *Poor understanding of condition and care of condition*

   Possible treatment: patient education

6. *Decreased sense of well-being/depression*

   Possible treatments: patient support groups; psychological and/or psychiatric assessment and treatment

   What features of restrictive lung diseases are reversible by physical therapy?

# CHRONIC OBSTRUCTIVE PULMONARY DISEASE

## Definitions

COPD is a chronic respiratory condition characterized by progressive airways obstruction that is not fully reversible. The processes of chronic bronchitis and emphysema usually cause it. *Chronic bronchitis* is defined clinically as excess mucus production with expectoration most days for 3 months for at least 2 consecutive years. *Emphysema* is a pathological diagnosis—ie, it is defined by examination of the lung tissue, not the clinical presentation of the client. It is defined as destruction of the airspaces distal to the terminal bronchiole with destruction of the alveolar septa.

## Epidemiology

Approximately 2.9% of Canadians and 6.2% Americans have been diagnosed with COPD.[11,12] This figure may under-represent the actual prevalence of COPD because many individuals with early symptoms to not seek medical help and certain groups such as the elderly and women can be misdiagnosed. COPD is the fourth-leading cause of death in the world and the only leading cause of death that is increasing.

## Etiology and Pathophysiology

Smoking is the major cause of COPD although environmental pollutants can play a minor role. *Alpha-1-antitrypsin deficiency* is a genetic disorder that can result in very severe form of emphysema at a very young age. A chronic inflammatory process of the airways, parenchyma, and pulmonary vasculature follows. Increased oxidative stress and an imbalance of proteinases and antiproteinases may also contribute to lung damage. Enlargement of mucous glands and excessive mucus secretions layer the epithelial surfaces of the airways. Bronchial wall inflammation, edema, bronchospasm, and scarring occur. The most severe changes occur in the bronchi and bronchioles. Destruction of alveolar septa occurs, which includes both the alveoli and the pulmonary capillary vascular bed.

Airways obstruction is worse during expiration. During inspiration, the negative pleural pressure tends to pull both the alveoli and the compliant small airways open during inflation of the lungs. During expiration, however, the positive pleural pressure results in deflation of the alveoli and compression of the small airways. In COPD, some of the small airways may collapse during expiration, resulting in air trapping in the alveoli.

The air trapping results in overfilling of the lungs such that they become hyperinflated or have larger volumes both at functional residual capacity and total lung capacity. Larger lung volumes or hyperinflation causes the diaphragm to be in a more flattened position at end-expiration. This decreases its mechanical advantage and decreases its potential for excursion and pumping. Thus, abnormal pathology in the lungs results in abnormal respiratory muscle function.

COPD results in airways obstruction, ventilation-perfusion mismatch, and shunting. Secondary changes are hyperinflation that places the inspiratory muscles at shortened lengths and a mechanical disadvantage further increasing their workloads. Destruction of the pulmonary vascular bed and hypoxic vasoconstriction results in increased pulmonary vascular resistance, leading to pulmonary hypertension and cor pulmonale. Also, impaired bronchial hygiene due to poor ciliary function and increased mucus secretion results in an increased incidence of infection.

## Clinical Presentation and Course

The patient usually presents with progressive shortness of breath and a smoking history. Not all patients have a history of cough and sputum. Other features include: hypercapnia, hypoxia, and cyanosis. The emphysematous patient is often described as being very thin (*pink puffer*) and the bronchitic as being overweight and edematous (*blue bloater*), however, this is an oversimplification of his or her physical appearance.

### Physical Signs at Rest and During Exercise That Might Be Predictive of COPD

- Coughing and/or expectoration during exercise or recovery
- Dyspnea that is disproportionate to workload extending into recovery
- Borg's Rating of Perceived Exertion that is disproportionate to workload
- Audible wheezing

- Bracing of shoulder girdle during exercise
- Prolonged expiration, pursed lip breathing, braced position
- Accessory muscle use during inspiration and expiration
- Exercise desaturation with cyanosis

Symptoms change or worsen at the time of exacerbation such as increased dyspnea, sore throat, cough, and cold symptoms; an acute exacerbation does not correlate well with lung function. Recovery after a COPD exacerbation is lengthy and often incomplete.[13]

## Medical and Surgical Interventions

The medical interventions are directed to early detection, accurate diagnosis, managing stable COPD, and treating exacerbations. Managing stable COPD includes health education especially directed toward smoking cessation, bronchodilator medications for symptomatic relief, glucocorticosteroids for select patients, promotion of exercise training, and oxygen therapy. Details of medications are provided in Table 18-2. Other pharmacologic treatments can include annual influenza vaccines, pneumovax (vaccine against pneumococcal infection), and antibiotics as indicated.

Surgical interventions include bullectomy, lung volume reduction surgery, and lung transplantation. Select patients who meet strict criteria to identify severe lung disease but are healthy enough to survive extensive surgery can benefit from these procedures but their success can be limited.

Exacerbations are commonly caused by lung infection and hence, antibiotic therapy is often implemented. Bronchodilator and glucocorticoid therapy can be effective. The patient may require noninvasive or invasive mechanical ventilation to maintain adequate gas exchange.

## Physical Therapy Interventions

Problems and possible treatments for *stable* COPD include:

1. *Dyspnea*

   Possible treatments: breathing control and relaxation positions

2. *Poor gas exchange and may desaturate with exercise*

   Possible treatments: ensure using oxygen properly (if prescribed), monitor $SpO_2$ during exercise, and may modify flow rate if prescribed; may position in order to maximize $SpO_2$

3. *Poor nutrition*

   Possible treatments: slow progression of exercise program; consult with dietician

4. *Poor exercise tolerance*

   Possible treatments: ensure safe to exercise—ie, $SpO_{2;}$ rule out cardiac abnormalities and other limitations to exercise; devise exercise program which may incorporate flexibility, strength and endurance components; educate in modification of ADL and conservation of energy techniques; walk with devices that support upper body—ie, wheeled walker, shopping cart, wheelchair; may include specific inspiratory muscle training exercises[9]

5. *Poor understanding of conditions and care of condition*

   Possible treatments: patient education; self-initiated care—ie, when to go to the Emergency Room or to the doctor, or when to start antibiotics

6. *Increased use of accessory muscles*

   Possible treatments: neck, upper extremity, and thoracic mobility exercises; relaxation positions

7. *Possibly increased secretions*

   Possible treatments: airway clearance techniques

8. *Decreased sense of well-being/depression*

   Possible treatments: patient support groups; psychological and/or psychiatric assessment and treatment

   What features of COPD are reversible by physical therapy?

Further details about the evidence to support components of COPD rehabilitation are outlined in by Celli,[14] ACCP/AACVPR,[15] and Lacasse et al.[16] Clinical competency guidelines for pulmonary rehabilitation professionals are outlined by Southard et al.[17]

Table 18-2

## Examples of Common Medications Used in Asthma and COPD

| Medication Trade Name (Generic Drug Name) | Route of Delivery | Medication Effect | Physical Therapy Considerations |
|---|---|---|---|
| Ventolin (salbutamol), Serevent (salmeterol) Bricanyl Turbuhaler (terbutaline) | Metered-dose inhaler | Bronchodilators (ß2-adrenergic agonist) | With high dosage, patient may complain of tremor, anxiety, dizziness, and muscle cramps. Use care with mobilization when patients show these signs and symptoms. |
| Atrovent (ipratropium bromide) | Metered-dose inhaler | Anticholinergic bronchodilators | Dry mouth. |
| Theodur (theophylline) | Oral tablet | Anti-inflammatory and bronchodilatory effects Increases myocardial and diaphragmatic contractility | Patients may complain of nausea, vomiting, and headache. Requires routine check on serum theophylline level because high serum levels can cause toxicity. |
| Prednisone Medrol (methyl-prednisolone) | Oral tablet | Corticosteriod. Anti-inflammatory effect | Water retention, osteoporosis, and tendency to have fractures with minimal trauma |
| Beclovent (beclometh-asone dipropionate) Pulmicort (budesonide) Flovent (fluticasone) | Metered-dose inhaler or dry powder inhaler | Corticosteriod. Anti-inflammatory effect | Due to lower systematic effects, side effects are less than oral tablets. |
| Intal (cromolyn) Tilade (nedocromil) | Metered-dose inhaler or dry powder inhaler | Non-steroidal. Anti-inflammatory and broncho-dilatory effects | Unpleasant taste in mouth and headache. |
| Singulair (montelukast) Accolate (zafirlukast) | Oral tablet | Leukotriene modifiers. Anti-inflammatory effect | Patients may complain of dizziness, stomach ache, cough, and headache. |

# ASTHMA

## Definition

*Asthma* is a chronic inflammation of the lungs characterized by variable airflow limitation and airway hyper-responsiveness associated with paroxysmal or persistent symptoms of dyspnea, chest tightness, wheeze, and cough.

## Epidemiology

8.7% of Canadians and 9.7% of Americans have been diagnosed with asthma and the prevalence of self-reported asthma is increasing. The numbers appear to be greater in elite athletes—10% to 15% of Olympic athletes have exercise-induced asthma (EIA).

## Etiology and Pathophysiology

A variety of stimuli can trigger increased airway responsiveness in asthma including allergens, cool or dry air, emotions, and work-related agents. Those with atopy have a predisposition and other factors such as smoking during pregnancy and childhood, respiratory infections, and air quality appear to contribute to asthma. Triggers stimulate occlusion of bronchi and bronchioles by thick tenacious mucus plugs, edematous bronchiolar walls, hypertrophy of mucus glands, and smooth muscle hypertrophy and spasm.

## Clinical Presentation and Course

Between attacks the patient may be asymptomatic although some have a component of chronic bronchitis. Rarely, the patient may experience a state of unremitting attack that will prove to be fatal known as status asthmatics. Signs and symptoms include labored respiration, wheezing, acute hyperinflation, hypoxia, and hypercapnia. Asthmatics have a larger decline in $FEV_1$ over time than healthy subjects (a decline of 38 ml/year compared to 22 ml/year, respectively). Among asthmatics, those who have chronic mucous hypersecretion have an even higher decline in $FEV_1$ than those without.[18]

EIA is common. A 15% drop in $FEV_1$ or PEFR after exercise is indicative of EIA. *Asthmogenic exercises* are cycling, basketball, long distance running, and soccer. Those activities that require high ventilatory rates in cool, dry air can be especially asthmogenic including cross-country skiing, hockey, and speed skating.

## Physical Signs During Exercise That Might Be Predictive of Exercise Induced Asthma— Prescreening for Exercise Induced Asthma

- May have coughing, wheezing, prolonged expiration, accessory muscle use, dyspnea, and/or chest pain during exercise
- Signs and symptoms vary with seasons and other aspects of environment

### After Exercise

- Cough, chest tightness or pain, shortness of breath, nausea, stomachache

## Medical Interventions

Well-developed guidelines for asthma management have been developed in many countries and a global initiative on asthma (GINA) was implemented in 2002. Management includes an accurate diagnosis; education to improve self-management; avoidance and control of triggers; and medication to *relieve* the symptoms for those with mild asthma, supplemented by medication to *control* symptoms for those with more frequent and severe symptoms. (*Relievers* are short acting bronchodilators and *controllers* are inhaled and oral corticosteroids.) Details of medications are provided in Table 18-2. Optimal management should result in minimal night wake-ups and exacerbations.

## Physical Therapy Interventions

Considering how common the condition is, *when treating all clients*, physical therapists should actively screen for asthma so those who show relevant symptoms can be referred to physicians for adequate management and follow-up.

Problems and possible treatments for *asthma during an acute exacerbation* include:
1. Dyspnea

   Possible treatments: breathing control and relaxation positions
2. *Poor gas exchange*

   Possible treatments: ensure using oxygen properly; monitor $SpO_2$; ensure taking medication (bronchodilators) properly; position to maximize $SpO_2$ if necessary
3. *Increased use of accessory muscles*

   Possible treatments: neck and thoracic mobility exercises; relaxation positions
4. *Possibly increased secretions*

   Possible treatments: modified airway clearance techniques
5. *Poor understanding of condition and care of condition*

   Possible treatments: patient education, self-initiated care—ie, when to go to Emergency Room or to physician when condition worsens

What features of asthma are reversible by physical therapy?

# BRONCHIECTASIS

## *Definition*

Bronchiectasis is a chronic necrotizing infection of the bronchi and bronchioles leading to or associated with abnormal dilation of these airways.

## *Etiology and Pathophysiology*

The cause is usually due to a necrotizing infection and less often due to aspiration of a foreign body. Destruction of bronchial mucosa occurs and there may be lung collapse distal to obstruction. This disease often affects the lower lobes, particularly those air passages that are vertical. It can be sharply localized if the bronchiectasis was due to aspiration of a foreign body.

## *Clinical Presentation and Course*

- Two thirds have had a previous history of respiratory infection
- Often have a severe cough producing copious amounts of foul-smelling, sometimes blood-stained sputum
- May have clubbing of fingers
- Increased incidence of cor pulmonale

## *Medical Interventions*

Medical interventions are measures to control infection including antibiotics and annual influenza vaccination. Good pulmonary hygiene including adequate hydration and airway clearance techniques are promoted.

## *Physical Therapy Interventions*

Problems and possible treatments for this condition include:
1. *Greatly increased secretions*

   Possible treatments: airway clearance techniques
2. *Poor exercise tolerance*

   Possible treatments: ensure safe to exercise; devise exercise program that may incorporate both strength and endurance components. Exercise can be used as an adjunct to precede airway clearance techniques
3. *Poor understanding of conditions and care of condition*

   Possible treatments: patient education

What features of bronchiectasis are reversible by physical therapy?

# CYSTIC FIBROSIS

## Definition

Cystic fibrosis (CF) is a hereditary disease that affects all exocrine glands resulting in abnormal mucus production. The most common problems are bronchopulmonary infection and pancreatic insufficiency leading to malabsorption; however, exocrine glands in several other organ systems can be affected.

## Epidemiology

It is an autosomal, recessively inherited disorder with a carrier frequency in Whites of 1 in 20 to 25. In America, Western Europe, and Australia, 1 in 2,500 births are homozygous for the CF gene. CF is rare in Blacks and in Asians. Most children are diagnosed with CF by the age of 5. Most live until 20 years of age but an increasing number live until later decades of life.

## Etiology and Pathophysiology

The primary abnormality is in ion transport that is reflected by a high sweat sodium and chloride concentration. Progressive obstruction of the exocrine ducts by thick secretions seems to occur in almost all clinical manifestations. Thick tenacious secretions are not efficiently cleared in the lungs resulting in recurrent lung infections. Over time fibrosis and scarring can occur. Malabsorption results in poor growth and skeletal abnormalities.

## Clinical Presentation and Course

- *Respiratory symptoms* are usually the presenting feature; CF is the most common cause of recurrent bronchopulmonary infection in childhood. As the disease progresses, hypercapnia, hypoxemia, and cor pulmonale can develop. Hemoptysis often occurs.
- *Finger clubbing* is universal.
- *Breathlessness* occurs in the later stages as airflow limitation develops. Patients are often not as distressed by this symptom compared to patients who develop other respiratory disorders later in life.
- *Delayed puberty and skeletal maturity.*
- *Infertility in males* due to failure of development of the vas deferens and the epididymis. There is reduced fertility in females.
- *Symptomatic steatorrhea* (thick fatty stools) occurs in 85% of patients owing to pancreatic dysfunction.
- *Diabetes mellitus* is common in this patient group.
- *Liver disease*.
- *Osteoporosis* may contribute to kyphosis and increased fractures.

## Medical Interventions

A major goal of medical interventions is to prevent and treat pulmonary disease including infections by promoting airway clearance techniques, and administering antibiotics, mucolytics, and bronchodilators as indicated. Pancreatic insufficiency is managed by enzyme replacement and increased caloric intake.

## Physical Therapy Interventions

Problems and possible treatments for this condition include:
1. *Greatly increased secretions that are thick and tenacious, leading to frequent recurrent infections*

   Possible treatments: vigorous airway clearance techniques; time physical therapy sessions after bronchodilator use; or other techniques that may facilitate loosening of secretions
2. *Poor posture*

   Possible treatments: thoracic mobility and extension exercises
3. *Dyspnea*

   Possible treatments: often don't appear as anxious as patients with other chronic respiratory conditions who show a similar degree of respiratory distress

4. *Poor gas exchange and may desaturate with exercise*

   Possible treatments: ensure using oxygen properly, monitor $SpO_2$ during exercise, and may modify flow rate if prescribed; may position in order to maximize $SpO_2$

5. *Poor understanding of conditions and care of condition*

   Possible treatments: patient education but often very aware of their condition because it is a life-long illness. If patient education is provided, it should be focused

6. *Poor exercise tolerance*

   Possible treatments: ensure safe to exercise; design appropriate exercise test; devise exercise program that may incorporate both strength and endurance components

7. *Poor nutrition*

   Possible treatments: slow progression of exercise regime

8. *Presence of other medical conditions—ie, diabetes mellitus and osteoporosis*

   Ensure proper precautions are taken during prescription and performance of exercise program and other physical therapy interventions.

9. *Decreased sense of well-being/depression*

   Possible treatments: CF support groups; psychological assessment and treatment; ensure issues around death, terminal illness, and grieving are addressed

What features of CF are reversible by physical therapy?

# LUNG CANCER

## Epidemiology

Lung cancer is the leading cause of death due to cancer in Canada and the United States. Approximately 30% of cancer deaths in men and 20% of cancer deaths in women are due to lung cancer.[19] The incidence in women is rising. Because of the high case-fatality rates, the incidence and mortality are almost equivalent. During 1992 to 1998, the age-adjusted incidence rates were 54 per 100,000 in the United States.[20]

## Etiology and Pathophysiology

Smoking accounts for 80% of lung cancer cases in women and 90% in men. Other environmental factors such as occupational hazards and air pollution appear to increase risk. High intake of fresh vegetables and fruits decrease the risk.

## Medical and Surgical Treatment

Treatment can include surgical resection, chemotherapy, and radiation therapy to remove or control the tumor growth.

## Physical Therapy Interventions

Problems and possible treatments for this condition depends on the medical treatment selected and if surgery is required. These might include:

1. *Poor gas exchange and may desaturate with exercise*

   Possible treatments: ensure using oxygen properly, monitor $SpO_2$ during exercise, and may modify flow rate if prescribed; may position in order to maximize $SpO_2$. Deep breathing exercises especially following surgery

2. *Increased secretions/recurrent infections*

   Possible treatments: airway clearance techniques

3. *Poor exercise tolerance*

   Possible treatments: ensure safe to exercise; devise exercise program that may incorporate both strength and endurance components. The therapist should aim for increased or maintained function especially in advanced cases

4. *Poor posture*

   Possible treatments: thoracic mobility and shoulder range-of-motion exercises especially post-thoracotomy

5. *Dyspnea*

   Possible treatments: breathing control and relaxation positions

6. *Poor nutrition*

   Possible treatments: slow progression of exercise regime

# AGING

Many changes related to aging of the respiratory system begin at 20 years of age.

## Epidemiology

- 20% of Canadians are aged 50 to 70 years and 9% are over the age of 70 years.

## Physiology

- Changes occur in the chest wall, lung tissue, and pulmonary blood vessels.
- Aging results in a breakdown of elastin in all tissues, including the lungs, making the lungs more compliant. This leads to decreased elastic recoil and increased dynamic compression causing increased airway closure at or near FRC.
- The chest wall is more rigid due to an increase in cross-linking of collagen fibers contributing to tissue stiffness and resistance to movement. There may also be calcification of chondral cartilages and kyphoscoliosis.
- FRC and RV are increased. TLC does not change and VC decreases.
- *Alveolar surface area* decreases at a rate of about 2.7 sq. M/decade contributing to a decreased $PaO_2$. Between 70 to 80 years of age, a normal $PaO_2$ is 75 to 80 mmHg.
- Endurance and strength of the respiratory muscles decreases with age.
- Ventilatory response to hypoxia and hypercapnia decreases with age.
- May have decreased cough and laryngeal reflexes, making the elderly more susceptible to aspiration.

## Clinical Implications

- The elderly have a decreased respiratory reserve capacity
- This population is at greater risk when the respiratory system is further compromised by such conditions as bed rest, surgical procedures especially those involving general anesthesia, lung pathology, and/or thoracic trauma.

# SMOKING

## Epidemiology

In 2000, 20% of adults in Canada smoked on a daily basis and an additional 5% smoke occasionally. Twenty-five percent of children under the age of 12 were exposed to second-hand smoke daily or almost every day.[19]

## Pathophysiology

- Acutely, can increase airways resistance. Eg, single inhalation can increase airways resistance 2 to 3 times
- Chronic effects
  - Decreased activity of cilia, mucus gland hypertrophy, inhibition of phagocytic activity leading to an increased incidence of infection
  - Increased risk of complications during surgery under general anesthetic
  - Inhibits exercise performance

## Clinical Presentation and Course

- 15% of smokers develop COPD. If smokers stop by age 45, they are less likely to develop symptomatic COPD[21]
- Significantly increases risk of lung cancer and heart diseases

## Medical Interventions

Active promotion of smoking cessation by all health professionals is paramount to reduce its deleterious effects. In the Lung Health study, 35% of subjects were able to quit smoking for an extended period of time and 22% of subjects quit for at least 5 years.[22,23]

## Physical Therapy Interventions

Physical therapists should be aware of the smoking cessation programs available in their regions and convey relevant information to patients when they are receptive to this information.

What aspects of smoking are reversible by physical therapy?

# OBESITY

## Definition

Obesity is defined as a body weight greater than 20% more than the ideal body weight.

## Etiology and Pathophysiology

- Decreased compliance of chest wall from the shear weight of it and increased abdominal mass
- Decreased diaphragmatic excursion against abdominal mass
- Increased minute ventilation because of the larger mass of tissue
- Regional ventilation can be altered to preferential ventilation of lung apices and thus, dependent regions are at greater risk of airway closure
- Ventilation-perfusion mismatch and hypoxemia can occur

## Clinical Presentation and Course

- *Postoperatively*—the obese have a much greater risk of hypoventilation and respiratory failure.
- A greater incidence of sleep apnea occurs in the obese.

## Medical Interventions

Diet, exercise, life style change, and medication. Surgery is used in some morbidly obese patients.

## Physical Therapy Interventions

Physical therapy can be directed toward weight loss and treating the consequences of obesity such as arthritis, back problems, and cardiovascular problems.

What features of obesity are reversible by physical therapy?

# EXERCISE

1. Photocopy Table 18-3, Problems and Associated Outcome Measures, and complete 1 table for acute respiratory conditions and 1 table for chronic respiratory conditions by identifying outcome measures that could be used by a physical therapist to evaluate whether improvement has occurred after treatment for a specific problem. The problems are grouped because often outcome measures do not distinctly reflect 1 problem but may reflect similar or related problems.

Table 18-3

## *Problems and Associated Outcome Measures*

| *Problem* | *Outcome Measure* |
|---|---|
| • Poor gas exchange in affected regions especially at low lung volumes ($\uparrow PaCO_2$ and $\downarrow PaO_2$) | |
| • May desaturate with exercise/mobility | |
| • Poor cardiovascular function | |
| • Myocardial ischemia | |
| • Decreased cardiac output | |
| • Decreased oxygen transport/circulation to periphery | |
| • Pain—incisional or trauma | |
| • Chest or musculoskeletal or peripheral vascular | |
| • Decreased mobility/poor exercise tolerance | |
| • Decreased fitness | |
| • Decreased strength and endurance | |
| • Retained/increased secretions | |
| • Recurrent infections | |
| • Dyspnea | |
| • Increased work of breathing | |
| • Increased use of accessory muscles | |
| • Deep vein thrombosis | |
| • Altered cognitive status | |
| • Altered coordination and/or balance | |
| • Ileus | |
| • Urinary retention | |
| • Poor posture | |
| • Decreased ROM of shoulder and other related joints | |
| • Sternal limitations | |
| • Poor nutrition | |
| • Poor understanding of condition, care of condition, and self-management | |
| • Decreased sense of well-being/depression | |
| • Discharge planning needs | |

# REFERENCES

1. Drakulovic MB, Torres A, Bauer TT, et al. Supine body position as a risk factor for nosocomial pneumonia in mechanically ventilated patients: a randomized trial. *Lancet.* 1999;354:1851-1858.

2. Mahul P, Auboyer C, Jospe R, et al. Prevention of nosocomial pneumonia in intubated patients: respective role of mechanical subglottic secretions drainage and stress ulcer prophylaxis. *Intensive Care Med.* 1992;18:20-25.

3. Shorr AF, O'Malley PG. Continuous subglottic suctioning for the prevention of ventilator-associated pneumonia: potential economic implications. *Chest.* 2001;119:228-35.

4. Halm EA, Fine MJ, Kapoor WN, et al. Instability on hospital discharge and the risk of adverse outcome in patients with pneumonia. *Arch Intern Med.* 2002;162:1278-1284.

5. Ntoumenopoulos G, Presneill JJ, McElholum M, et al. Chest physiotherapy for the prevention of ventilator-associated pneumonia. *Intensive Care Med.* 2002;28:850-856.

6. Shaker R, Easterling C, Kern M, et al. Rehabilitation of swallowing by exercise in tube-fed patients with pharyngeal dysphagia secondary to abnormal UES opening. *Gastroenterology.* 2002;122:1314-1321.

7. Shaker R, Kern M, Bardan E, et al. Augmentation of deglutitive upper esophageal sphincter opening in the elderly by exercise. *Am J Physiol.* 1997;272:G1518-1522.

8  Hudson LD, Steinberg KP. Epidemiology of acute lung injury and ARDS. *Chest.* 1999;116:74S-82S.

9. Reid WD, Sharma A. Respiratory muscle training in people with chronic obstructive pulmonary disease. *Physiotherapy Singapore.* 2000;3:113-126.

10. American Thoracic Society and European Respiratory Society. Idiopathic pulmonary fibrosis: diagnosis and treatment. International Consensus statement. *Am J Respir Crit Care Med.* 2000;161:646-664.

11. Stewart PJ, Sales P. *The prevention and management of asthma in Canada.* A report of the National Asthma Control Task Force. 2000.

12. National Lung Health Education Program Executive Committee. Strategies in preserving lung health and preventing COPD and associated diseases. *Chest.* 1998;113(Supple):123S-163S.

13. Seemungal TA, Donaldson GC, Bhowmik A, et al. Time course and recovery of exacerbations in patients with COPD. *Am J Respir Crit Care Med.* 2000;161:1608-1613.

14. Celli B. Is pulmonary rehabilitation an effective treatment for chronic obstructive pulmonary disease? Yes. *Am J Respir Crit Care Med.* 1997;155:781-783.

15. ACCP/AACVPR Pulmonary Rehabilitation Guidelines Panel. Pulmonary rehabilitation. Joint ACCP/AACVPR Evidence-based guidelines. *Chest.* 1997;112:1363-1396.

16. Lacasse Y, Guyatt GH, Goldstein RS. The components of a respiratory rehabilitation program. A systematic overview. *Chest.* 1997;1111:1077-1088.

17. Southard DR, Cahalin LP, Carlin BW, et al. Clinical competency guidelines for pulmonary rehabilitation professionals. American Association of Cardiovascular and Pulmonary Rehabilitation position statement. *Journal of Cardiopulmonary Rehabilitation.* 1995;15(3):173-8.

18. Lange P, Parner J, Vestbo J, et al. A 15-year follow-up study of ventilatory function in adults with asthma. *N Eng J Med.* 1998;339:1194-1200.

19. Canadian Institute for Health Information. Respiratory Diseases in Canada. Canadian Lung Association. Health Canada, Statistics Canada. September 2001. Available from: http://www.hc-sc.gc.ca/pphb-dgspsp/ or http://www.statcan.ca/. Accessed on April 15, 2004.

20. Alberg AJ, Sarnet JM. Epidemiology of lung cancer. *Chest.* 2003;123(1Suppl):21S-49S.

21. Murray RP, Gerald LB, Lindgren PG, Connett JE, Rand CS, Anthonisen NR. Characteristics of participants who stop smoking and sustain abstinence for 1 and 5 years in the Lung Health Study. *Preventive Medicine.* 2000;30(5):392-400.

22. Anthonisen NR, Connett JE, Enright PL, Manfreda J. Lung Health Study Research Group. Hospitalizations and mortality in the Lung Health Study. *Am J Respir Crit Care Med.* 2002;166(3):333-9.

23. Kanner RE, Anthonisen NR, Connett JE. The Lung Health Study Research Group. Lower respiratory illnesses promote FEV(1) decline in current smokers but not ex-smokers with mild chronic obstructive pulmonary disease: results from the lung health study. *Am J Respir Crit Care Med.* 2001;164(3):358-64.

# BIBLIOGRAPHY

Ajemian MS, Nirmul GB, Anderson MT, et al. Routine fiberoptic endoscopic evaluation of swallowing following prolonged intubation: implications for management. *Arch Surg.* 2001;136:434-437.

Australia National Asthma Council. On-line publications on asthma management. Available at: http://www.nationalasthma.org.au/publications.html. Accessed on April 15, 2004.

Cahalin LP, Sadowsky HS. Pulmonary medications. *Phys Ther.* 1995;75:397-414.

Craig TJ. Drugs to be used with caution in patients with asthma. *Am Fam Physician.* 1996;54:947-953.

Goodman G. *The Pharmacological Basis of Therapeutics.* New York: McGraw-Hill; 1996.

Kapsali T, Permutt S, Laube N, et al. Potent bronchoprotective effect of deep inspiration and its absence in asthma. *J Appl Physiol*. 2000;89:711-720.

Pauwels RA, Buist AS, Claberley PMA, Jenkins CR, Hurd S on behalf of the COLD Scientific Committee. Global strategy for the diagnosis, management and prevention of chronic obstructive pulmonary disease. *Am J Respir Crit Care Med*. 2001;163:1256-1276.

Poole PJ, Black PN. Oral mucolytic drugs for exacerbations of chronic obstructive pulmonary disease: systematic review. *BMJ*. 2001;322:1271-1274.

Stewart PJ, Sales P. National action plan for the prevention and management of chronic obstructive pulmonary disease. *Canadian Chronic Obstructive Pulmonary Disease Alliance*. July 2000.

World Health Organization. Global Initiative for Asthma: Global Strategy for Asthma Management and Prevention NHLBI/WHO Report. *National Institutes of Health*. January 1995.

http://www.merck.com/pubs/mmanual/

http://www.nlm.nih.gov/medlineplus/druginformation.html

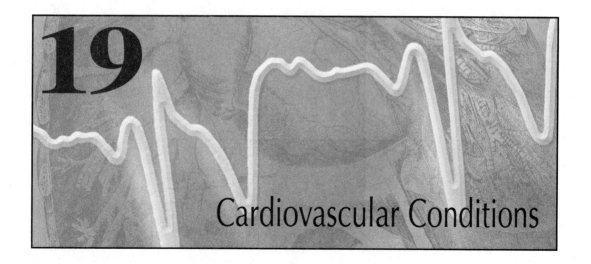

Cardiovascular Conditions

# OBJECTIVES

Upon completion of this chapter, the reader should be able to describe:

1. The definition, etiology, pathophysiology, presentation and medical management of cardiac conditions including: congestive heart failure, hypertension, angina, acute coronary syndrome, atrial fibrillation, cardiomyopathy, cardiac effusion, cardiac tamponade, peripheral vascular disease, and pulmonary embolism

2. Common physical therapy managements in these cardiac conditions including:
   - Congestive heart failure, hypertension, angina, acute coronary syndrome, atrial fibrillation, cardiomyopathy, cardiac effusion, cardiac tamponade, peripheral vascular disease, and pulmonary embolism

3. Medications frequently prescribed in these cardiac conditions including:
   - Congestive heart failure, hypertension, angina, acute coronary syndrome, atrial fibrillation, cardiomyopathy, peripheral vascular disease, and pulmonary embolism

This chapter describes common cardiac conditions, clinical information, and medications that pertain to physical therapy management.

# CONGESTIVE HEART FAILURE

## Definition

Congestive heart failure (CHF) is defined as the inability of the heart to pump sufficient amounts of oxygenated blood to meet the metabolic demands of the body both at rest and during activity.

## Etiology and Pathophysiology

*Right-sided heart failure* is characterized by blood backing up in the systemic circulation resulting in systemic venous hypertension and edema. Chronic left heart failure is a common cause of right heart failure. Other causes are: increased left atrial pressure, right ventricular infarct, pulmonary hypertension, pulmonary emboli, COPD, tricuspid valve regurgitation (Table 19-1), and pulmonary regurgitation. Another term for right-sided heart failure is cor pulmonale.

Left heart failure is characterized by blood backing up in the pulmonary circulation leading to pulmonary congestion. It can be classified as:

- *Diastolic dysfunction*—inability of the ventricle to relax completely resulting in high left ventricular end diastolic pressure and pulmonary edema. Left ventricular hypertrophy is also a frequent finding. Examples of causes include: restrictive cardiomyopathy, ischemic heart disease, pericardial tamponade, mitral valve regurgitation (see Table 19-1), and stenosis.

Table 19-1

## Overview of Congenital Heart and Valve Diseases

| Definition | Prevalence/ Incidence | Etiology and Pathophysiology | Clinical Presentation and Course |
|---|---|---|---|
| *Congenital Heart Disease*: Anatomic defects of the heart and great vessels present at birth | The incidence is 1/120 live births. Some common causes are: chromosomal defects (eg, trisomy 13 or 18), maternal illness (eg, diabetes mellitus, fetal alcohol syndrome, rubella), medication (eg, thalidomide). | Many congenital cardiac defects do not produce significant hemodynamic alteration. Others cause abnormal ventricular volume load, ventricular pressure load, and atrial emptying; venous admixture; or inadequate systemic cardiac output. | Heart murmurs due to turbulent flow are common. Signs of heart failure, cyanosis, and hepatomegaly may be present in the newborn. Long-standing hypoxemia can lead to clubbing, polycythemia, and other signs of inadequate systemic perfusion. Dilation and hypertrophy of cardiac chambers may result from the increased cardiac workload. |
| *Mitral Valve Disease*: A bulging of one or both mitral valve leaflets into the left atrium during systole | Between 1% and 6% in otherwise normal populations. It is higher in persons with Duchenne muscular dystrophy, myotonic dystrophy, sickle cell disease, atrial septal defect, and rheumatic heart disease. About 25% of patients have joint laxity, a high-arched palate, or other skeletal abnormalities. | Complete myxomatous degeneration of the valve can lead to severe mitral regurgitation, or floppy valve syndrome. | In mild cases, patients are asymptomatic. Patients might have a crisp systolic sound or click and a delayed or late systolic mitral regurgitation murmur. In more severe cases, can present with arrhythmias, palpitations, syncope, fatigue, lightheadedness, transient ischemic attacks, dyspnea, and hemoptysis and abnormal EKG findings despite normal coronary angiograms. |
| *Aortic Valve Disease*: Retrograde flow from the aorta into the left ventricle through incompetent aortic cusps | Incidences of aortic regurgitation usually increases with age. Common causes are: idiopathic degeneration of the aortic valves or root, rheumatic heart disease, infective endocarditis, and trauma. Less common causes are: severe hypertension and some autoimmune diseases. | LV volume and LV stroke volume are increased because the LV receives blood regurgitated in diastole in addition to the normal blood flow from the pulmonary veins. LV hypertrophy occurs proportionally with dilation in order to maintain pressure. | Dyspnea on exertion, orthopnea, and paroxysmal nocturnal dyspnea develop. Palpitations may occur because of the awareness of the heart due to LV enlargement. Angina is especially common at night. |

Table 19-1 continued

## Overview of Congenital Heart and Valve Diseases

| Definition | Prevalence/ Incidence | Etiology and Pathophysiology | Clinical Presentation and Course |
|---|---|---|---|
| *Tricuspid Valve Disease*: Retrograde flow of blood from right ventricle to right atrium due to inadequate apposition of the tricuspid valves | Due to a cleft tricuspid valve (eg, in endocardial cushion defects), blunt trauma, or carcinoid disease, in which the valve may be fixed in a semi-open position. Less common causes are: infective endocarditis, papillary muscle dysfunction, RV infarction, or the use of fenfluramine. | Severe pulmonary hypertension or RV outflow obstruction leads to RV dilation that frequently results in tricuspid valve regurgitation. | Fatigue, cold skin, dyspnea, edema, and the sensation of pulsations in the neck due to the high jugular regurgitant are common. Right upper quadrant abdominal discomfort due to hepatic congestion may occur. Atrial fibrillation or flutter, which usually occurs when the right atrium enlarges, further decreases the cardiac output and may precipitate sudden, severe heart failure. |

Abbreviation: LV: left ventricle; RV: right ventricle

- *Systolic dysfunction*
  - *Reduced inotrophy* (myocardial contractility) results in decreased ejection fraction, cardiac output, and oxygen transport. Examples of causes are: CAD and dilated cardiomyopathies.
  - *Increased afterload* —increased resistance to flow down stream. Examples of causes are: aortic stenosis or regurgitation, systemic hypertension, coarctation of the aorta, and left-to-right shunt.

## Clinical Presentation and Course

CHF classically manifests itself with shortness of breath and frothy pinkish sputum. Clinical signs of left heart failure and associated pulmonary edema are:
- Dyspnea—related to pulmonary edema. Initially happens during activity and can progress to occur at rest.
- Orthopnea—dyspnea when lying down flat because of an increase in venous return. Sometimes it is accompanied by a dry hacking cough, which is relieved by sitting up.
- Adventitious breath sounds—cardiac asthma (which consists of wheezes) and moist crackles.
- Frothy sputum (white/pink)
- Abnormal heart sound—murmurs, $S_3$ (decompensatory heart failure), $S_4$ (cardiac hypertrophy results in a stiff ventricle)
- Decreased exercise capacity
- Radiographic changes—see Case 10 for example

Additional clinical signs commonly associated with systolic dysfunction:
- Tachycardia, decreased pulse pressure
- Syncope, lightheadedness, lethargy
- Skin can be cold and clammy

Table 19-2

## Classification of Blood Pressure for Adults Age 18 Years and Older

| Category | Systolic BP (mmHg) | | Diastolic BP (mmHg) |
|---|---|---|---|
| Normal | <120 | and | <80 |
| Prehypertension | 120 to 139 | or | 80 to 89 |
| Hypertension | | | |
| Stage 1 | 140 to 159 | or | 90 to 99 |
| Stage 2 | >160 | or | >100 |

Adapted from: www.nhlbi.nih.gov/guidelines/hypertension; Chobanian AV, Bakris GL, Black HR, et al. The seventh report of the joint national committee on prevention, detection, evaluation, and treatment of high blood pressure: the JNC 7 report. *JAMA*. 2003; 289:2560-2571.[1]

## Medical and Surgical Intervention

Medical treatments involve reversing or optimizing the underlying problem, using of diuretics, pneumovax (pneumococcal vaccination), properly balancing fluids, controlling hypertension, and improving cardiac function.[2]

# HYPERTENSION

## Definition

Arterial hypertension is the elevation of systolic and/or diastolic BP that can be termed either primary (unknown etiology) or secondary (associated with a known underlying cause) hypertension.

Table 19-2 provides the classification of hypertensive and normal BP for adults aged 18 years or older.[1]

## Prevalence

It is estimated that nearly 50 million Americans and about 1 billion worldwide are hypertensive (systolic BP >140 mmHg and/or diastolic >90 mmHg, or taking antihypertensive medication). The prevalence of hypertension increases with age (Figure 19-1).[3]

## Etiology and Pathophysiology

In *primary* or *essential* hypertension, the etiology is unknown. The cause is likely multifactoral, leading to diverse hemodynamic and pathophysiologic dysfunctions.[1] The condition may be hereditary and lifestyle factors such as increased salt intake, obesity, and stress can further aggravate the condition. *Secondary* hypertension is associated with conditions such as renal parenchymal disease, Cushing's syndrome, primary aldosteronism, hyperthyroidism, or coarctation of the aorta. It is also associated with the use of excessive alcohol,[4] sympathomimetics, corticosteroids, cocaine, or licorice.

## Clinical Presentations and Course

No early pathologic changes occur in primary hypertension. Hypertension is also called a silent killer. Patients are usually asymptomatic until complications develop in target organs. Over time, generalized arteriolar sclerosis develops and is characterized by medial hypertrophy and hyalinization. Patients often develop left ventricular hypertrophy in order to overcome increased peripheral vascular resistance. This can eventually progress to dilation of the left ventricle. Coronary, cerebral, aortic, renal, and peripheral atherosclerosis are more common in hypertensive patients. Hypertension is a more important risk factor for stroke than for atherosclerotic heart disease.

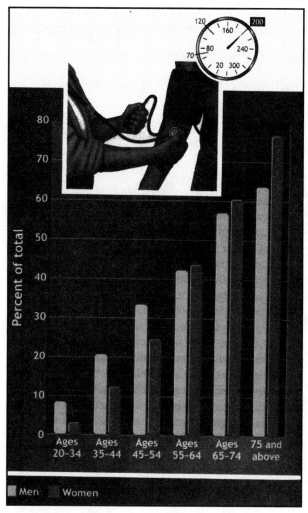

**Figure 19-1.** Prevalence of hypertension in the United States based on studies from 1988 to 1994. (Reprinted from McArdle WD, Katch KI, Katch VL. *Exercise Physiology. Energy, Nutrition, and Human Performance.* 5th ed. Philadelphia: Lipincott, Williams & Wilkins. 2001;316, with permission.)[3]

## Medical and Surgical Intervention

### Antihypertensive Drug Therapy[1,5]

For prehypertension, antihypertensive drugs are usually prescribed if lifestyle modificaitons do not normalize BP. For stage 1 and 2 hypertension, drug therapy should be initiated promptly when target organ damage or other risk factors are present. In patients with heart failure, symptomatic coronary atherosclerosis, cerebrovascular disease, and renal failure, immediate and judicious antihypertensive therapy is required. For more details see the consensus recommendations for the management of hypertension.[1,5]

### Lifestyle Modifications[6-9]

Lifestyle modifications include weight reduction in obese individuals; increase in physical activities; dietary changes—selecting foods that are rich in potassium and calcium but low in sodium, and saturated and total fat content; increase in intake of fruit and vegetables; and moderation of alcohol consumption. Patients with uncomplicated hypertension are not required to restrict their activities so long as their BP is controlled. Dietary restrictions can help control coexisting diabetes mellitus, obesity, and blood lipid abnormalities in addition to facilitating the control of hypertension in some individuals.

Table 19-3

### Differentiating Characteristics of Chest Pain

| Characteristics | Angina | Pericarditis | Musculoskeletal |
|---|---|---|---|
| Location | Sternal, substernal | Left sided, substernal | Variable over chest wall |
| Radiation | Jaw, left arm, neck | Neck, trapezius ridge | None |
| Quality | Heavy pressure, tightness, squeezing feeling | Sharp, stabbing, deep | Sharp |
| Alleviating factors | Rest, nitroglycerin | Lean forward sitting, shallow breathing | Rest, anti-inflammatory or analgesia medications |
| Aggravating factors | Exercise, stress, cold weather | Inspiration, supine lying, laughter, cough | Muscle movement and contraction, palpation |
| Duration | 5 to 10 minutes | Hours | Variable |

# ANGINA

## Definition

Angina is pain in the chest arising from myocardial ischemia that is initially precipitated by myocardial oxygen supply not meeting demand. It is a common cardiac symptom. Resting EKG is unchanged and troponin I levels are normal; however, reversible ischemia EKG changes can be seen during a spontaneous attack. Not all chest pain is angina. Table 19-3 shows differentiating characteristics of chest pain.

### Etiology and Pathophysiology

Stable angina is caused by myocardial oxygen supply not meeting demand. The imbalance is reversible and is relieved with rest and nitroglycerin. Coronary spasm is frequently associated with stable angina with no intimal disruption or thrombus. Atherosclerotic segments in coronary arteries tend to have a decreased response to vasodilators, an increased response to vasoconstrictors, and sometimes paradoxical vasoconstriction when exposed to vasodilators. Increased platelet reactivity and platelet aggregates further contribute to vessel lumen narrowing and release chemicals that can trigger vasoconstriction.

An episode of angina is not a heart attack although it is an indication of underlying CHD. The pain is caused by the transient ischemia, which is reversible. Thus, episodes of angina seldom cause permanent damage to the heart muscle. When patients have repeating but stable patterns of angina, an episode of angina does not mean that a heart attack is imminent. However, they are at an increased risk of heart attack compared to those who have no symptoms of CAD. Patients with angina and who subsequently developed coronary events are likely to have many vulnerable lesions throughout the coronary tree. In contrast, when the pattern of angina changes— if episodes become more frequent, last longer, or occur without exercise—the risk of heart attack in subsequent days or weeks is much higher. Specifically, the levels of markers of acute inflammation[10,11] such as C-reactive protein and fibrinogen are higher in patients with unstable coronary disease than in those with stable coronary disease. Moreover, persistent elevation of C-reactive protein in patients with unstable angina is predictive of future myocardial ischemia and infarction. The New York Heart Association Angina Classification is a scale used to indicate the severity of angina according to symptoms.

### New York Heart Association Angina Classification

- Class I—No limitation of physical activity (ordinary physical activity does not cause symptoms).
- Class II—Slight limitation of physical activity (ordinary physical activity does cause symptoms).
- Class III—Moderate limitation of physical activity (comfort at rest but less than ordinary physical activity cause symptoms).
- Class IV—Unable to perform any physical activity without discomfort (may be symptomatic even at rest).

## Medical and Surgical Intervention

The use of medication to relieve symptoms, lifestyle modification, and risk reduction is frequently used to slow the progression of disease and to reduce future adverse events.[12,13] Exercise can increase the level of pain-free activity, relieve stress, improve the heart's blood supply, and help control weight. Sedentary patients should build up their activity level gradually. For example, they should start with a short walk to tolerance and increase by 1 minute per day over days or weeks. The idea is to gradually increase fitness level by working at a steady pace and avoiding sudden bursts of effort.

# ACUTE CORONARY SYNDROME

## Definition

Acute coronary syndrome (ACS) consists of a spectrum of clinical presentations of acute myocardial ischemia and infarct.[14] ACS is suspected when chest pain is accompanied with ischemic changes in the EKG or elevated troponin I from a blood sample.

## Etiology and Pathophysiology

ACS is caused by the myocardial oxygen supply not meeting the demand. The imbalance is reversible or could progress to a nontransmural or transmural myocardial infarct. Common examples of supply ischemia are from functional or structural disruption of the coronary artery circulation such as vasospasm, nonocclusive thrombus, and significant coronary artery stenosis. Common examples of demand ischemia are associated with increased work of the heart such as during exercise and stress.

## Cardiovascular Disease Risk Factors With Coronary Artery Disease[15-23]

Risk factors that cannot be changed:
- Age—cardiovascular risk increases with age
- Gender—cardiovascular risk is higher in males
- Family history—cardiovascular risk increases with a family history

Risk factors that can be changed:
- Smoking—is extremely harmful
- Diabetes—should be aggressively managed
- Elevated serum cholesterol—proper diet is important
- Hypertension—should be closely regulated. Exercise has a slightly beneficial effect in lowering the systolic BP by about 4 mmHg and diastolic BP by about 3 mmHg
- Obesity—weight loss is beneficial
- Left ventricular hypertrophy

Protective factors:
- Elevated HDL cholesterol
- Active lifestyle
- Estrogen replacement therapy
- Moderate alcohol use

Having multiple risk factors can drastically increase the cardiovascular disease (CVD) risk. There are many models using CVD risk factors to predict the probability of cardiovascular disease. One study[20] reported that the use of antihypertensive medication or diabetes can double the CVD risk over 5 years while cigarette smoking may increase the risk by 50%. A more practical way to see the effects of combinations of CVD risk factors on the risk score (level of risk of having CVD in the future) is to use a CVD risk calculator. Below are some cardiovascular risk calculators located on different Web sites:

http://hin.nhlbi.nih.gov/atpiii/calculator.asp
http://livingheart.com/main/riskmain.asp
http://www.americanheart.org/presenter.jhtml?identifier=3003499

Table 19-4

### Differentiating Characteristics Between Q-Wave and Non Q-Wave Myocardial Infarcts

| Characteristics | Q-Wave | Non-Q Wave |
|---|---|---|
| Prevalence | 47% | 53% |
| Incidence of coronary occlusion | 80% to 90% | 15% to 25% |
| In-hospital mortality | High | Low |
| 1-month mortality | 10% to 15% | 3% to 5% |
| 2-year mortality | 30% | 30% |
| Infarct size | Big | Small |
| Acute complications | Frequent | Infrequent |

Adapted from Fus RV, Alexander RW, O'Rourke RA. *Hurst's the Heart*. New York: McGraw Hill; 2001.

## Clinical Presentations and Course

ACS consists of 3 levels:

1. *Unstable angina*, which is caused by the myocardial oxygen supply not meeting the demand. The imbalance is reversible or could progress to the next 2 levels. The pain is usually longer, variable, and not completely relieved by nitroglycerin. Nausea, sweating, and dyspnea are other commonly associated symptoms. In progressing to unstable angina, patients who formerly had stable angina usually recognize new symptoms or a change in symptoms. The EKG taken, while pain-free, is usually normal. The EKG taken while having angina shows signs of ischemia (ST segment depression, peaked or inverted T waves).

2. *Non-ST elevation MI or non Q-wave MI*. This is also termed a non-transmural infarct. Early spontaneous reperfusion may occur (Table 19-4). Troponin I is elevated.[12,24]

3. *ST elevation MI or Q-wave MI*. This is also termed a transmural infarct. The Q-wave might appear as early as 10 hours post infarct or take as long as 1 to 2 days. It is a sign of myocardial death (see Table 19-4). The EKG findings and clinical presentations depend on the site or sites of coronary artery blockage (Table 19-5). Troponin I is elevated.[24,25]

Sometimes EKG findings are not conclusive, especially in patients with an old infarct or bundle branch block. Variations between EKG findings and site of infarct also exist. Additional laboratory tests are used:

- Echocardiogram is used to evaluate wall motion abnormalities and overall ventricular function. This also can identify complications of an acute MI (eg, valvular insufficiency, ventricular dysfunction, pericardial effusion).
- Technetium-99m sestamibi scan (MIBI). The radioisotope is taken up by the myocardium in proportion to the blood flow and is redistributed minimally after injection.
- Thallium scanning: thallium accumulates in the viable myocardium.
- Coronary angiography is usually done prior to percutaneous transluminal coronary angioplasty (PTCA) especially in patients who have failed to respond to previous thrombolytics.

## Common Complications With an Acute Myocardial Infarction

- Arrhythmias—Most common complication but tends to be self-limiting. Ventricular ectopy may lead to more serious arrhythmias; supraventricular ectopy is more benign. Sinus bradycardia and sinus tachycardia, especially the former, can be medication related.
- Infarct expansion—Frequently occurs a week after a large transmural anterior MI
- Heart failure—Common with elderly or patients with a large infarct of the left ventricle
- Angina—Usually associated with ongoing ischemia or infarct extension
- Infarct extension—Associated with increased CK-MB beyond the normal time frame
- Cardiogenic shock—Frequently occurs with a large left ventricular infarct or patients with a previous MI

Table 19-5

### Site of Myocardial Infarct, Diagnosis and Clinical Significance

| Site of infarction | Vessel Involved | Hyperacute EKG Findings | Clinical Presentations |
| --- | --- | --- | --- |
| Anterior | Left anterior descending coronary artery | ST-segment elevation in V1 to V4 | Heart failure, AV block, sinus tachycardia, mural thrombi, BBB, septal rupture |
| Inferior | 80% right coronary artery (posterior descending branch). 20% left circumflex artery | ST-segment elevation in II, III, aVF Reciprocal changes in I, aVL, V2, V3 | Sinus block, atrial arrhythmia, 2-degree AV block, hiccup, nausea, vomiting indigestion, sinus bradycardia, hypotension, papillary muscle rupture |
| Posterior | Posterior interventricular artery or posterior descending artery | ST-segment depression in V1 to V4 | Usually associated with a lateral or inferior MI. Serious rhythm disturbances, left ventricular failure |
| Lateral | Left circumflex artery | ST-segment elevation in I, aVL, V5, V 6 Reciprocal changes in V1 to V4 | Conduction abnormality, arrhythmia, heart failure, ventricular aneurysm |
| Right ventricle | Right coronary artery | ST-segment elevation in III more than II with ST-segment depression in lead I. Right-sided EKG to be done when associated with inferior MI | Usually associated with inferior-posterior infarct. Right heart failure, thrombus/emboli, atrial fibrillation, indigestion |

- Pericarditis—Usually associated with a transmural MI. In rare occasions, this can lead to cardiac tamponade.

## Medical and Surgical Intervention

Management involves treating the underlying cause of the ischemia and restoring perfusion to the myocardium with treatments such as thrombolytic therapy, angioplasty, or coronary artery bypass grafts (CABG).[26,27] Cardiac medications are used to optimize the cardiac function and to reduce future adverse events.[15] Pneumovax (pneumococcal vaccination) is recommended as the condition becomes more chronic. Lifestyle modifications to minimize cardiac risk factors are important.[6-9,28-34] Primary and secondary risk factor reduction accounted for more than the 70% decline in mortality in patients with coronary disease in the United States between 1980 and 1990. Some examples of lifestyle modification included reduced intake of red meat, diet that included nuts, weight loss in overweight patients, low to moderate alcohol intake, regular exercise, and smoking cessation. The use of vitamin (vitamin E, vitamin C, and multivitamin) supplements, however, have not been shown to be effective in lowering cardiovascular disease risk.[35]

### Coronary Artery Bypass Graft

When cardiac patients have unrelenting chest pain, unstable angina, or other serious cardiac symptoms that are refractory to medical management and angioplasty, invasive surgery such as CABG is considered.[36] Under

**Figure 19-2.** Coronary arteries.

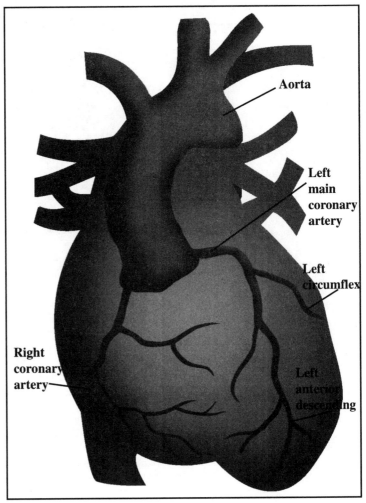

Aorta

Left main coronary artery

Left circumflex

Right coronary artery

Left anterior descending

general anesthesia, the chest is opened through the midline of the sternum (sternotomy). In order to maintain blood flow to the heart muscle beyond blockages, blood is bypassed onto the same artery beyond the blockage with a graft (Figure 19-2). In order to attach the grafts, the heart is cooled with iced physiologic salt solution, while a preservative solution is injected into the heart arteries. This process minimizes damage caused by reducing blood flow during surgery. The heart is stopped and placed on a bypass pump to allow attachment of the graft to the artery. The blockage is left in place, and blood is simply shunted around it. After the grafts are connected, the heart is disconnected from the bypass machine and restarted. Once the cardiac circulation has resumed, the chest wall layers are wired and sutured. The whole procedure lasts several hours depending on the number of vessels involved.

Graft vessels are usually obtained from:
- The internal mammary arteries
- Saphenous vein graft with an associated leg incision

Physical therapy intervention during the postoperative period:
- Patients will be transferred to the intensive care unit. Ventilator, chest drainage tubes, and other invasive lines (eg, arterial line, pulmonary catheter) are usually removed the next morning. Postoperative physical therapy routine usually involves thoracic expansion exercises, coughing, and mobilization.
- By the second day, patients are usually transferred to the step down cardiac unit. The patient may attend exercise class if stable and continue with breathing exercises and ambulation.
- Up to 25% of patients develop atrial fibrillation within the first 3 or 4 days after CABG surgery. It is related to the trauma during surgery and responds well to medication.[37-38]

- By day 3 or 4, patients may start walking 1 to 2 flights of stairs.
- Patients are usually ready for discharge home on day 5 postoperatively.

## Recovering at Home

At this stage, it is important for the patient to get sufficient rest and gradually increase his or her activity level. Patients are encouraged to participate in stage 2 cardiac rehabilitation. The patients are instructed to continue to follow sternal precautions (see Answer Guide for Case 12) for 6 to 8 weeks. It is normal for patients to be emotional after heart surgery or any health crisis. Feelings of depression, anger, and fear are rather common. This is a normal part of the healing process and will resolve with time. The patient should be encouraged to try to resume regular nonexertional activities that he or she enjoys.

# ATRIAL FIBRILLATION

## Definition

Atrial fibrillation (AF) is when the atria quiver instead of beating in a coordinated rhythm. This results in a very fast, uncontrolled heart rhythm of the ventricles. During AF, the atrial rate could be as high as 600 beats per minute.

## Etiology and Pathophysiology

Common causes of AF are:
- Medical related conditions such as: aging, post MI (especially right ventricle infarction, or diseases that result in atrial wall distension), heart failure, open heart surgery, hyperthyroidism, alcoholism, hypertension, and diabetes
- Drug related problems such as: illicit drug abuse or digoxin toxicity. The use of calcium channel blockers might increase the level of digoxin in the blood. The use of calcium channel blockers with amiodarone can cause bradycardia and decrease cardiac output. When used concurrently with beta-blockers, they can increase cardiac depression

During AF, the pumping action of the atria is fast and not synchronized with the ventricles such that the blood is not completely emptied from the atrial chambers. Blood clots are frequently formed. In about 5 percent of patients with AF, clotted blood dislodges from the atria and results in a stroke. AF with a concurrent diagnosis of hypertension, cardiac valve problems, or MI can increase the risk of stroke or heart failure. The American Heart Association estimates that in the United States, AF is responsible for over 70,000 strokes each year.

## Clinical Presentations and Course

- Palpitations, arrhythmias, dyspnea, chest discomfort, and dizziness
- Feelings of weakness caused by decreased cardiac output
- Anxiety from the awareness of a rapid and/or irregular heart beat
- Patients with underlying heart disease are generally less able to tolerate AF without complications
- Symptomatic AF implies poor overall cardiac function resulting in conditions such as angina, CHF, hemodynamic dysfunction, and embolism

### Types of Atrial Fibrillation

1. Paroxysmal AF is characterized by brief episodes of the arrhythmia, which can resolve on its own
2. Persistent AF—the episodes require some form of intervention to return the heart rhythm back to normal
3 Permanent AF—intervention (if successful at all) only restores normal heart rhythm for a brief time

## Medical and Surgical Intervention

Management involves treating the underlying cause of the fibrillation, cardioverting (converting using medications or electric shocks) back to normal sinus rhythm, rate control with medication, and the use of anticoagulation. Ablations (surgical removal) of the focal triggers of AF are sometimes used on selected patients.

Table 19-6

## Functional Classification and Clinical Signs of Cardiomyopathies

| Name | Dilated Congested Cardiomyopathy | Hypertrophic Cardiomyopathy | Restrictive Cardiomyopathy |
|---|---|---|---|
| Common causes | Idiopathic, hypertension, viral infection, immuno-logic disorders and toxic effects from chemical agents. | Genetic disorders and hypertension. | Idiopathic, amyloido-sis, and endomyocar-dial fibrosis. |
| Heart char-acteristics | Dilatation of both vent-ricles frequently with systolic dysfunction and increased myocardial mass. | Massive ventricular hypertrophy with small ventricular cavities. There are obstructive and non-obstructive types. The obstructive type is caused by the hypertrophic ventricular septum restricting mitral valve motions leading to the obstr-uction of blood flow during systole. | Decreased compliance and size of the ventric-ular cavities. |
| Heart function | The grossly enlarged ventricles resulted in myocardial contractile dysfunction. | The most important feature is diast-olic dysfunction. The massive vent-ricular wall results in a small vent-ricular space with a reduced end diastolic volume. The ejection vol-ume is above normal (sometimes approaching 90%) and end systolic ventricular volume is markedly de-creased. | The most important feature is decreased myocardial compli-ance leading to dias-tolic dysfunction. Systolic function and ejection fraction is usu-ally normal. |
| Clinical manifestation | Similar to that of left and right heart failure. Dyspnea, nocturnal dry cough, pulmonary and peripheral edema might occur. | Dyspnea, chest pain, and ventri-cular arrhythmia are common. Sudden death in young athletes is frequently associated with hyper-trophic cardiomyopathy. | Dyspnea with exertion and may progress to nocturnal dyspnea. The decrease in ven-tricular compliance usually leads to pul-monary and systematic congestion. |
| Diagnostic tests | Coronary angiography and left heart catheter-ization. | Echocardiography, radionuclide imaging, and angiography. | Radionuclide imaging, angiography and myocardial biopsy. |

# CARDIOMYOPATHY

## Definition

Cardiomyopathy is a disease of the heart muscle. The contractile function of the heart is affected resulting in decreased cardiac output.

## Etiology and Pathophysiology

This can be one of many varieties (Table 19-6). It can arise because of genetic causes, a viral infection, or consumption of toxins (lead, alcohol, etc.). In many cases, the condition is idiopathic. Ventricular remodeling occurs when the myocardium undergoes structural reorganization, usually resulting in a loss of wall motion and decreased contractile function. Ventricular remodeling is a common adverse effect of ACS.

## Clinical Presentation and Course

The disorder is usually chronic and common clinical features are:
- Dyspnea with exertion
- Fatigue
- Normal or low blood pressure
- Sinus tachycardia
- Basal crackles on lung auscultation
- Jugular venous distension
- Peripheral pitting edema
- In severe cases, hepatomegaly, ascites, and skeletal muscle wasting occur

## Medical and Surgical Intervention

Management involves treating the underlying cause, improving cardiac output, controlling heart failure, pneumovax (pneumococcal vaccination), and minimizing complications and future adverse events. Appropriate rest and stress avoidance are important. Physical exercise within the limits imposed by symptoms improves overall well being. Surgical procedures involving removal of strips of myocardium to remodel the dilated ventricle can be useful in selected patients.[2]

# CARDIAC EFFUSION AND CARDIAC TAMPONADE

## Definition

Cardiac effusion is an abnormal fluid accumulation in the pericardial space between the myocardium and pericardium. *Cardiac tamponade* occurs when fluid accumulation in pericardial space compresses the heart.[39-40]

## Etiology and Pathophysiology

The pericardium has an outer fibrous layer and an inner serous layer. The fibrous layer is a flask-shaped with a tough outer sac. It is attached to the diaphragm, sternum, and costal cartilages. The thin serous layer lies next to the surface of the heart. The pericardium protects the heart from the spread of infection or inflammation from other areas.

Inflammation of the pericardium, known as pericarditis, may occur in conditions such as malignant disease, cardiac surgery, post MI and tuberculosis. Fluid accumulates in the pericardial space resulting in a cardiac effusion. The pericardial space normally contains approximately 20 ml of fluid but can accommodate an extra 120 ml of fluid without deleterious effects. Cardiac tamponade is caused by further increases in fluid in pericardial space that compresses the heart. Hemodynamic effects such as a decreased venous return and decreased diastolic filling leads to decreased cardiac output and shock.

## Clinical Presentation and Course

### Clinical Presentation of Pericarditis
- Chest pain but it differs from angina (see Table 19-3)
- Dyspnea and pericardial friction rub (heard on auscultation)
- Low-grade fever is common
- Premature atrial and ventricular contractions occasionally are present

### Clinical Presentation of Cardiac Tamponade
- Jugular venous distension, hypotension, and muffled heart sounds
- *Pulsus paradoxus.* The first sphygmomanometer reading is recorded at the point when beats are audible during expiration and disappear during inspiration. The second reading is taken when each beat is audible during the respiratory cycle. A difference of more than 10 mmHg defines pulsus paradoxus.
- Cyanosis, decreased level of consciousness, shock.

- In patients with slow fluid accumulation > 200 mL, the chest x-ray can show an enlarged cardiac silhouette. However, with rapid fluid accumulation, the cardiac silhouette may be normal.

## Medical and Surgical Intervention

EKG, echocardiography, and CT scan are useful in the diagnosis of pericardial effusion and tamponade. Management involves treating the underlying cause, providing adequate pain control, and drainage of the fluid with a chest tube or creating a pericardial window with surgery.[2,38,39]

# PERIPHERAL VASCULAR DISEASE

## Definition

The arterial system can be affected by processes such as atherosclerosis and/or the venous system can be affected by processes such as thrombo-embolism, which can result in impeded blood supply to the muscles or venous return to the heart.

## Etiology and Pathophysiology

Common causes of arterial insufficiency are atherosclerosis, thrombo-embolism, and trauma (eg, compartment syndrome). Common causes of chronic venous insufficiency are obesity, ascites, lymphatic obstruction or destruction, malignant disease, surgery and radiation therapy. Deep vein thrombosis (DVT) is common after limb surgery (eg, total knee replacement) and immobilization (eg, bed rest, casted limb, paralysis). It can progress to chronic insufficiency with a large clot or repeated episodes (see Answer Guide for Case 17).

## Clinical Presentations and Course

### Arterial Occlusive Disease

Peripheral arterial diseases usually are present in patients with atherosclerosis and coronary artery disease. Both of the conditions share similar risk factors. Common clinical signs and symptoms are pain, minimal swelling, and a cold dusky appearance. A decrease or absence of pulses in the affected limb is the main distinguishing factor from venous insufficiency. In chronic cases, symptoms of claudication—a pain, ache, cramp, or tired feeling that occurs when walking—are most common in the lower leg. Claudication is aggravated by walking rapidly or uphill but is usually alleviated by rest. Delayed wound healing, skin ulcers, and gangrene are common in more severe cases. Doppler ultrasound is frequently used to check for peripheral pulses. An arteriogram is diagnostic.

### Venous Insufficiency

The condition is usually chronic except in the case of DVT. Common clinical presentations are redness, warmth, and a swollen calf muscle with pain and tenderness on palpation. Passive dorsiflexion of ankle (Homan's sign) also increases the pain. Doppler ultrasound or venogram is used for the diagnosis of DVT.

## Medical and Surgical Intervention

Medications, proper foot care and fitting shoes, and smoking cessation are essential for patients with arterial insufficiency. Complete arterial occlusion requires immediate medical or surgical attention to limit cell damage or death. DVT requires anticoagulation therapy (eg, heparin and warfarin) while chronic venous insufficiency management involves treating the cause and supportive treatment such as medication to decrease edema and the use of compression stockings. Ambulation has been shown to be beneficial in patients with claudication from peripheral vascular disease. Table 19-7 provides a brief description of an outpatient exercise program.[41]

# COMMON MEDICATIONS PRESCRIBED IN CARDIAC PATIENTS

A brief summary of some common medications for management of hypertension, congestive heart failure, angina, myocardial infarct, and blood clots is presented (Table 19-8). However, a comprehensive list is beyond the scope of this book. The Web sites in the references at the end of this chapter provide detailed up-to-date information about medical conditions and medical treatment.

Table 19-7

## Ambulation Program for Patients With Claudication From Peripheral Vascular Disease

*How to Do*

- Warm-up and cool-down periods of 5 to 10 minutes each

*Intensity*

- Treadmill walking or track walking with initial workload set to a speed and grade that elicits claudication symptoms within 3 to 5 minutes
- Patients may rest briefly in standing or sitting to permit symptoms to decrease
- Resume ambulation when able

*Duration*

- Cycles of ambulation with rest periods in between
- Exercise to tolerance initially
- Increase the time by 5 minutes per session until 50 minutes of intermittent ambulation is reached

*Frequency*

- 3 to 5 times per week

Adapted from Stewart KJ, Hiatt WR, Regensteiner JG, et al. Exercise training for with claudication from peripheral vascular disease. *N Eng J Med.* 2002:347;1941-1951.[41]

Table 19-8

## Examples of Common Medication Prescribed to Cardiovascular Patients

| Medication Trade name (Drug name) | Medication Effect | Physical Therapy Considerations |
|---|---|---|
| *Diuretics* Spironolactone, (Aldatone), Lasix (Furosemide). | "Water pill," which reduces plasma volume. Antihypertensive effect. | Patients may complain of feeling dizzy, and lightheaded with postural change, light sensitive and frequent voiding. Bedside commode or urinal is useful in mobility-impaired individuals especially at night. |
| *Beta-blocker* Inderal (propranolol), Lopressor (metoprolol), Sotacor (sotalol), Atenolol (tenormin). | Decreases the work of the heart. Has antianginal, anti-hypertensive, anti-arrhythmic, antiadrenergic effects, and prevents additional heart attacks. | Not suitable for asthmatics and restricts heart rate response to exercise. |
| *Calcium channel blocker* Cardizem, (diltiazem), Isoptin (verapamil), Plendil (felodipine), Procardia (nifedipine). | Has anti-anginal, antihypertensive, anti-arrhythmic effects. It affects the movement of calcium into the cells of the heart and blood vessels, relaxes blood vessels, and increases the supply of blood and oxygen to the heart while reducing its workload. | Patients may complain of dizziness, coughing, wheezing, and swelling of the lower limbs. |

Table 19-8 continued

## *Common Medication Prescribed to Cardiovascular Patients*

| Medication Trade name (Drug name) | Medication Effect | Physical Therapy Considerations |
|---|---|---|
| *ACE-inhibitor* Accupril (quina-pril), Altace (ramipril),Capo-ten (captopril), Monopril (fosin-opril),Vasotec (enalapril). | Antihypertensive, vaso-dilator and used in pat-ients with congestive heart failure or with an MI. | Light headedness and dizziness especially with exer-cise or hot weather. Frequent dry irritating cough. |
| *Angiotensin II Receptor blocker* Lorsartan (coz-aar), Valsartan (diovan). | Similar to ACE-inhibitor but more specific action with fewer side effects. | |
| Nitrol (nitro-glycerin), Isordil (isosorbide) | Lowers systolic BP and dilates systemic veins, thus reducing myocardial wall tension, a major de-terminant of myocardial oxygen need. Used for treatment of angina. | Ensure patients carry their nitro with them if they have frequent angina. |
| Streptokinase, anistreplase, alteplase, and reteplase. | Thrombolytic frequently used in MI patients. | Increased risk of bleeding. Follow specific protocol in coronary care unit. |
| Aspirin Plavix (clopid-ogrel) | Prevents thrombus form-ation by inhibition of platelet aggregation. | Bleeding. |
| Heparin Coumadin (warfarin). | Anticoagulation therapy (clot-preventing medication) consists of intravenous infusion of heparin initially, follow by oral warfarin. | Patient is prone to bruising and bleeding. |

Abbreviations: ACE: angiotensin-converting enzyme

# EXERCISES

Photocopy Table 18-3, Problems and Associated Outcome Measures, and complete a table for cardiac con-ditions by identifying outcome measures that could be used by a physical therapist to evaluate whether improve-ment has occurred after treatment for a specific problem. The problems are grouped because often outcome measures do not distinctly reflect 1 problem but may reflect similar or related problems.

# REFERENCES

1. Chobanian AV, Bakris GL, Black HR, et al. The seventh report of the joint national committee on prevention, detection, evaluation, and treatment of high blood pressure: the JNC 7 report. *JAMA*. 2003; 289:2560-2571.

2. Ahya SN, Flood K, Paranjothi S. *The Washington Manual of Medical Therapeutics*. Philadelphia: Lippincott Williams & Wilkins; 2001.

3. McArdle WD, Katch KI, Katch VL. Exercise physiology. *Energy, Nutrition, and Human Performance*. 5th ed. Philadelphia: Lipincott Williams & Wilkins; 2001;316.

4. Thadhani R, Camargo CA, Stampfer MJ, et al. Prospective study of moderate alcohol consumption and risk of hypertension in young women. *Arch Intern Med*. 2002;162:569-574.

5. McAlister FA, Zarnke KB, Campbell NR, et al. The 2001 Canadian recommendations for the management of hypertension: Part two—Therapy. *Can J Cardiol*. 2002;18:625-641.

6. Hinderliter A, Sherwood A, PhD, Gullette ECD, et al. Reduction of left ventricular hypertrophy after exercise and weight loss in overweight patients with mild hypertension. *Arch Intern Med*. 2002;162:1333-1339.

7. NIH. Sixth report of the Joint Committee on Prevention, Detection, Evaluation, and Treatment of High Blood Pressure (JNVI), Public Health Service, National Institutes of Health, National Heart, Lung Blood Institute. NIH Publication no 98-4080, Nov 1997.

8. Padwal R, Straus SE, McAlister FA. Evidence based management of hypertension. Cardiovascular risk factors and their effects on the decision to treat hypertension: evidence based review. *BMJ*. 2001;322:977-980.

9. Whelton SP, Chin A, Xin X, et al. Effect of aerobic exercise on blood pressure: A meta-analysis of randomized, controlled trials. *Ann Intern Med*. 2002;136:493-503.

10. Buffon A, Biasucci LM, Liuzzo G, et al. Widespread coronary inflammation in unstable angina. *N Engl J Med*. 2002;347:5-12.

11. Keaney JF Jr, Vita JA. The value of inflammation for predicting unstable angina. *N Engl J Med*. 2002;347:55-57.

12 Braunwald E, Antman E, Beasley J, et al. ACC/AHA 2002 guideline update for the management of patients with unstable angina and non-ST-segment elevation myocardial infarction-summary article. A report of the American College of Cardiology/American Heart Association task force on practice guidelines (Committee on the Management of Patients With Unstable Angina). *J Am Coll Cardiol*. 2002;40:1366-1374.

13. Gibbons RJ, Chatterjee K, Daley J, et al. ACC/AHA/ACP-ASIM guidelines for the management of patients with chronic stable angina: executive summary and recommendations. A Report of the American College of Cardiology/American Heart Association Task Force on Practice Guidelines (Committee on Management of Patients with Chronic Stable Angina). *Circulation*. 1999;99:2829-2848.

14. Rosamond TL. Initial appraisal of acute coronary syndrome: understanding the mechanisms, identifying patient risk. *Postgrad Med*. 2002;112:29-42.

15 Braunstein JB, Cheng A, Fakhry C, et al. ABCs of cardiovascular disease risk management. *Cardiol Rev*. 2001;9:96-105.

16. Franklin B, Bonzheim K, Warren J, et al. Effects of a contemporary, exercise-based rehabilitation and cardiovascular risk-reduction program on coronary patients with abnormal baseline risk factors. *Chest*. 2002;122:338-343.

17. Gordon NF, English CD, Contractor AS, et al. Effectiveness of three models for comprehensive cardiovascular disease risk reduction. *Am J Cardiol*. 2002;89:1263-1268.

18. Hunink MGM, Goldman L, Tosteson ANA, et al. The recent decline in mortality from coronary heart disease, 1980-1990. The effect of secular trends in risk factors and treatment. *JAMA*. 1997;277:535-542.

19. Jousilahti P, Vartiainen E, Tuomilehto J, et al. Sex, age, cardiovascular risk factors, and coronary heart disease: a prospective follow-up study of 14 786 middle-aged men and women in Finland. *Circulation*. 1999;99:1165-1172.

20. Simons LA, Simons J Friedlander Y, et al. Risk functions for prediction of cardiovascular disease in elderly Australians: the Dobbo Study. *Med J Aust.* 2003;178:113-116.

21. Tonkin AM, Lim SS, Schirmer H. Cardiovascular risk factors: when should we treat? *Med J Aust.* 2003;178:101-102.

22. Wilson PW, D'Agostino RB, Levy D, et al. Prediction of coronary heart disease using risk factor categories. *Circulation.* 1998;97:1837-1847.

23. Daviglus ML, Stamler J. Major risk factors and coronary heart disease: much has been achieved but crucial challenges remain. *J Am Coll Cardiol.* 2001;38:1018-1022.

24. Meier MA, Al-Badr WH, Cooper JV, et al. The new definition of myocardial infarction. Diagnostic and prognostic implications in patients with acute coronary syndromes. *Arch Intern Med.* 2002;162:1585-1589.

25. Vacek JL. Classic Q wave myocardial infarction: aggressive, early intervention has dramatic results. *Postgrad Med.* 2002;112:71-77.

26. Ryan TJ, Antman EM, Brooks NH, et al. 1999 update: ACC/AHA guidelines for the management of patients with acute myocardial infarction. A report of the American College of Cardiology/American Heart Association Task Force on Practice Guidelines (Committee on Management of Acute Myocardial Infarction). *J Am Coll Cardiol.* 1999;34:890-911.

27. Santiago P, Tadros P. Non-ST-segment elevation syndromes: pharmacologic management, conservative versus early invasive approach. *Postgrad Med.* 2002;112:47-68.

28. Albert CM, Gaziano JM, Willett WC, et al. Nut consumption and decreased risk of sudden cardiac death in the physicians' health study. *Arch Intern Med.* 2002;162:1382-1387.

29. Fedder DO, Koro CE, L'Italien GJ. New National Cholesterol Education Program III guidelines for primary prevention lipid-lowering drug therapy: projected impact on the size, sex, and age distribution of the treatment-eligible population. *Circulation.* 2002;105:152-156.

30. Gould KL, Ornish D, Scherwitz L. Changes in myocardial perfusion abnormalities by positron emission tomography after long-term, intense risk factor modification. *JAMA.* 1995;274:894-901.

31. Ito MK, Delucca GM, Aldridge MA. The relationship between low-density lipoprotein cholesterol goal attainment and prevention of coronary heart disease—related events. *J Cardiovasc Pharmacol Ther.* 2001;6:129-135.

32. Jones PH. Lipid-lowering treatment in coronary artery disease: how low should cholesterol go? *Drugs.* 2000;59:1127-1135.

33. Ornish D, Scherwitz LW, Billings JH. Intensive lifestyle changes for reversal of coronary heart disease. *JAMA.* 1998;280:2001-2007.

34. Menotti A, Lanti M. Coronary risk factors predicting early and late coronary deaths. *Heart.* 2003;89:19-24.

35. Muntwyler J, Hennekens CH, Manson JE, et al. Vitamin supplement use in a low-risk population of US male physicians and subsequent cardiovascular mortality. *Arch Intern Med.* 2002;162:1472-1476.

36. Eagle KA and Guyton RA. ACC/AHA guidelines for CABG surgery. *J Am Coll Cardiol.* 1999;34,1262-1347.

37. Jayam VK, Flaker GC, Jones JW. Atrial fibrillation after coronary bypass: etiology and pharmacologic prevention. *Cardiovasc Surg.* 2002;10:351-358.

38. Taylor AD, Groen JG, Thorn SL, et al. New insights into onset mechanisms of atrial fibrillation and flutter after coronary artery bypass graft surgery. *Heart.* 2002;88:499-504.

39. Aikat S, Ghaffari S. A review of pericardial diseases: clinical, EKG and hemodynamic features and management. *Cleve Clin J Med.* 2000;67:903-914.

40. Valley VT. Pericarditis and cardiac tamponade. *E Medicine Journal.* 2001;2(6).

41. Stewart KJ, Hiatt WR, Regensteiner JG, et al. Exercise training for with claudication from peripheral vascular disease. *N Eng J Med.* 2002:347;1941-1951.

# BIBLIOGRAPHY

Beasley B, West M. *Understanding 12-Lead EKGs. A Practical Approach*. Upper Saddle River, NJ: Prentice Hall; 2001.

Beers MH, Berkow R. *The Merck Manual of Diagnosis and Therapy*. 17th ed. Internet Edition provided by Medical Services, USMEDSA, USHH. © 1999-2004 by Merck & Co, Inc. http://www.merck.com/pubs/mmanual/

EMedicine. © 2003 eMedicine.com, Inc. http://www.emedicine.com/

Fuster V, Alexander RW, O'Rourke RA. *Hurst's The Heart*. New York: McGraw Hill; 2001.

Goodman & Gilman. *The Pharmacological Basis of Therapeutics*. New York: McGraw-Hill, 1996.

MedlinePlus. US National Library of Medicine and the National Institute of Health. Patient Drug Information database provides information copyrighted by the American Society of Health-System Pharmacists, Inc., Bethesda, Md; 2001. http://www.nlm.nih.gov/medlineplus/druginformation.html

National Heart, Lung, and Blood institute and National Institute of Health Third Report of the Expert Panel on Detection, Evaluation, and Treatment of High Blood Cholesterol in Adults (Adult Treatment Panel III) http://www.nhlbi.nih.gov/guidelines/cholesterol/index.htm

Otto CM, Shavelle DM. *Approach to cardiovascular patient*. Scientific America. WebMD Corp; 2001.

Rifai N, Burling JE, Lee IM, et al. Is C-reactive protein specific for vascular disease in woman? *Ann Inten Med*. 2002;136:529-533.

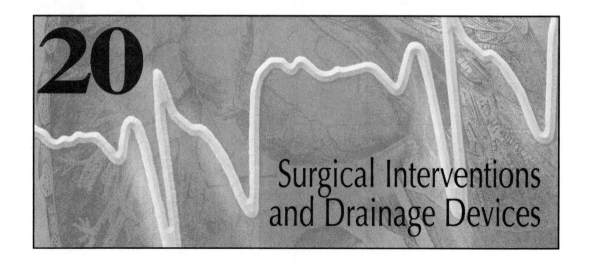

**20**

# Surgical Interventions and Drainage Devices

## OBJECTIVES

Upon completion of this chapter, the reader should be able to describe:

1. Anesthetics risk factors and effects related to major abdominal or thoracic surgery
2. The effects of upper abdominal or thoracic incisions on the pulmonary system
3. Perioperative physical therapy management
4. The pathophysiology that is reversible by physical therapy and other health professionals in surgical patients
5. Various fluid drainage devices, fluid access devices, analgesic devices, and monitoring devices

Risk factors and effects related to anesthesia, location of surgical incision and their effects on the physical therapy management of these patients are discussed. Clinical trials on postoperative physical therapy management are reviewed. Fluid drainage devices, fluid access devices, analgesic devices, and monitoring devices that are frequently used in medical and surgical patients are also described in this chapter.

## ANESTHETICS RISKS FACTORS AND EFFECTS RELATED TO MAJOR ABDOMINAL AND THORACIC SURGERY

The American Society of Anesthesiologists' physical status classification (ASA class) is frequently used to stratify the risk of mortality from anesthetics (Table 20-1). Other than the surgical condition, those patients who are otherwise healthy are considered to be low risk while seriously ill patients are considered to be at high risk of death. It is recommended in the absence of major contraindications, beta-blockers should be given to patients with an intermediate or high risk of cardiac complications.[1-3]

Additional factors that will predispose patients to develop *cardiac* complications are[1-4]:

- High risk surgical procedures (eg, intraperitoneal, intrathoracic, or aortic surgery, emergency surgery)
- History of ischemic heart disease, myocardial infarction in the preceding 6 months
- History of congestive heart failure
- History of cerebrovascular disease
- Preoperative treatment with insulin
- Preoperative serum creatinine concentration greater than 2.0 mg per deciliter

Factors that will predispose patients to develop *pulmonary* complications are[5-7]:

- Type of surgery and technique. The highest risk is with abdominal aortic aneurysm repair, thoracic (noncardiac), and upper abdominal surgeries
- Older age

Table 20-1

### Risk of Mortality With the American Society of Anesthesiologists' Physical Status Classification

| ASA Class | Definition | Mortality (%) |
|---|---|---|
| 1 | Otherwise healthy patient | <0.3 |
| 2 | Mild systematic disease | <0.6 |
| 3 | Severe systematic disease but not incapacitating | <2.0 |
| 4 | Incapacitating systemic disease | <8.0 |
| 5 | Moribund | 34 |

- Low preoperative functional status
- Weight loss greater than 10% during the past 6 months
- History of COPD

General anesthesia carries higher risk while epidural and spinal anesthesia carry lower risk.

Anesthetics tends to suppress the cardiopulmonary and neuromuscular function of the patients. Women have a lower overall quality of recovery from anesthesia. Women also had a 25% slower rate of return to the preoperative health status and experienced more postoperative complications than men.[8]

The effects of anesthetics on the *cardiovascular system* are:
- Depressed myocardial function
- Hypotension
- Decreased myocardial contractility
- Decreased cardiac output

The effects of anesthetics on the *respiratory system* are:
- Up to 90% of patients and one-quarter of the dependent lung region will develop atelectasis
- Increased respiratory rate
- Decreased tidal volume
- Lack of sighing
- Decreased ventilatory drive
- Decreased functional residual capacity
- Closing capacity occurring at a higher lung volume

The effects of anesthetics on *psychomotor function* (especially in combination with hypocapnia)[9] are:
- Increased time to regain consciousness
- Decreased higher intellectual functions
- Personality changes

These effects are more profound in elderly and adverse effects may last up to 6 days.

# EFFECTS OF UPPER ABDOMINAL OR THORACIC INCISIONS ON THE PULMONARY SYSTEM

The upper abdominal or thoracic surgical incisions often lead to postoperative atelectasis. The effects of upper abdominal and thoracic surgical incisions are:
- Decreased maximum inspiratory pressure (a measure of inspiratory muscle strength).
- Diaphragmatic dysfunction and altered breathing pattern resulting in a shift of ventilation to the upper lung zones. The diaphragmatic dysfunction is thought to be due to sympathetic vagal or splanchnic/abdominal receptor stimulation from the surgery causing inhibition of either the central drive and/or phrenic nerve output.[10,11]

- Decreased ventilation in the dependent lung zones leading to hypoxemia.
- The lowering of the functional residual capacity such that the dependent (atelectatic) lung zones are on the flat lower portion of the "pressure-volume" curve (see Chapter 13, Figure 13-1). Because the ability to inhale deeply is inhibited, the subsequent submaximal inspiratory effort will generate lesser volume changes in the dependent lung zone and most of the ventilation will be distributed to the already expanded upper lung zones.
- Pain and splinting leading to the use of accessory muscles during tidal breathing instead of the diaphragm; this might preferentially distribute the ventilation to the nondependent lung zones as well.[12]

Other compounding clinical factors are:

- Deep breathing can eliminate atelectasis in postoperative patients. However, when patients were breathing 40% of oxygen, up to 25% of the lung bases can become atelectatic in 40 minutes. Furthermore, when patients were on 100% oxygen, atelectasis can recur in 5 minutes.[13]
- Applying manual percussion and vibration techniques, especially on inappropriate patients, can further increase atelectasis. Emphasis on coughing without thoracic expansion exercises can further accentuate atelectasis.
- Improper positioning or prolonged immobility promotes atelectasis.
- Insufficient and infrequent pain control will decrease the ability of the patient to inspire deeply and cooperate with breathing exercises and mobilization.[12,14,15]
- Overuse of sedation, narcotics and analgesics results in a decreased level of consciousness, delirium, and hypotension in some patients. This can result in decreased compliance with the postoperative exercise routine and mobility.
- Improper use of incentive spirometer and excessive accessory muscle use might distribute ventilation to the already ventilated areas due to the rapid inspiratory flow that is required to raise the ball.
- Fasting before and after surgery resulting in malnutrition can result in general weakness.
- Malnutrition coupled with rapid shallow breathing with infrequent sighing has a negative impact on surfactant and lung mechanics making lung expansion more difficult.[11] It is due to the formation of nonfunctional aggregated surfactant, which has a decreased ability to lower surface tension of the alveoli.[16,17] This results in alveoli having a lower compliance such that a larger inspiratory pressure is needed to inflate the collapsed lung.
- Secretions in the airways might increase the airway resistance and decrease the airflow. The ability to cough is reduced due to pain inhibition. This can cause mucus retention in some patients and increase the risk of developing infection.

# EVIDENCE-BASED PRACTICE: PERIOPERATIVE PHYSICAL THERAPY MANAGEMENT

Recent clinical trials on the perioperative physical therapy management are summarized in Appendix V. The number of patients needed to treat (NNT) to prevent pulmonary complications ranges from 3 to 8 (Table 20-2). It can be beneficial to see patient preoperatively in the preadmission clinic to assess and familiarize the patient with perioperative routine.[7]

Purposes of physical therapy preoperative session are to:

- Develop a rapport between therapist and patient
- Assess the patient
- Explain to the patient the reasons for physical therapy interventions
- Go through physical therapy routines such as: slow deep inspiration with end-inspiratory hold; gentle and unforced expiration to FRC; coughing; circulatory exercises, position change, transfer technique; and mobilization
- Perform breathing exercises a minimum of 10 breaths and should be repeated hourly when awake
- Instruct the use of incentive spirometry and obtain the best value preoperatively to use as a target following surgery

Table 20-2

## Number Needed to Treat With Physical Therapy to Prevent Complications After Abdominal Surgery

| Journal Reference | Complication Type | Complication Rate | | NNT[a] |
|---|---|---|---|---|
| | | Control % | Treatment % | |
| Acta Anesth Scand. 1991; 35:97-104[18] | Pneumonia | 29 | 6 | 4.3 |
| | Needed supplemental $O_2$ | 47 | 29 | 5.6 |
| Arch Phys Med Rehabil. 1998; 79:5-9[19] | Pulmonary complications* | 19.5 | 7.5 | 8.3** |
| Br J Surg. 1997; 84: 1535-8[20] | Pulmonary complications* in low risk group | 27 | 6 | 4.8** |
| | Pulmonary complications* in high risk group | 51 | 15 | 2.8** |

* Pulmonary complications include increased temperature, productive cough, new findings on chest x-ray, pneumonia, respiratory failure, prolonged ventilation, bronchospasm.
** Statistical significance (P<0.05)
[a] The number of patients that need to be treated to avoid 1 adverse event

Brooks et al[21] reported discharge criteria for postoperative physical therapy care. It is composed of 5 categories: the ability to mobilize, the quality of breath sounds, the ability to clear airway secretions, the level of oxygen saturation, and the respiratory rate. The score for the postoperative physical therapy discharge scoring tool (POP-DST) ranges from 6 to 15, with a score of > 13 indicating readiness for discharge.

## Physical Therapy Management in Postoperative Patients

- Teach the patient how to do deep breathing exercises properly and frequently. Breath-stacking may be useful in some patients (see Chapter 12 for details). Avoid forced exhalation below FRC.
- Frequent position change and deep breathing in different positions is encouraged. Studies have been shown that sitting in the upright position and standing will increase the FRC and the VC. If the patient has to rest in bed, side lying is best to preserve the FRC. Slumped sitting and supine tend to decrease the FRC.
- Perform lower extremity exercises to stimulate circulation and venous return.
- Promote early ambulating and sitting at the edge of the bed. Intermittent suction resulting from disconnecting chest tube from wall suction and utilizing water seal only for ambulation might decrease the duration of air leak. Intermittent versus continuous wall suction has been shown to decrease the number of days for the air leak to resolve.
- When the patient is congested and unable to expectorate by deep breathing and positioning alone, manual techniques should be used concurrently with deep breathing and must finish with deep breathing exercises to ensure full expansion of the treated area.
- Coordinate treatment with pain medication. Ensure sufficient pain control prior to intervention. Keeping patients warm might also help to decrease infection.[22-25]

## Summary on Physical Therapy Intervention in Upper Abdominal Surgery

1. The pulmonary complication rates ranges from 27% to >50%.
2. Respiratory physical therapy interventions including deep breathing, coughing, and mobilization is better than no treatment.[18-20]

3. The routine use of incentive spirometer in conjunction with respiratory physical therapy is questionable. Incentive spirometry may be useful in high-risk cases or patients with restricted mobility.[26]

4. The use of the positive expiratory mask might be useful.[27,28]

5. Preoperative assessment can be valuable.[7]

## Summary on Physical Therapy Intervention in Open Heart Surgery

1. The pulmonary complication rate is <10%.

2. Respiratory physical therapy interventions including deep breathing, coughing and mobilization are better than no treatment.[29-31]

In addition, Brooks et al[32] in the clinical practice guideline on perioperative cardiorespiratory physical therapy recommended the use of transcutaneous electrical nerve stimulation for pain relief in thoracic and abdominal surgery patient. They also recommended the use of inspiratory muscle training 2 to 4 weeks before cardiac surgery.[32]

# MEDICAL DEVICES FREQUENTLY USED IN MEDICAL AND SURGICAL PATIENTS

## Fluid Drainage Devices

### Suctioning[33-34]

This section describes suction techniques used in patients that have significant mucus congestion that they are unable to clear. Patients might have an ineffective cough, altered upper airways function, or the presence of artificial airways. Suctioning can be done:

- Orally with the use of an oral airway. Lubrication is required when going through the oral airway
- Nasal pharynx with the use of a nasal airway. Lubrication is required when going through the nasal airway
- Via endotracheal tube typically using in-line suction (see Chapter 17, Figure 17-2)
- Via tracheostomy tube typically using in-line suction (see Chapter 17, Figure 17-3)

*Preparation Prior to Suctioning*

- Patient is positioned or treated with the appropriate airway clearance technique to localize the mucus within reach of the suction catheter especially in those patients with a weak or absent cough.
- Check to see if the suction pressure is set at the appropriate range (80 to 120 mmHg) and there is sufficient suction pressure at the catheter tip.
- Ensure the in-line suction is ready to use or alternatively, the suction kit with glove, catheter, and lubricant are within easy reach.
- Ensure the normal saline for instillation and to flush the catheter is set up.
- Hyperoxygenate the patient prior to suctioning. Wait for 1 to 2 minutes or until the oxygen saturation starts to rise.
- Be aware of the vital signs and the clinical status of the patient prior to suctioning.

*Suctioning Technique*

- Estimate how far the suction catheter will need to be advanced.
- Instilling the patient with 5 to 10 ml of normal saline prior to suction can be helpful in loosening thick secretions.
- Insert the suction catheter gently using your dominant hand. Do not force the catheter down.
- Apply counterpressure with your other hand holding onto the airway/breathing tube.
- When the estimated length of the catheter is inserted and resistance is felt, withdraw the catheter for a few millimeters, start suctioning and gradually withdraw catheter.
- To avoid contamination especially when the in-line suction system is not in use, the caregiver should NOT stand directly in front of the patient's airway. Use of the face shield is recommended.

**Figure 20-1.** Jackson-Pratt drain. The end of the drainage tubing containing the suction ports is flattened whereas the remaining part of the drainage tubing is round and smooth. The flattened end is positioned inside the wound of the patient and the fluid from the wound is collected into the spherical collection chamber, which is attached to the patient's gown with a safety pin.

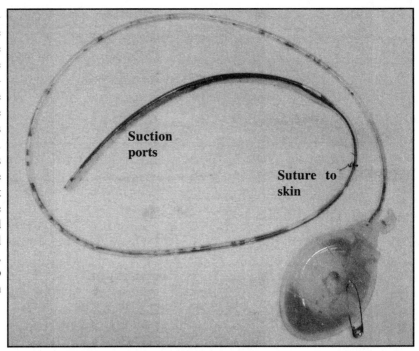

- Flush the suction catheter after use.
- When needed, allow a few minutes until the patient has recovered before repeating suctioning.
- Stay and observe the patient until their status has stabilized. Let the appropriate team member know if the patient's condition deteriorates after treatment.

*Adverse Side Effects of Suctioning*

The therapist frequently has to weigh the risks and benefits of suctioning for each patient. Adverse effects are:

- Airway trauma and bleeding. The caregiver might consider lowering the suction pressure, using a smaller size or softer catheter, gentle insertion, or decreasing the frequency of suctioning.
- Pulmonary problems such as bronchospasm, hypoxemia, or laborious breathing. The caregiver might consider suctioning after the use of asthma medications, adequate hyper-oxygenation, or decreasing the frequency of suctioning.
- Cardiovascular instability such as arrhythmia, a decrease or increase in heart rate and blood pressure. In patients with increased cardiovascular responses, increased sedation, analgesia or cardiac medication might be required. In patients with decreased cardiovascular responses, atropine, inotropic drugs or decreased frequency of suction might be required.
- Increased restlessness and agitation. An increase in sedation or analgesia might be required.

## Abdominal or Wound Drainage

See Figure 20-1 (Jackson-Pratt drain).

- *Purposes:* to drain blood, pus or other abnormal body fluid. Usually the drain is put in during surgery or using ultrasound, CT, or laparoscopic guidance in other cases.
- *Common conditions:* postabdominal surgery, organ or a pocket of fluid collection, cyst, abscess, or pockets of infection.
- *Handling tips:* avoid traction or kinking of the tube. Pin the drain to the patient's gown when patient is up in chair or ambulating.

## Chest Drainage

See Figure 20-2.

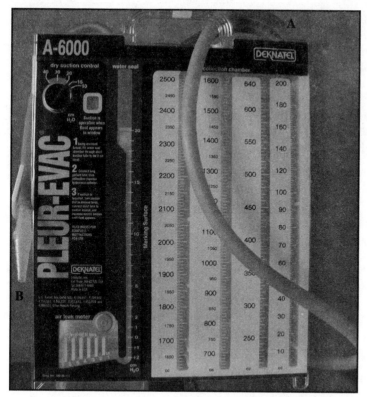

**Figure 20-2.** Chest tube drainage system. The tube from drainage system labeled (A) is connected to chest tube for drainage of fluid or air from the pleural, mediastinal, or pericardial space. The tube that is labeled (B) is connected to wall suction.

- *Purposes:* to evacuate air, blood, and other body fluid. The fluid drained from the insertion site is collected via tubing connected to a collection chamber with a water seal to prevent reflux of the drainage fluid back into the chest cavity.
- *Insertion sites:* pleural, pericardial, or mediastinal area.
- *Common conditions:* pneumothorax, pleural effusion, hemothorax, empyema, pericardial effusion, post-thoracic, or cardiac surgery.
- *Handling tips:* Avoid traction or kinking of the tube. The chest tube collection chamber should be kept lower than the chest tube insertion site to avoid drainage of fluid back into the patient. Disconnect from wall suction unit (if permissible) to mobilize patient.[35]

## Nasogastric Tube (NG)

See Figure 20-3.
- *Purposes:* to remove fluid and gas from stomach especially in patients with gastrointestinal dysfunction and immediately following major abdominal surgery. NG drainage also helps to relieve nausea and vomiting.
- *Handling tips:* avoid traction or kinking of the tube. Disconnect from wall suction (if permissible) and pin the drain to the patient's gown when up in chair or ambulating.

## Urinary Catheter

- *Purpose:* to drain urine from bladder. Commonly used after major surgery or in patients with urinary retention.
- *Handling tips:* avoid traction and kinking of the catheter. Keep the catheter bag lower than the bladder of the patient to avoid draining urine back into the bladder.

**Figure 20-3.** Nasogastric tube. The end with the suction ports is inserted into the stomach of the patient. Black markers along this end of the tubing denote distance to the tip of the last suction port. The plug is inserted into the other end when mobilizing the patient; however, this end is usually connected to wall suction while the patient is resting in bed.

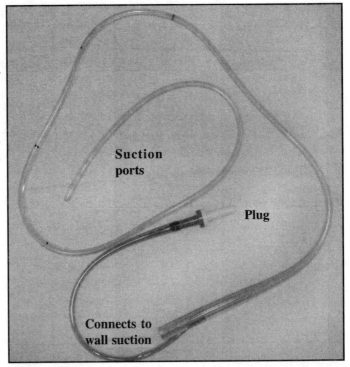

## Fluid Access Devices

### Feeding Tube
- *Purposes:* to provide food intake directly to the stomach or duodenum. It is usually through a nasogastrointestinal or percutaneous route.
- *Handling tips:* avoid traction or kinking of the tube. Keep head of bed elevated to at least 45 degrees during and immediately after feeding.

### Intravenous Access
- *Purposes:* to maintain or replenish body fluid, electrolytes, chemical and acid-base balance. It is also used to administer medications, blood products, and nutrition.
- *Signs of complications related to IV lines are:* redness, swelling and discomfort; signs of infection (increased temperature, chills, elevated white blood cell count etc); hemorrhage; and occlusion and venous thrombosis.

### Peripheral Line
See Figure 20-4.
- *Access:* Via peripheral vein

Central line
See Figure 20-5.
- *Access:* It is threaded through the subclavian vein or internal jugular into the superior vena cava (SVC). Tip location is at the lower one-third of the SVC. An alternative route is to thread the central line through the femoral vein to the upper one-third of inferior vena cava. The central line consists of multiple lumens allowing administration of multiple medications, nutrition, and hemodynamic monitoring.

### IV Access for Dialysis
- *Peritoneal dialysis:* indwelling catheter inserted into the peritoneal cavity

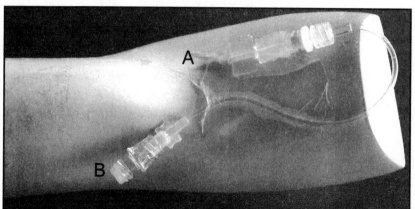

**Figure 20-4.** Peripheral intravenous line inserted into a model of a person's arm. (A) insertion into a peripheral vein. (B) connection to intravenous bag that might contain medication or fluid.

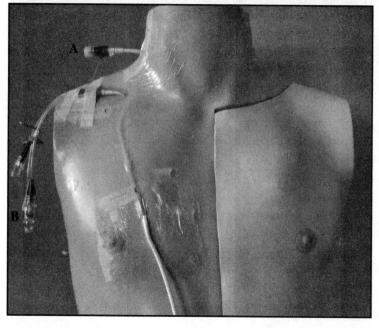

**Figure 20-5.** Central line. (A) a single lumen central line using jugular vein approach. (B) triple lumen central line using subclavian vein approach.

- *Hemodialysis:* Some of the common access routes are to:
  - o Create an arteriovenous fistula by connecting a vein directly to an artery.
  - o Use of a central venous catheter.
  - o Create an arteriovenous graft by using a saphenous vein or from polytetrafluoroethylene material.
- *Handling tips:* avoid traction and kinking of the IV. Avoid movement at the insertion site.

## Analgesia Devices

### Patient-Controlled Analgesia
- *Purpose:* patients can self-medicate as required. There is a lockout control to prevent inadvertent overdose of narcotics.
- *Handling tips:* avoid traction and kinking of the IV. Avoid movement at the insertion site.

### Epidural Analgesia
- *Purpose:* local pain control by injecting narcotics into the epidural space and minimizing systematic effects.
- *Common complications:* nausea, dizziness, decreased sensation, and motor weakness.

- *Handling tips*: avoid traction and kinking of the epidural catheter. Avoid movement at the insertion site. Check for lower limb function before mobilizing patients.

## Monitoring Devices

### Hemodynamic Monitoring
- A: Arterial line: usually inserted into the radial artery at the wrist. It is connected to a transducer and then to a processor and monitor.
  - *Purpose*: to monitor arterial pressure
  - *Handling tips*: avoid movement near the insertion site
- B: Pulmonary artery pressure monitoring: See central line.
  - *Purpose*: to monitor cardiac output, and from the right atrium, right ventricle, pulmonary artery, left atrium, and the ventricular filling pressure
  - *Handling tips*: avoid movement near the insertion site. Patient is on bed rest when the balloon at the catheter tip is inflated

### Cardiac Pacing
The heart rate is controlled by an external (temporary) or internal (permanent) pacemaker when the heart's own pacemaker is not functioning properly. The pacemaker can be set to fire at a fixed rate or to fire when the natural heart rate drops below a certain level (on demand). More advanced devices can be triggered to fire by some events such as atrial impulses, exercise or stress. The pacemaker can stimulate the right atrium, the 2 ventricles, or both in sequence.
- *Handling tips*: With temporary pacemakers, avoid traction to the wires and movement at the insertion site. With permanent pacemakers, avoid percussion and vibrations at or near the pacemaker. Physical modalities involving diathermy are contraindicated.

# REFERENCES

1. Lee TH. Reducing cardiac risk in noncardiac surgery. *N Eng J Med*. 1999:341;1838-1840.
2. Lee TH, Marcantonio ER, Mangione CM, et al. Derivation and prospective validation of a simple index for prediction of cardiac risk of major noncardiac surgery. *Circulation*. 1999;100:1043-1049.
3. Poldermans D, Boersma E, Bax JJ, et al. The effect of bisoprolol on perioperative mortality and myocardial infarction in high-risk patients undergoing vascular surgery. *N Eng J Med*. 1999;341:1789-1794.
4. Goldman L, Caldera DL, Nussbaum SR, et al. Multifactorial index of cardiac risk in noncardiac surgical procedures. *N Eng J Med*. 1977;297:845-850.
5. Arozullah AM, Khuri SF, Henderson WG, et al. Development and validation of a multifactorial risk index for predicting postoperative pneumonia after major noncardiac surgery. *Ann Intern Med*. 2001;135:847-859.
6. Lawrence VA. Predicting postoperative pulmonary complications: the sleeping giant stirs. *Ann Intern Med*. 2001;135:919-921.
7. Smetana GW. Preoperative pulmonary evaluation. *N Eng J Med*. 1999;340:937-944.
8. Myles PS, McLeod ADM, Hunt JO, et al. Sex differences in speed of emergence and quality of recovery after anaesthesia: cohort study. *BMJ*. 2001;322:710-711.
9. Laffey JG, Kavanagh BP. Hypocapnia. *N Engl J Med*. 2002;347:43-53.
10 Dureuil B, Viires N, Caantineau JP, et al. Diaphragmatic contractility after upper abdominal surgery. *J Appl Physiol*. 1986;61:1775-1780.
11. Ford GT, Whitelaw WA, Rosenal TW, et al. Diaphragm function and upper abdominal surgery in humans. *Am Rev Respir Dis*. 1983;127:431-436.
12. Vassilakopoulos T, Mastora Z, Paraskevi P, et al. Contribution of pain to inspiratory muscle dysfunction after upper abdominal surgery. A randomized controlled trial. *Am J Respir Crit Care Med*. 2000:161;1372-1375.
13. Rothen, et al. Prevention of atelectasis during general anesthesia. *Lancet*. 1995;345:1387-1391.

14. Blanchard AR. Sedation and analgesia in intensive care: medications attenuate stress response in critical illness. *Postgrad Med.* 2002;111:59-74.

15. Mann C, Pouzeratte Y, Boccara G, et al. Comparison of intravenous or epidural patient-controlled analgesia in the elderly after major abdominal surgery. *Anesthesiology.* 2000;92:433-441.

16. Paul GW, Sanders RL, Harsett RJ. Kinetics of film formation and surface activity of lamellar bodies, extracted lipids, tubular myelin figures and alveolar surfactant from rat lung. *Fed Proc.* 1977;36:615.

17. Thet LA, Alvarez H. Effect of hyperventilation and starvation on rat lung mechanics and surfactant. *Am Rev Respir Dis.* 1982;126:286-290.

18. Christensen EF, Schultz P, Jensen OV, et al. Postoperative pulmonary complications and lung function in high risk patients: a comparison of three physiotherapy regimens after upper abdominal surgery in general anesthesia. *Acta Anaesthesiol Scand.* 1991;35:97-104.

19. Chumillas S, Ponce JL, Delgado F. Prevention of postoperative pulmonary complications through respiratory rehabilitation: a controlled clinical study. *Arch Phys Med Rehabil.* 1998;79:5-9.

20. Olsen MF, Hahnn I, Nordgren S, et al. Randomized controlled trial of prophylactic chest physiotherapy in major abdominal surgery. *Br J Surg.* 1997;84:1535-1538.

21. Brooks D, Parson J, Newton J, et al. Discharge criteria from perioperative physical therapy. *Chest.* 2002:121:488-494.

22. Kurz A, Sessler DI, Lenhardt R. Perioperative normathermia to reduce the incidence of surgical wound infections and shorten hospitalisation. *N Engl J Med.* 1996;334:1209-1216.

23. Melling AC, Ali B, Scott EM, et al. Effects of preoperative warming on the incidence of wound infection after clean surgery: a randomised controlled trial. *Lancet.* 2001;358:876-880.

24. Sheffield CW, Sessler DI, Hunt TK. Mild hypothermia during isolurane anesthesia decreases resistance to E coli dermal infection in guinea pigs. *Acta Anaesthesiol Scand.* 1994;38:201-205.

25. Sheffield CW, Sessler DI, Hunt TK. Mild hypothermia during halothane induced anaesthesia decreases resistance to Staphlyococcus aureus dermal infection in guinea pigs. *Wound Repair Regeneration.* 1994;2:48-56.

26. Hall JC, Tarala RA, Tapper J, et al. Prevention of respiratory complications after abdominal surgery: a randomised clinical trial. *BMJ.* 1996;312:148-153.

27. Denehy L, Carroll S, Ntoumenopoulos G, et al. A randomized controlled trial comparing periodic mask CPAP with physiotherapy after abdominal surgery. *Physiother Res Int.* 2001;6:236-250.

28. Richter Larsen K, Ingwersen U, Thode S, et al. Mask physiotherapy in patients after heart surgery: a controlled study. *Intensive Care Med.* 1995;21:469-474.

29. Gosselink R, Schrever K, Cops P, et al. Incentive spirometry does not enhance recovery after thoracic surgery. *Crit Care Med.* 2000;28:679-683.

30. Stiller K, Montarello J, Wallace M, et al. Efficacy of breathing and coughing exercises in the prevention of pulmonary complications after coronary artery surgery. *Chest.* 1994;105:741-747.

31. Westerdahl E, Lindmark B, Almgren SO, et al. Chest physiotherapy after coronary artery bypass graft surgery-a comparison of three different deep breathing techniques. *J Rehabil Med.* 2001;33:79-84.

32. Brooks D, Crow J, Kelsey CJ, Lacy JB, Parsons J, Solway S. A clinical practice guideline on peri-operative cardiorespiratory physiotherapy. *Physiotherapy Canada.* 2001;Winter:9-25.

33. Brooks D, Anderson CM, Carter MA, et al. Clinical practice guidelines for suctioning the airway of the intubated and nonintubated patient. *Can Respir J.* 2001;8:163-181.

34. Brooks D, Solway S, Graham I, et al. A survey of suctioning practices among physical therapists, respiratory therapists and nurses. *Can Respir J.* 1999;6:513-520.

35. Marshall MB, Deeb ME, Bleier JIS, et al. Suction vs water seal after pulmonary resection. *Chest.* 2002;121:831-835.

# BIBLIOGRAPHY

Nettina SM. *The Lippincott Manual of Nursing Practice.* 7th ed. Philadelphia: Lippincott Williams & Wilkins; 2000.

Wood M, Wood AJJ. *Drugs and Anesthesia.* Baltimore: Williams & Wilkins; 1990.

# Section 2

# Case Histories

These cases were formulated to reflect typical clinical presentations of patients that reflect a spectrum of the most common patient scenarios treated at entry-level practice. They are usually a combination of information from a variety of sources and do not reflect the clinical manifestations of a single patient. Names of clinics, dates, and other identifying features have been removed and replaced by fictitious names or labels. Any resemblance to an individual, institution, or location is coincidental.

# ABBREVIATIONS USED IN HISTORY/CHART NOTES OF CASES

ABGs: arterial blood gas values
ACBT: active cycle breathing techniques
bilat: bilateral
BP: blood pressure
bpm: beats per minute
br: breaths
C: centigrade
CABG: coronary artery bypass graft
CHF: congestive heart failure
CK: creatine kinase
dL: deciliter
Dx: diagnosis
EKG: electrocardiogram
F: fahrenheit
ft: feet
$HCO_3^-$: bicarbonate ion
Hgb: hemoglobin
HPI: history of present illness
HR: heart rate
Hx: history
IV: intravenous
L: liter
lbs: pounds
meas: measured
MI: myocardial infarct
ml: milliliter
mmol/L: millimole per liter
mmHg: millimeters of mercury
mph: miles per hour
NYD: not yet diagnosed
O/A: on auscultation
OR: operation
PCA: patient-controlled analgesia
PMH: past medical history
ppd: packages per day
pred: predicted
prn: according to circumstances as required
$pCO_2$ or $PaCO_2$: arterial carbon dioxide partial pressure
$pO_2$ or $PaO_2$: arterial oxygen partial pressure
physio: physical therapy
pred: predicted
R/O: rule out
RR: respiratory rate
mg/L: microgram per liter
WBC: white blood cell count
% Prd: percent predicted

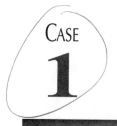

CASE
1

# Atelectasis Postoperatively in an Older Patient

## HISTORY/CHART NOTES

*HPI:* This is a 73-year-old female who had an abdominal aortic aneurysm (AAA) resection and grafting yesterday. Her AAA was 8 cm in size. She spent 3 hours on the OR table in the supine position, 2 hours of this was under general anesthetic.

*PMH:* Includes bladder cancer (untreated) and a transient ischemic attack (TIA) 2 years ago. In addition, she has smoked 1 package of cigarettes per day for 47 years.

*Medications:* None at admission. Postoperatively, she is on an epidural morphine infusion.

*Social Hx:* She lives in Delta with her husband and has 1 flight of stairs to get into the house.

*On examination:* She is awake, alert, and oriented. She is breathing shallowly and rapidly. There is a nasogastric (NG) tube, central line, right radial arterial line, epidural infusion, and urinary catheter in situ. Her RR is 30 BPM, HR is 95 BPM in normal sinus rhythm, BP is 146/70, and she has a temperature of 38.2°C (100.8°F.). She is on 35% oxygen via face mask and her oxygen saturation is 96%. On auscultation: decreased breath sounds, especially in the bases. Her ABG's are:

pH 7.51        $pCO_2$ 27        $pO_2$ 146        $HCO_3^-$ 21

An activity as tolerated order has been written but she has not yet mobilized.

### Questions

1. Identify several factors that place this patient at high risk for postoperative cardiopulmonary complications. List those related to the patient and those related to the procedures performed on her.

## CHEST X-RAY

- Refer to Figure 1-1. The X-ray is fairly good quality but it is slightly underexposed (too white).
- *Begin* by looking at the *soft tissues*.
- Is the heart more central than usual? Yes, the cardiothoracic index is greater than 0.5, indicating an enlarged heart.
- Are there sharp cardiophrenic and costophrenic angles? Look especially on the right.
- Is the trachea deviated more so to the right than usual?
- *Now* look at the *lungs*.
- Can you see increased opacity anywhere in the lung fields?
- Can you see an oblique fissure?
- These are indicative of a loss of volume on which side? Is there any blurring of borders? In which part of the lung fields?
- What are the x-ray signs consistent with atelectasis?

## PULMONARY FUNCTION TESTS

Results from an elderly woman are shown in Table 1-1.

Note the predicted values, the values the women achieved for her best test, the percent predicted of those values and the predicted values for a women of the same height but 20 years of age.

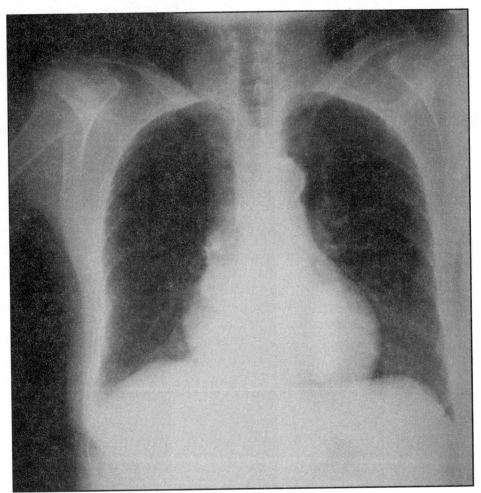

**Figure 1-1.** Chest x-ray of older patient with atelectasis.

Table 1-1

## UNIVERSITY CITY HOSPITAL—RESPIRATORY MEDICINE
## PULMONARY FUNCTION REPORT

| | | | |
|---|---|---|---|
| Name: | | ID#: | |
| Age: | 73 Years | Smoking history: | |
| Sex: | F | | Pack-years: |
| Height: | 160 cm | Race: | C |
| Weight: | 71 kg | | Doctor: |
| | | Tech: | ZXY |
| Test set started: June 21st 15:45:18 | | Report printed: June 21st 15:58:34 | |

(Pre-:    June 21st              08:00:23)

*Best* (±5%)

| Function | Pred | Meas | %Prd | Predicted Values for Age 20 Years Old |
|---|---|---|---|---|
| FVC (L) | 2.69 | 2.67 | 101% | 3.92 |
| FEV$_1$ (L) | 1.90 | 1.70 | 87% | 3.18 |
| FEV$_1$/FVC | 0.71 | 0.64 | 84% | .81 or 81% |

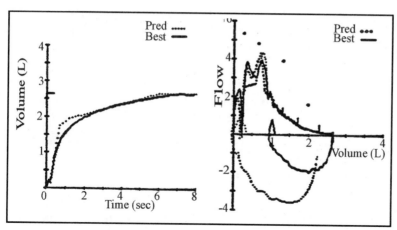

**Figure 1-2.** Spirometric tracing and flow-volume loop for older patient.

## Questions—Most Important Points to Note

1. Do these values indicate any lung pathology?
2. How do the values compare to someone of similar height and gender but a much younger age?
3. How are the predicted values determined?
4. How are the percent predicted values calculated?

## Other Questions

5. What is some of the other information that can be derived from this Pulmonary Function Report regarding patient characteristics and test information?
6. What do the 2 sets of tracings in Figure 1-2 show?

# ARTERIAL BLOOD GASES

This 73-year-old woman has had an abdominal aortic aneurysm resection and grafting yesterday. She is found to be breathing shallowly and rapidly. She is on 35% oxygen via a facemask. Her diagnosis is postoperative atelectasis. Her ABGs are:

pH 7.51          $PaCO_2$ 27          $PaO_2$ 146          $HCO_3^-$ 21

What is the primary acid-base disturbance? Look at the pattern of changes in the pH, $PaCO_2$, and $HCO_3^-$ to determine the primary acid-base disturbance?

Is the $PaO_2$ what you would expect in a healthy individual?

# PHYSICAL THERAPY MANAGEMENT

Develop a physiotherapy problem list and treatment plan for this patient. Identify any treatment outcomes to use for reassessment of the effectiveness of your treatment plan.

| Problem | Outcome Measure |
| --- | --- |
|  |  |
|  |  |
|  |  |
|  |  |
|  |  |

# CASE 2

# Atelectasis Postoperatively in a Smoker

## HISTORY/CHART NOTES

This 54-year-old woman apparently has been having vague epigastric discomfort. She is known to have alcohol abuse, but has no documented liver disease. Now she is admitted with a complete bowel obstruction, witnessed on abdominal x-ray. At the bedside, faint bowel sounds with a distended abdomen were observed. She went for emergency bowel surgery that night. I was able to talk to her husband the following day to confirm that she has smoked between 2 to 3 packs a day for over 30 years. She coughs every morning and expectorates yellowish, sometimes brownish mucus. She was told by the doctor that she has bronchitis but she seldom seeks medical attention. She drinks excessively by herself when she goes to her summer home on Gabriola Island.

She is febrile immediately postoperatively. Today, on day 3 after surgery, her temperature is 39°C (102.2°F).

On examination, the patient is diaphoretic and in moderate respiratory distress. Her breathing is rapid and shallow and she has a loose congested cough.

The patient is referred for intensive chest physiotherapy.

### Questions

1. Briefly describe the pertinent features related to her smoking history.
2. List the clinical signs of a chest infection and atelectasis in this patient. What would you expect to see on chest x-ray and to hear on auscultation?

## CHEST X-RAY

Concentrate on the soft tissues and lung fields in Figure 2-1. What are the x-ray signs consistent with atelectasis? What structures have shifted and in what direction? Is there part of a silhouette of a soft tissue structure that has been obliterated? Refer to the Table 6-1 and Figure 6-3 in Chapter 6 and describe the silhouette sign.

## AUSCULTATION

What are the breath sounds and the adventitious sounds that you would expect to hear from this patient?

## ARTERIAL BLOOD GASES

pH 7.50          $PaCO_2$ 32          $PaO_2$ 85          $HCO_3^-$ 24

What is the acid-base disturbance? Is there compensation? Is there hypoxemia and via which mechanisms?

## PULMONARY FUNCTION TESTS

Pulmonary function tests are not usually done in patients preoperatively for an emergency bowel surgery. Pulmonary function tests can be performed for early detection of lung disease in smokers; however, this is not done routinely.

The average $FEV_1$ and FVC are usually 5% to 10% lower than normal values in young smokers but these values will deteriorate more rapidly at older ages than non-smokers.

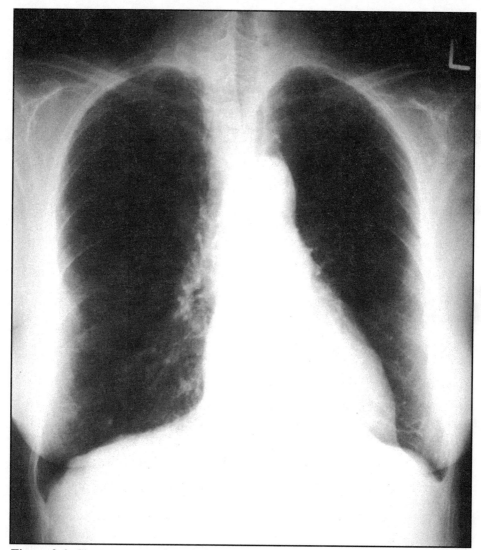

**Figure 2-1.** Chest x-ray—atelectasis in a smoker.

# PHYSICAL THERAPY MANAGEMENT

Formulate a problem list and treatment plan for this patient.

CASE

# 3       Aspiration Pneumonia—Elderly

## HISTORY/CHART NOTES

A 65-year-old man was found unconscious in his apartment with a suicide note. Apparently his wife just passed away suddenly and he was very depressed. A bottle of antifreeze was found next to him.

In the Emergency Room, he was found to be mumbling incoherently. He was foaming from the mouth. His respiration was spontaneous but erratic. A NG tube was inserted after the patient was restrained by 4 nurses. The patient had vomited about 300 ml of watery fluid and undigested food during NG tube insertion. Endotracheal tube insertion was attempted with success after 4 trials. His lungs cleared, oxygenation improved, he remains satisfactory at 96% with supplemental oxygen, and he was extubated yesterday.

The next morning, the patient is found to be febrile. He is drowsy but rousable. His respiratory rate is 26 BPM and receiving 40% of oxygen via facemask. He is using his neck accessory muscles on inspiration. Moist congestion is noted with tactile fremitus in the upper anterior chest.

Intensive chest physiotherapy is prescribed.

### Questions

1. List the sequence of events leading to gastric aspiration.
2. List the physical findings related to respiratory compromise.

## AUSCULTATION

What breath sounds and adventitious sounds would you expect to hear on auscultation?

## CHEST X-RAY

An unconscious man aspirated large amounts of gastric contents following attempted suicide by ingestion of a bottle of antifreeze. He was intubated and admitted to ICU. His chest x-ray is shown in Figure 3-1. Concentrate on the soft-tissues and the lung fields. There are 2 major pathological processes apparent on this CXR and more than one location for both of these pathologies. Describe these.

## ARTERIAL BLOOD GASES

An unconscious man was found in his apartment with a suicide note. A bottle of antifreeze was found next to him. He is referred to you because of aspiration of gastric contents. His ABGs on the mechanical ventilator were:

pH 7.2          PaCO$_2$ 40          HCO$_3^-$ 15          PaO$_2$ 60

Describe the acid-base disturbance. Is there compensation? Is there hypoxemia and via which mechanisms?

## PHYSICAL THERAPY MANAGEMENT

1. List the problems and treatment goals for this patient.
2. What aspects of this patient and his condition need to be considered when positioning him? How would you position him and how often would you recommend a position change?

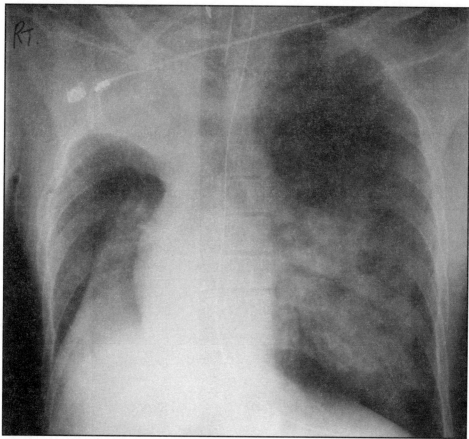

**Figure 3-1.** Chest x-ray of aspiration pneumonia.

CASE

# 4

# Chest Trauma—
# Pneumothorax/Fractured Ribs

## HISTORY/CHART NOTES

This 54-year-old man has a history of alcohol abuse. Yesterday he tripped and fell over the headboard of his bed and sustained trauma to the left side of his chest. On arrival to the Emergency Room, he was found to have multiple rib fractures on the left and a pneumothorax. A chest tube was inserted with good results. He is disabled, secondary to old musculoskeletal injuries sustained in a motor vehicle accident (MVA) in 1969. He is a smoker and although he denies heavy smoking, has marked nicotine stains on his fingers.

Since admission, he has required regular analgesic because of left-sided chest pain. On examination, he was mildly drowsy but oriented in all spheres. He was in moderate distress and experienced marked discomfort with movement or taking a big breath. Examination of thorax revealed subcutaneous emphysema on the left side of the chest with mild bruising on the lateral aspect of the left side of the chest. Abdominal examination was unremarkable.

He requires chest physio and regular use of an incentive spirometer. In addition, salbutamol was prescribed as he has some mild obstructive lung disease. To enhance deep breathing and mobility, bupivacaine was injected into the pleural space. The patient reported a moderate reduction in discomfort in response to this.

## Questions

1. Briefly describe the mechanism of injury and the medical management.
2. Describe the physical findings of this patient related to respiratory compromise.

# PHYSICAL EXAM

See Figure 4-1.
1. List the precautions and considerations when assessing the mobility of a patient with a chest tube.
2. List the structures that the chest tube pierces.

# AUSCULTATION

What are the breath sounds and the adventitious sounds that you would expect to hear when auscultating this patient?

# CHEST X-RAY

Examine Figure 4-2. Can you identify the pneumothorax? Which direction have the soft tissues shifted relative to the pneumothorax? Describe the x-ray signs consistent with a pneumothorax.

# ARTERIAL BLOOD GASES

The admission arterial blood gases for this smoker patient with multiple fracture ribs are:
pH 7.21        PaCO$_2$ 70        HCO$_3^-$ 27        PaO$_2$ 55
Describe the acid-base disturbance. Is there compensation? Is there hypoxemia and via which mechanisms?

# PULMONARY FUNCTION TESTS

Not usually done on in-patients after chest trauma.

# PHYSICAL THERAPY MANAGEMENT

1. List problems and treatment plan.
2. What aspects of medical care need to be carefully coordinated with physical therapy treatment?

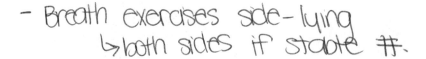
- Breath exercises side-lying
  ↳ both sides if stable #.

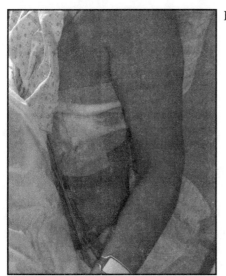

**Figure 4-1.** Photograph of chest tube inserted into patient.

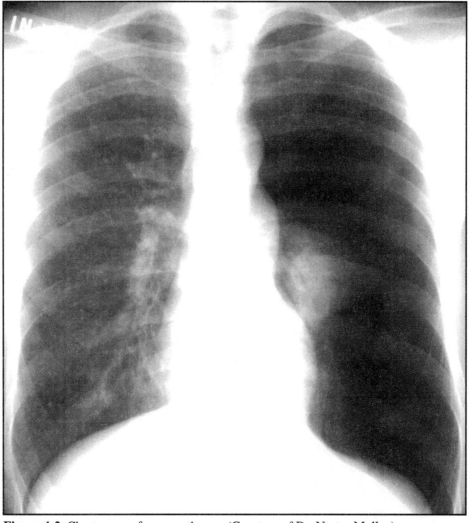

**Figure 4-2.** Chest x-ray of pneumothorax. (Courtesy of Dr. Nestor Muller.)

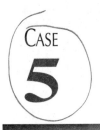

CASE

5

# Restrictive Lung Disease

## HISTORY/CHART NOTES

This 75-year-old man came to his physician 3 years ago complaining of increasing fatigue and shortness of breath during the last year. This fatigue and shortness of breath has progressively worsened over the last 3 years and is especially difficult when he does yard work, and some indoor activities like shaving. Although he smoked 2 ppd from age 13 to 65, he quit upon retirement.

*PMH:* He had his gall bladder removed at age 54. Otherwise, he has been relatively healthy.

*Occupation:* He retired 10 years ago but previously worked on a farm in Saskatchewan. Part of his work entailed shoveling grain in grain elevators during harvest season.

Because of increasing fatigue and limited ability to do daily activities, his family physician referred him to the Uptown Respiratory Rehabilitation Clinic for its outpatient rehabilitation program.

### Questions

1. What are some key features of his medical history that may have contributed to his lung disease?

## AUSCULTATION

1. What breath sounds and adventitious sounds would you expect to hear on auscultation?

## CHEST X-RAY

Refer to Figure 5-1. Concentrate on the soft tissues and the lung fields while considering the pathological changes that occur in restrictive lung disease. Are the lung fields smaller or larger than normal? What other changes do you observe over the lung fields? Describe the x-ray findings consistent with restrictive lung disease.

## ARTERIAL BLOOD GASES

On recent hospital admission, his arterial blood gases were as follows:

pH 7.32          $PaCO_2$ 60          $HCO_3^-$ 30          $PaO_2$ 47          $SaO_2$ 82

What is the primary acid-base disturbance? Is compensation present? Is the patient hypoxemic? If so, is the hypoxemia due to hypoventilation or other causes?

## PULMONARY FUNCTION TESTS

1. Examine the spirometric values: $FEV_1$, FVC, and $FEV_1/FVC$ in Table 5-1. Are these values abnormal? If so, what major category of chronic lung disease are they consistent with? The $FEF_{25-75}$, PEFR, $FEF_{50}$, and $FIF_{50}$ are other values that can be obtained from the forced expiratory and inspiratory maneuvers. Ignore these for now.

2. Look at the lung volumes. SVC is the abbreviation for slow vital capacity. The other abbreviations are all standard abbreviations for lung volumes. With the exception of the ERV, all the lung volumes exhibit changes consistent with what major category of lung disease?

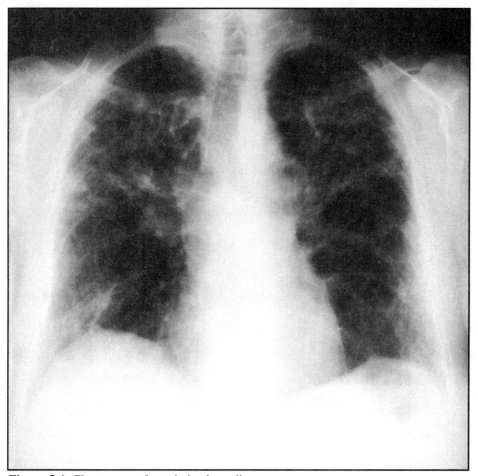

**Figure 5-1.** Chest x-ray of restrictive lung disease.

3. Look at the flow-volume loop (Figure 5-2 left panel). This information is derived from a forced expiration followed by a forced inspiration. Are the inspiratory or expiratory flows low, high, or normal? What would you expect in this patient? Is the vital capacity (horizontal dimension) in this patient low, high, or normal? What would you expect in this patient?

# PHYSICAL THERAPY MANAGEMENT

1. What are some of his major complaints that might be addressed by physiotherapy and respiratory rehabilitation?

Table 5-1

## Pulmonary Function Report for Patient With Restrictive Lung Disease

PULMONARY FUNCTION LABORATORY - REPORT

| Patient: | | Height: | 69 in or 174 cm | Sex: | M |
|----------|--|---------|-----------------|------|---|
| ID Number: | | Weight: | 187 lb or 85 kg | BSA: | 2.00 |
| Date: | | Age: | 75 | BP: | 768 |
| Time of day: | 1300 | Temp: | 22°C, 71.6°F | ATPS: | .917 |
| Physician: | | Referring Physician: | | Therapist: | |
| Ex-Smoker | 1 pack/day | 10 years not Smoking | | | |

| (BTPS) | Pre-dilator | | | Post-dilator | | |
|--------|-------------|--------|------|--------------|--------|----------|
| Spirometry | Actual | % Pred | Pred | Actual | % Pred | % Change |
| FVC (L) | 3.21 | 77 | 4.18 | 3.22 | 77 | 0 |
| FEV-1 (L) | 2.75 | 86 | 3.18 | 2.78 | 87 | 1 |
| FEV-1/FVC (%) | 86 | | 76 | 86 | | 1 |
| FEF$^{25\text{-}75}$ (L/S) | 3.61 | 127 | 2.83 | 3.99 | 141 | 11 |
| PEFR (L/S) | 14.35 | 185 | 7.74 | 13.04 | 168 | -9 |
| FEF$^{50}$ (L/S) | 6.94 | 166 | 4.18 | 7.07 | 169 | 2 |
| FIF$^{50}$ (L/S) | 7.37 | 176 | 4.18 | 6.07 | 145 | -18 |

| (BTPS) | Pre-dilator | | |
|--------|-------------|--------|------|
| Lung Volumes | Actual | % Pred | Pred |
| SVC (L) | 3.12 | 74 | 4.18 |
| IC (L) | 1.96 | 59 | 3.31 |
| ERV (L) | 1.16 | 132 | 0.88 |
| RV (L) | 1.17 | 46 | 2.53 |
| FRC (L) | 2.33 | 68 | 3.40 |
| TLC (L) | 4.29 | 64 | 6.71 |
| RV/TLC (%) | 27 | | 38 |

| Diffusion | Pre-dilator | | |
|-----------|-------------|--------|------|
| | Actual | % Pred | Pred |
| DLCO (SB) | 12.74 | 58 | 22.11 |
| DL/VA | 3.12 | 69 | 4.53 |
| VA (BTPS) | 4.08 | 61 | 6.71 |

✱ Table 7.1

**Figure 5-2.** Flow-volume loop of patient with restrictive lung disease.

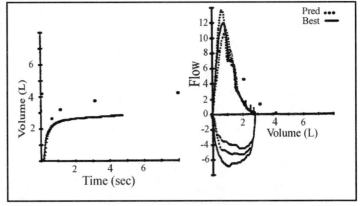

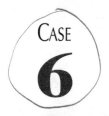

CASE
6

# Stable Chronic Obstructive Pulmonary Disease

## HISTORY/CHART NOTES

The patient is a pleasant 70-year-old woman. She has had progressive shortness of breath over the last few years. At present, she has difficulty walking the 2 blocks to the community center. She does not drive, cannot manage stairs at all, and does not really get out of her house. She has a homemaker to help with her laundry and with some of the heavier housework.

Patient has a modest cough. She occasionally brings up one teaspoon of sputum every day. She has been a heavy smoker in the past. She used to smoke 2 packs of cigarettes per day since age 20 and she quit smoking approximately 6 years ago. She uses salbutamol intermittently and she does not notice improvement with this.

Patient presents symptoms suggestive of chronic airflow obstruction and emphysema. Patient might benefit from the respiratory rehabilitation program but I think we would best leave this until after the hot weather of the summer is over.

*broncho- dilator (eg. ventilator)*
*△ 14-15% = lung disease is reversible*

### Questions

1. Describe the functional history of this patient.
2. Describe the smoking history of this patient.

## AUSCULTATION

Describe the breath sounds and adventitious sounds that you would expect to hear on auscultation.

## CHEST X-RAY

Concentrate on soft tissues and lung fields in Figure 6-1. Are the lungs bigger or smaller than usual? Which soft tissues are drastically altered? Describe the x-ray findings that are consistent with COPD.

## ARTERIAL BLOOD GASES

pH 7.32        $PaCO_2$ 60        $PaO_2$ 51        $HCO_3^-$ 31

What is the primary acid-base disturbance? Is compensation present? Is the patient hypoxemic? If so, is the hypoxemia due to hypoventilation or other causes?

## PULMONARY FUNCTION TESTS

See Table 6-1 for the patient's data.
1. Look at the $FEV_1$, FVC and $FEV_1$/FVC ratio. Of what pattern of disease are these results suggestive? Why? Is there a significant bronchodilator response? How do you know?
2. Look at the lung volumes. What pattern of lung disease are these results suggestive of? What pathophysiologic factors contribute to such large lung volumes?

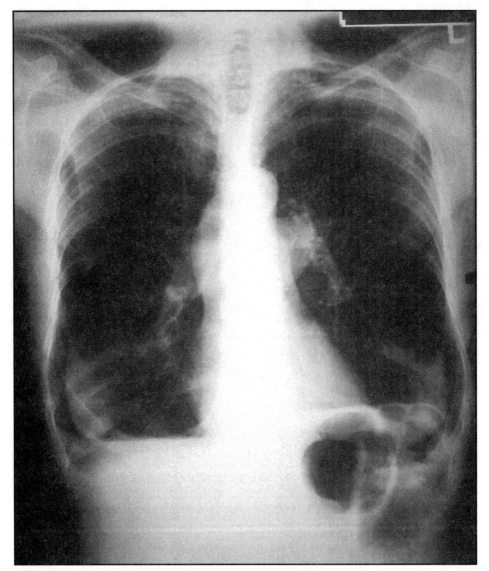

**Figure 6-1.** Chest x-ray of COPD patient.

# PHYSICAL THERAPY MANAGEMENT

1. List the problem list and treatment plan for this patient.
2. What challenges or obstacles do you think this woman will need to overcome to regularly attend a respiratory rehabilitation program? What support would facilitate her ability to attend the rehabilitation program?

Table 6-1

## Pulmonary Function Report for Patient With COPD

(Pre- vs. Post- Comparison)

Name:    Age: 70  Sex: F    Height: 167 cm    Weight: 57 kg
Predicted:                                                    Report: FULL PFT

### FVC

Pre-: 13:55:48                              Post-:14:15:56

| Function | Pred | Pre- Meas | % Prd | Post- Meas | % Prd | % Change |
|---|---|---|---|---|---|---|
| FVC (L) | 3.10 | 2.18 | 70 | 2.44 | 79 | 12 |
| $FEV_1$ (L) | 2.35 | 0.57 | 24 | 0.78 | 33 | 37 |
| $FEV_1$/FVC | 0.75 | 0.26 | 35 | 0.32 | 43 | 23 |
| PEFR (L/s) | 5.70 | 2.71 | 48 | 2.57 | 45 | -5 |
| $FEF_{50}$ (L/s) | 4.49 | 0.06 | 1 | 0.38 | 8 | 533 |
| $FEF_{25-75}$ (L/s) | 6.36 | 0.18 | 3 | 0.34 | 5 | 89 |
| FIVC (L) | 3.10 | | | 2.40 | 77 | |
| $FIF_{50}$ (L/s) | | | | 3.89 | | |

### FRC/SVC

(Pre-: 06-25-2001        14:11:23)

(No Post-FRC/SVC performed)

| Function | Pred | Pre- Meas | % Prd |
|---|---|---|---|
| SVC (L, BTPS) | 3.10 | 3.22 | 104 |
| ERV (L, BTPS) | 0.72 | 1.44 | 200 |
| FRC (L, BTPS) | 3.05 | 4.60 | 151 |
| RV(L, BTPS) | 2.33 | 3.16 | 136 |
| TLC (L, BTPS) | 5.32 | 6.38 | 120 |
| RV/TLC | 0.43 | 0.50 | 115 |
| IC (L, BTPS) | 2.27 | 1.78 | 78 |

### DLCO

(Pre-: 06-25-2001        14:42:49)

(No Post-DLCO performed)

| Function | Pred | Post- Meas | % Prd |
|---|---|---|---|
| DLCO (ml/m/mm Hg) | 21.21 | 9.19 | 43 |
| DLCO/VA | 4.21 | 1.63 | 39 |
| DLCO Hgb corr | | | |
| DLCO/VA Hgb corr | | | |
| VA (L, BTPS) | 5.35 | 5.63 | 105 |
| Hgb (g/100ml) | | | |

Test performed post bronchodilator.

# CASE
# 7
# Cystic Fibrosis

## HISTORY/CHART NOTES

This is a 22-year-old male who was diagnosed with cystic fibrosis at 6 months of age. He had 2 older brothers with cystic fibrosis who have since died of respiratory complications. He is unemployed and is on social assistance. This patient is considered to have moderate to severe disability and is undergoing testing to determine his eligibility for transplant. He presents to the hospital complaining of a 3-week history of a worsening productive cough, dyspnea, occasional hemoptysis, extreme fatigue, and weight loss. He is colonized with *staphylococcus aureus* and is resistant to most antibiotics. He also has an asthmatic component to his disease and takes salbutamol via puffer q4h prn. He claims to be coughing up one-half to one-third cup of dark green, thick sputum per day. He usually uses autogenic drainage and exercise to keep his chest clear.

### Questions

1. What other information besides that shown for this case would you want on your initial assessment?
2. Examine Figure 7-1 to observe some of the features of a 22-year-old man with cystic fibrosis. List the features of this man that are consistent with respiratory compromise and cystic fibrosis.

## AUSCULTATION

Describe the breath sounds and adventitious sounds that you would expect to hear on auscultation.

## CHEST X-RAY

Observe the chest x-ray in Figure 7-2. Concentrate on the bony skeleton, soft tissues, and lung fields. There are definite abnormalities in each of these 3 categories. Describe the x-ray findings consistent with cystic fibrosis.

## ARTERIAL BLOOD GASES

Shown below are the arterial blood gases of this person with cystic fibrosis during an acute exacerbation. What is the primary acid-base disturbance? Is compensation present? Is the patient hypoxemic? If so, is the hypoxemia due to hypoventilation or other causes?

pH 7.30          $PaCO_2$ 110          $HCO_3^-$ 52          $PaO_2$ 45

## PULMONARY FUNCTION TESTS

Examine the patient's data in Table 7-1.
1. What kind of lung disease pattern is shown by the $FEV_1$, FVC, and $FEV_1$/FVC ratio?
2. Which curve is the flow-volume loop? What characteristic shape is shown on the flow-volume loop?
3. Look at the flow-time curve in Figure 7-3. Why do you think the flow-time curve terminated between 9 and 10 seconds?

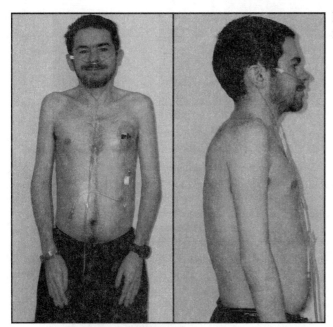

**Figure 7-1.** Frontal view and side profile of patient with cystic fibrosis.

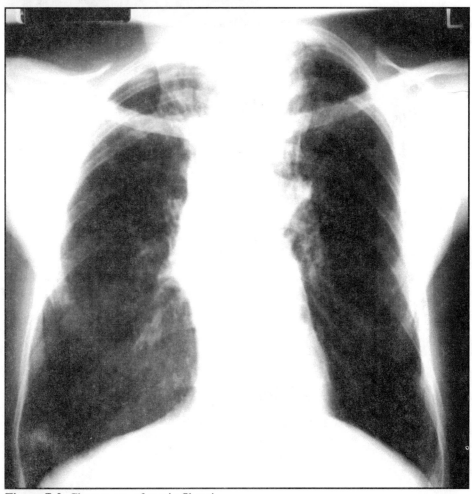

**Figure 7-2.** Chest x-ray of cystic fibrosis.

Table 7-1

## Pulmonary Function Report of Patient With Cystic Fibrosis

CITY HOSPITAL RESPIRATORY SERVICES
BEDSIDE SPIROMETRY

| PT: | Height: | 178 cm | Weight: | 64.2 kg |
|-----|---------|--------|---------|---------|
| PT#: | Sex: | M | Age: | 22 |
| Date: Feb 15th | Time: | 13:37:15 | Smk Hx: | |
| Occ: | Race: | C | | |
| Physician: | Tech: | XYZ | | |

| | | Post-Drug | | |
|---|---|---|---|---|
| *Spirometry* | *Predicted* | *Post* | *% Post* | |
| FVC (L) | 5.46 | 2.11 | 38 | |
| $FEV_1$ (L) | 4.32 | 1.08 | 25 | |
| $FEV_1/FVC$ (%) | 79 | 51 | 65 | |
| $FEF_{25-75}$ (L/S) | 4.59 | 0.40 | 8 | |
| FEFmax (L/S) | 9.66 | 5.14 | 53 | |
| $FEF_{50}$ (L/S) | 6.15 | 0.52 | 8 | |
| $FIF_{50}$ (L/S) | | 4.01 | | |

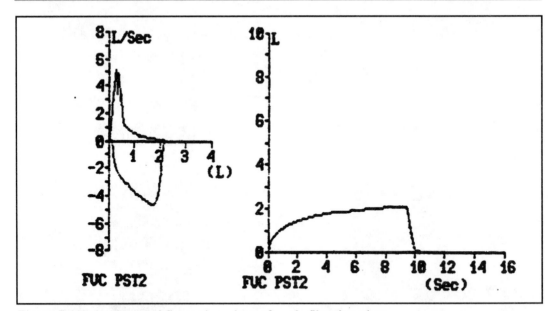

**Figure 7-1.** Spirometry and flow-volume loop of cystic fibrosis patient.

# PHYSICAL THERAPY MANAGEMENT

1. What other health professionals would you expect to see involved with this patient? Why?
2. List the problem list and treatment plan.

## CASE

# 8

# Asthma—Acute Exacerbation

## HISTORY/CHART NOTES

A 20-year-old female was transported on a stretcher to the medical and physiotherapy facility at a national track meet. Her teammates report that she collapsed at the end of the 4 x 800 M. They stated that she does this all the time and has done so after other 800-M heats and practices. She becomes grey and extremely short of breath and usually is not able to speak during the first 5 minutes after the race. It usually takes approximately 25 minutes before she recovers. To their knowledge, she has never received medication or treatment for this but it has been described as "panic attacks."

You are the only physiotherapist in the facility. The physician has gone across the track to deal with another injury. The woman is still very out of breath but her teammates state that she is doing better.

### Questions

1. What assessment parameters should you monitor?
2. What factors would be indicative of worsening or improvement of her respiratory and cardiovascular status?
   Her PEFR is 3.81 L/sec. The age predicted PEFR for a person the same age and height is 8.87 L/sec.
   Do you think this person is having a panic attack?

## AUSCULTATION

What are the breath sounds and adventitious sounds that you would expect to hear on auscultation?

## CHEST X-RAY

After a similar event, she went to Emergency Room and had a chest x-ray (Figure 8-1). Identify the characteristic features of this x-ray. What do you think it will look like when the patient is feeling well and her pulmonary function is near normal?

## ARTERIAL BLOOD GASES

Her arterial blood gases at the Emergency Room were
pH 7.25      $PaCO_2$ 59      $HCO_3^-$ 26      $PaO_2$ 60
What is the primary acid-base disturbance? Is compensation present? Is the patient hypoxemic? If so, is the hypoxemia due to hypoventilation or other causes?

## SPIROMETRY AND EXPIRATORY FLOW RATES

Her spirometry and PEFR before and after the use of bronchodilators are shown in Table 8-1. Her height is 180 cm. Interpret the spirometric values. What pattern of lung pathology is shown? Complete the table and calculate the % predicted values and the % improvement after bronchodilator administration.

## PHYSICAL THERAPY MANAGEMENT

What health professionals would you advise this woman to see?

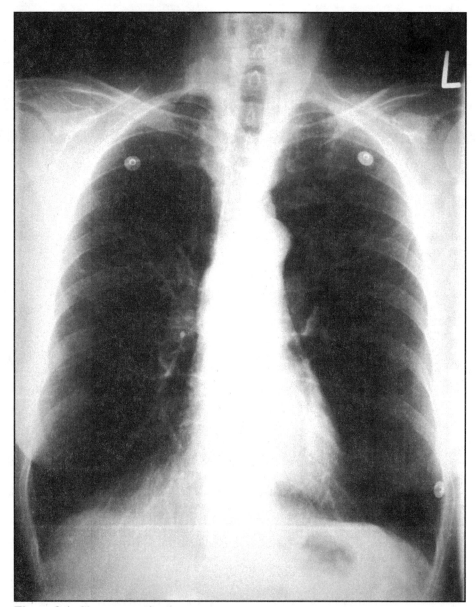

**Figure 8-1.** Chest x-ray of asthma.

Table 8-1

*Spirometry and Peak Expiratory Flow Rates*

|  | Pre BD | Pred | % Predicted | Post BD | % Improvement |
|---|---|---|---|---|---|
| FEV$_1$ | 1.8 | 3.8 L |  | 3.0 |  |
| FVC | 3.2 | 4.7 |  | 4.2 |  |
| FEV$_1$/FVC | 56% | 80% |  | 71% |  |
| PEFR | 3.81 | 8.87 |  |  |  |

# CASE 9

# Chronic Obstructive Pulmonary Disease and Pneumonia

## HISTORY/CHART NOTES

This 60-year-old man complains of feeling feverish, increased shortness of breath. and general weakness. He went to see his family doctor 2 days ago and was prescribed antibiotics. He said that his breathing has not improved and he is having diarrhea. He says that he is not coughing up much mucus at this time. This morning, he felt more short of breath and had to be admitted to hospital. Dx: COPD/emphysema with pneumonia. An arterial blood sample was taken in the emergency department. The results were:

pH   7.22      $PaCO_2$ 50          $HCO_3^-$ 20       $PaO_2$ 50

On examination, his face is flushed and diaphoretic. His forehead is warm to touch. He is predominately a mouth breather with obvious accessory muscle use during inspiration. He has to pause every sentence to catch his breath during the interview and prefers to sit up rather than lie down. There is an increased A-P diameter in his chest with decreased rib cage movements during inspiration. Slight indrawing of the intercostal muscles is also noted during inspiration. Lateral costal expansion is decreased especially on the right base. There are obvious nicotine stains on his fingers. Minimal edema is noted in both of his ankles. He is referred to you for assessment.

### Questions

1. List the relevant features pertinent to the history of his acute exacerbation.
2. List the pertinent physical findings related to worsening of his respiratory status.

## PHYSICAL FEATURES

Observe the physical features of the gentleman in Figure 9-1. List the physical features of this man that are consistent with respiratory compromise and COPD.

## AUSCULTATION

What breath sounds and adventitious sounds would you expect to hear on auscultation?

## CHEST X-RAY

What features of the chest x-ray are consistent with COPD and what features are consistent with pneumonia in Figure 9-2? Considering the silhouette sign, can you determine which lobe(s) the pneumonia is located? Can you see tubing crossing the patient's chest? What do you think this tubing is?

## ARTERIAL BLOOD GASES

These are the ABGs of a man with COPD admitted to hospital:

PH 7.22        $PaCO_2$ 50          $HCO_3^-$ 20        $PaO_2$ 50

What is the primary acid-base disturbance? Is compensation present? Is the patient hypoxemic? If so, is the hypoxemia due to hypoventilation or other causes?

**Figure 9-1.** Frontal and side views of COPD patient with pneumonia.

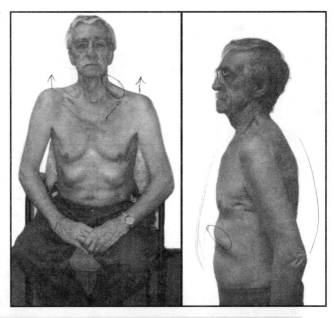

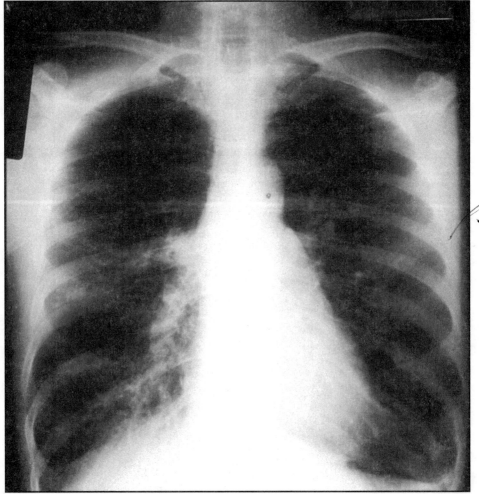

**Figure 9-2.** Chest x-ray of COPD patient with pneumonia.

# PHYSICAL THERAPY MANAGEMENT

1. List the problem list and treatment plan for this patient.
2. Would your treatment plan be different for this patient compared to a young adult with a similar pneumonia? Why or why not?

CASE

# 10

# Left-Sided Congestive Heart Failure—Pulmonary Edema

## HISTORY

This is a 62-year-old man who was admitted into the hospital 3 days ago for a mitral valve replacement. He had his surgery yesterday afternoon.

- *HPI:* Mitral valve replacement for a prolapsed mitral valve yesterday. 3 hours after surgery, he was returned to OR for arrest of postoperative bleed. Extubated this morning at 7:00 am.
- *PMH:*
  o 35 pack/year history of smoking
  o No known respiratory condition
  o Osteoarthritis of left hip, walks with a limp
- *Social History:*
  o Lives with wife in 2-story house in Ladner, B.C.
  o Works in a plant as a foreman
  o Likes to play golf and walk along the dikes

The nurse informs you that this patient has been referred for a physiotherapy consult.

## *On Examination*

*Patient status 12 hours postoperatively:*
- $SaO_2$ 93% on 40% via facemask
- LOC: easily rousable, follows commands well
- BP 162/76
- HR 135 BPM, RR: 27/minute
- Temperature 37.1°C (98.8°F)
- Skin: cool and clammy
- Pain Level: 6/10
- Hgb: 6.5 g/dL
- O/A: A/E t/o, ↓ bilat bases with fine late inspiratory crackles in sitting
- In the chart, you also find the following doctor's orders: "patient on bed rest, physio to see"

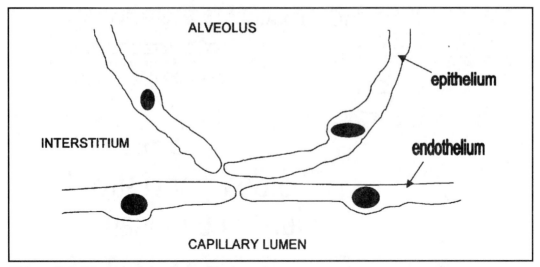

**Figure 10-1.** Diagram of alveolar-capillary membrane.

## Questions

1. Why does mitral valve prolapse lead to regurgitation? What are some of the causes of mitral valve prolapse leading to regurgitation? What are some of the signs and symptoms of mitral valve prolapse?

2. Examine Starling's equation (under section titled Pulmonary Edema in Chapter 18, Respiratory Conditions) and the description of the factors that contribute to capillary exchange and the net outflow of fluid from the capillaries. Which is the primary factor that increases the interstitial fluid level in left-sided heart failure? Incorporate the factors outlined in this equation in Figure 10-1. Use different-sized arrows to indicate the relative contribution of each factor.

*2 Days Postoperatively:* You have now been seeing the patient for 1 day. The bed rest order was lifted today. You assess the patient and receive the following information:

- $SaO_2$ 96% on 2L/min $O_2$ via nasal prongs
- LOC: Awake, alert & oriented
- BP: lying—128/67; sitting HOB increased to 75°—90/50
- HR 85 RR: 26
- Temp 36.9°C 98.4°F
- Skin: warm and dry
- Pain Level: 3/10 at rest, 7/10 with coughing
- Cough: strong with minimal production of sputum
- Hgb: 12.5 g/dL
- O/A: ↓ to LLL with fine late inspiratory crackles in sitting
- Subjective: weak, fatigues easily, decreased energy, light headedness when HOB—with nausea

3. Has the patient improved or deteriorated? On what information do you base your answer?

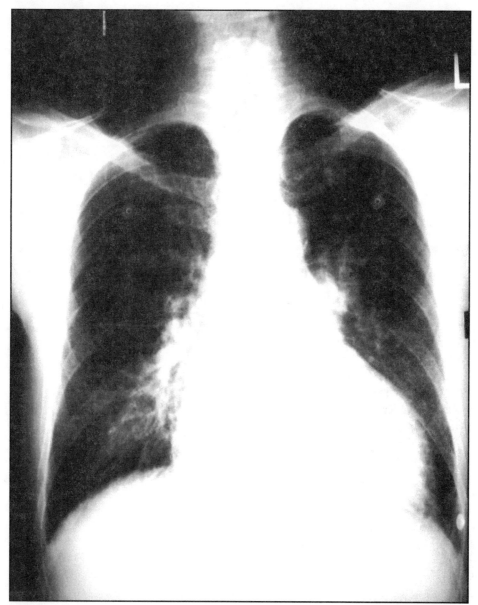

**Figure 10-2.** Chest x-ray of heart failure and pulmonary edema.

# CHEST X-RAY

Examine the chest x-ray closely (Figure 10-2). What is the most dramatic soft tissue change? Can you see one or more pathological patterns on the lung fields? Describe them.

# PHYSICAL THERAPY MANAGEMENT

How will your treatment approach change? How will you progress your treatment as the patient improves?

# REFERENCES

1. Harrison TR. *Harrison's principles of internal medicine*. New York: McGraw-Hill; 2001.
   (A good text to derive information about mitral valve prolapse)

2. http://www.merck.com/pubs/mmanual/

CASE

# 11

# Acute Myocardial Infarction—Good Recovery

## HISTORY/CHART NOTES

- *HPI:* Mr. G is a 75-year-old man complaining of left-sided chest pain radiating to his axillary area. The chest discomfort was described as if somebody was sitting on his chest. The pain came on just after supper about an hour ago.
- *Dx:* Non Q-wave anterior myocardial infarct.
- *Investigation:* Serial EKG showed ST segment depression in the precordial leads. Serial troponin I showed an increase to 10 mg/L at 6 hours and 20 mg/L at 18 hours. HR is 112 and in sinus rhythm. BP is 145/100.
- *PMH:* Appendectomy. Cancer of the prostate.

Mr. G's cardiac risk factors:
- Smoker 4 cigarettes a day and up to a half a pack a day in the past
- Occasional glass of wine
- No diabetes
- No hypertension
- No known cholesterol problems
- Moderately obese and "does not like to work up a sweat"

### Questions

1. Assess the cardiac risk factors for this patient and outline your plan for secondary prevention.

## ELECTROCARDIOGRAM

Review the V2 and V3 leads in the EKG (Figure 11-1) of this patient. What are the main features consistent with an MI shown by these leads?

## PHYSICAL THERAPY MANAGEMENT

1. On day 2 post-MI, the patient is stable and transferred to the step down cardiac unit. You were asked to see Mr. G for rehabilitation. Outline your in-patient rehabilitation plan for this patient.

**Figure 11-1.** Electrocardiogram.

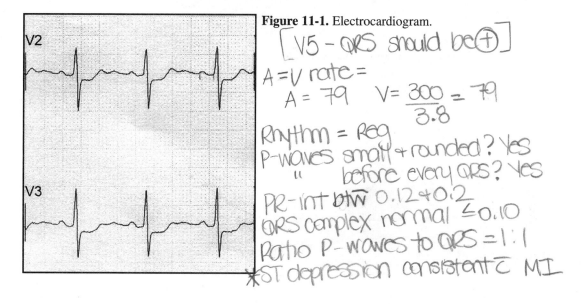

[handwritten annotations, right of figure:]

[V5 – QRS should be ⊕]

A = V rate =
  A = 79    V = 300 = 79
              3.8

Rhythm = Reg
P-waves small + rounded? Yes
  "    before every QRS? Yes
PR-int btw 0.12 + 0.2
QRS complex normal ≤0.10
Ratio P-waves to QRS = 1:1
*ST depression consistent c̄ MI

## CASE 12

# Acute Myocardial Infarction— Coronary Artery Bypass Graft (CABG)

## HISTORY/CHART NOTES

- *HPI:* Mr. F developed chest pain during an exercise stress test. He was subsequently transferred to the coronary care unit and then to the cardiac catheterization laboratory. Angioplasty and stenting were performed. However, the patient continued to have cardiac symptoms over night and emergency CABG x3 were done early this morning.

- *Stress test report:* Using the Bruce protocol, the patient exercised for 8 minutes reaching a target heart rate of 128 beats per minute which is submaximal of his age-predicted target. Three minutes into exercise, his ST segments began elevating in the inferior leads. He therefore had an acute inferior infarct. His stress test was stopped. He complained of vague chest pain.

### Questions

1. After CABG, what are the wound and sternal precautions taught to patients and why are these instructions provided?

## ELECTROCARDIOGRAM

1. Identify the acute EKG changes.

## PHYSICAL THERAPY MANAGEMENT

1. On day 2 post-CABG, the patient is stable and transferred to the step down cardiac unit. You were asked to see Mr. G for rehabilitation. Outline your in-patient rehabilitation plan for this patient.

**Figure 12-1.**
Electrocardi-
ogram.

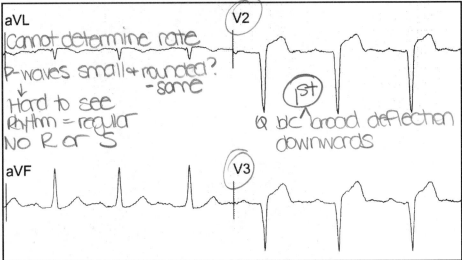

# CASE
# 13

# Chronic Heart Failure—
# Cardiomyopathy

## HISTORY/CHART NOTES

- *HPI:* Mr. C is a 59-year-old man complaining of progressive shortness of breath with exertion, dry cough, weight gain, and stiffness in hands and feet especially in the morning.
- *Dx:* SOB NYD
- *PMH:* Hypertension and appendectomy. Patient denied cardiac history and is a non-smoker. Consumes a few glasses of wine a week.
- *Social & Functional history:* Lives with wife in a 2-level house. He took early retirement from an auto assembly plant last year. Heavy housework and mowing the lawn is getting difficult. He has to take it easy with his gardening. Some days, he has to take it easy when climbing up stairs. He tries to keep active with morning walks with his wife but has been cutting back on the distance during the last month.
- *On examination:* Mr. C was sitting upright on the stretcher. His BP on admission to the Emergency Room was 151/95. Heart rate was 105. His respiratory rate was in the high 20's. He requires oxygen at 6 L/min to maintain oxygen saturation above 94%. Jugular veins were distended and ankle edema was marked. Inspiratory crackles were heard from the mid to lower lung zones posteriorly.
- *Investigations:* Initial blood work reviewed normal WBC and creatinine. Admitting CK estimate is 40 and troponin I is 0.1. Admitting electrocardiogram showed sinus tachycardia.

Subsequent investigation by coronary angiography and left heart catheterization reviewed idiopathic dilated cardiomyopathy.

### Questions

1. What are the differentiating features of acute coronary syndrome from this form of heart failure?
2. From the clinical information given, what is his pre-admission cardiac function?

## AUSCULTATION

What breath sounds and adventitious sounds would you expect to hear from this patient?

## PHYSICAL THERAPY MANAGEMENT

After the patient's medical condition is optimized and given the patient's functional history, what advice would you give to the patient in terms of activity and exercise?

<br>

CASE

# 14

# Chronic Heart Failure—Post Myocardial Infarct

## HISTORY/CHART NOTES

- *HPI:* Mrs. H is a 74-year-old woman with known CAD. She complained of flu-like symptoms, feeling tired, shortness of breath with minimal exertion, and dry cough especially at night for more than a week. Since yesterday, her shortness of breath has increased to the extent that she can no longer manage at home.

- *Dx:* CHF. R/O pneumonia

- *PMH:* Large anterior MI 2 years ago. She quit smoking 10 years ago. Frequent hospital admissions for pulmonary edema. Left ventricular ejection fraction was 25% 6 months ago. Mrs. H also has diabetes and uses insulin, 50 units in the morning and 40 units in the evening.

- *Social & functional history:* Lives alone in a ground floor apartment. Manages to look after self but needs help with house cleaning. She seldom goes out and can only walk 2 city blocks.

- *On examination:* Mrs. H was sitting upright on the stretcher. Her BP on admission to the Emergency Room was 121/90. Heart rate was 118. Her respiratory rate was in the mid 30s. She required 50% oxygen to maintain oxygen saturation above 92%. Jugular veins were distended and ankle edema was marked. The extremities were cold and clammy. Inspiratory crackles were heard from the mid to lower lung zones.

- *Investigations:* Initial blood work revealed normal WBC and creatinine. Admitting CK estimate is 40 and troponin I is 1.0. Admitting electrocardiogram showed left atrial enlargement and old anterior infarct with Q wave in leads V1 to V4, which were unchanged from the last report. ABGs are:

  pH 7.38 $\quad\quad\quad$ PaCO$_2$ 40 mmHg $\quad\quad\quad$ PaO$_2$ 64 mmHg $\quad\quad\quad$ HCO$_3^-$ 23 mmol/L

- *Medical management:* Mrs. H was given IV lasix and morphine. Nitroglycerin was given sublingually. Foley catheter was inserted. High flow oxygen was used to maintain oxygenation. Patient was subsequently transferred to the coronary care unit and put on bed rest.

### Questions

1. What are the differentiating features between pneumonia and acute heart failure?
2. From the clinical information given, what was her preadmission cardiac function level?

## ARTERIAL BLOOD GASES

Is there a primary acid-base disturbance? Is there hypoxemia?

pH 7.38                 $PaCO_2$ 40 mmHg                 $PaO_2$ 64 mmHg                 $HCO_3^-$ 23 mmol/L

## PHYSICAL THERAPY MANAGEMENT

Once the patient's medical condition is optimized and given the patient's functional history, what advice can you give to patient in terms of activity and exercise?

## CASE 15

# Exercising Outpatient— Arrhythmia and Hypotension

## HISTORY/CHART NOTES

A 54-year-old woman with "chronic fatigue syndrome" was referred for an exercise conditioning program. Her general practitioner has cleared her for exercise. When screened by the physical therapist using the Exercise ACSM Screening Questionnaire (see Chapter 9, Table 9-3), she answered negatively to all questions with the exception of some complaints of joint pain that come and go when she is feeling especially fatigued. Routine exercise testing is not performed for patients entering an exercise conditioning program in your department.

This is her second physical therapy session after the initial assessment.

After exercising on the treadmill for 5 minutes at a speed of 2.0 mph, flat grade, she complains of light-headedness and feeling dizzy. Her pulse, which had increased to 130 BPM during the first part of her exercise program, has decreased to a regular-irregular rhythm of 80 BPM.

### Questions

What should the therapist do?
1. What should the therapist's instructions be to the patient?
2. What should be monitored?
3. What should be communicated to nearby colleagues?

## ELECTROCARDIOGRAM

An EKG monitor is in the department, and the therapist immediately connects the patient to the monitor. The tracing from a modified V5 is shown in Figure 15-1.
1. What is the rate, rhythm, and aberrant conduction shown?
2. What should be done at this point in time before the patient leaves the department?
3. Will you refer the patient to another health professional before exercising her again in the physical therapy department?

**Figure 15-1.** EKG tracing from modified V5.

19

1a squares x0.2sec =3.8
7b7 3.8sec
Atrial

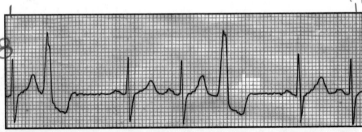

CASE
# 16

# Atelectasis—Postoperatively in an Older Patient—Hypotensive and Atrial Fibrillation

## HISTORY/CHART NOTES

- *HPI:* Mrs. H is a 78-year-old female who had a right hemicolectomy complicated by intraoperative bleeding. She spent 2.5 hours on the OR table in the supine position; 2 hours of this was under general anaesthetic.
- *PMH:* Hysterectomy, a MI 2 years ago, and atrial fibrillation.
- *Social Hx:* She lives in a senior's apartment with her husband and has one flight of stairs to get onto her floor.
- *On examination day one post-op:* She is awake, alert, and oriented. She is breathing shallowly and rapidly. There is a NG tube, central line, epidural infusion, and urinary catheter in situ. Her RR is 24 breaths per minute, HR is 90 BPM in normal sinus rhythm, BP is 148/92, and she has a temperature of 38.4. She is on 40% oxygen via facemask and her oxygen saturation is 97%. On auscultation: decreased breath sounds, especially in the bases. An activity as tolerated order has been written but she has not yet been out of bed.

### Questions

What are the common clinical findings of patients in atrial fibrillation?

## ELECTROCARDIOGRAM

Identify the acute EKG changes (Figure 16-1).

## PHYSICAL THERAPY MANAGEMENT

By day 2 postop, patient was able to mobilize with an IV pole and your assistance for 80 feet. On day 3 after surgery, however your patient complains of feeling tired, dizzy while in bed, and has had palpitations. What cardiopulmonary assessment procedures will you perform?

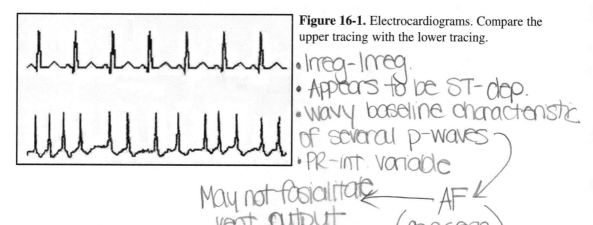

**Figure 16-1.** Electrocardiograms. Compare the upper tracing with the lower tracing.

- Irreg-Irreg.
- Appears to be ST-dep.
- Wavy baseline characteristic of several p-waves
- PR-int. variable

May not facilitate vent. output      AF (concern)

# CASE 17
# Atelectasis—Postoperatively in an Obese Patient—Pulmonary Embolus and Acute Arterial Insufficiency

## HISTORY/CHART NOTES

- *HPI*: Mrs. B is 55 years old and she called the emergency medical service (EMS) when she experienced sudden onset of intense abdominal pain with vomiting and diarrhea. She was transported to the hospital and underwent an emergency bowel resection for small bowel ischemia. She weighs 360 lbs.
- *PMH*: Previous myocardial infarctions x 2, unstable angina, and one previous admission for acute respiratory failure.
- *Meds*: Includes nitroglycerine and diltiazem (for BP). She is using patient controlled analgesia (PCA) for postoperative pain control.
- *Social Hx*: She lives alone in an apartment that has an elevator. She is a non-smoker.
- *On examination*: She is a morbidly obese individual observed lying supine with the head of the bed elevated to 30 degrees. She is very drowsy, but is rousable. She is noted to be mouth breathing with decreased diaphragmatic movement and decreased lateral costal expansions bilaterally. She has an IV in situ in her left forearm for PCA morphine. Her respiratory rate is 8 breaths per minute, with occasional apneic periods of >25 seconds. She is on oxygen at 3 L/min via nasal prongs and her oxygen saturation is 95%. Her HR is 110 BPM, BP 165/86, and temperature is normal at present. Her cough is strong, loose, and productive of a small amount of clear mucoid secretions. She is allowed activity as tolerated but she has not yet been out of bed since her surgery 3 days ago.
- *Entry from medical incident report*: On day 3 postoperative, as part of the routine postoperative management, the physical therapist instructed breathing exercises and ambulated the patient with an IV pole for 20 ft. The therapist then left the patient in a chair. Within 5 minutes, the patient complained of sudden onset of shortness of breath, profuse sweating, and feeling of general unwellness.

### Questions

1. What are the most common causes and presentations of pulmonary emboli (PE)?
2. How would you differentiate between an arterial insufficiency and venous insufficiency? What signs and/or symptoms would you examine for? Are there any tests that you would perform?

## PHYSICAL EXAMINATION

1. Relate the physical features of the subject to possible respiratory impairments.
2. List possible postoperative problems amenable to physiotherapy.

CASE

# 18  Lobar Pneumonia and Angina

## HISTORY/CHART NOTES

- *HPI:* Mrs. P is a 62-year-old female presented to the emergency department complaining of a 3-week history of a chest cold with increasing shortness of breath during activity, productive cough, malaise, decreased appetite, and recent weight loss. Initially her secretions were yellowish, but more recently they have become green. In addition, she has chest wall pain and abdominal discomfort from persistent coughing.

- *PMH:* CAD with angina. On wait list for coronary angiography.

- *Meds:* Nitroglycerin and blood pressure medication. She is now on an IV broad-spectrum antibiotic pending sputum C & S.

- *On examination:* She is a pale, sweaty (diaphoretic), elderly woman. She is observed sitting up in bed. There is a peripheral IV in situ in her right forearm. She is noted to have regular respirations, however, with decreased diaphragmatic movement. Her respiratory rate is 22 breaths per minutes. Her oxygen saturation is 96% while on 4 L/min oxygen via nasal prongs. She has a temperature of 38.5°C (101°F). She is suppressing her cough and wincing with pain. She is reluctant to mobilize secondary to fatigue, shortness of breath, and abdominal muscle discomfort.

### Questions

What is the common clinical presentation of angina?

## CHEST X-RAY

This woman was diagnosed as having pneumococcal pneumonia. Look at the chest x-ray (Figures 18-1A and 18-1B). What lobe is affected? What are the key features of pneumonia shown in this chest x-ray?

## AUSCULTATION

What breath sounds and adventitious sounds would you expect to hear on auscultation?

## PHYSICAL THERAPY MANAGEMENT

1. What advice will you give this patient to facilitate coughing and mobilization?
2. List the outcome measures you would use to reassess the treatment effectiveness.

The patient was in head down position and you were percussing the patient. The patient had a coughing spell earlier and is now complaining of chest pain.

3. How would you manage this patient?
4. How would you modify your subsequent treatment for this patient?

**Figure 18-1A.** Chest x-ray—PA view.

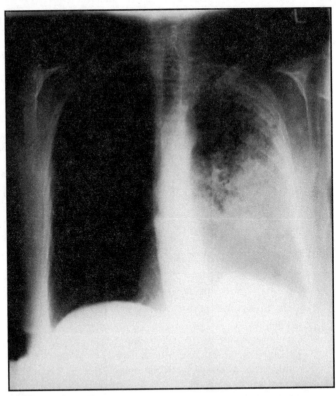

**Figure 18-1B.** Chest x-ray—lateral view.

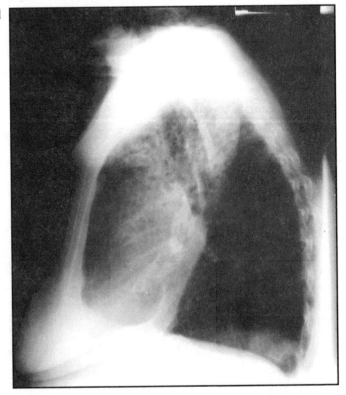

# Pleural Effusion Complicated By Cardiac Effusion and Cardiac Tamponade

CASE

## 19

## HISTORY/CHART NOTES

- *HPI:* Mr. P is an 80-year-old widower and a life-long smoker. He is diagnosed with cancer of the lung with malignant pleural and cardiac effusions. He is now in the palliative care unit waiting for drainage of effusions and other symptomatic control. You were asked to see this patient to assist with mobility and discharge planning.
- *Social and functional history:* He lives in a senior's apartment for independent living. He has to take the elevator and ambulate to the common dining room for meals.

### Question

1. What are the common clinical presentations of cardiac effusion and cardiac tamponade?

## CHEST X-RAY

Review the chest x-ray. What are the features consistent with pulmonary edema shown by the chest x-ray in Figure 19-1?

## AUSCULTATION

Describe the breath sounds you would expect to hear in patients with pleural effusion. How are the auscultatory findings of a pericardial rub different from a pleural rub?

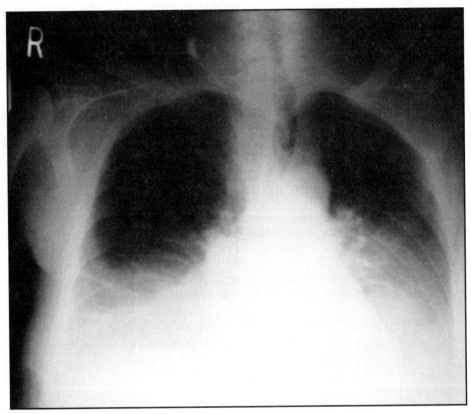

**Figure 19-1.** Chest x-ray.

# Section 3

# Answer Guides

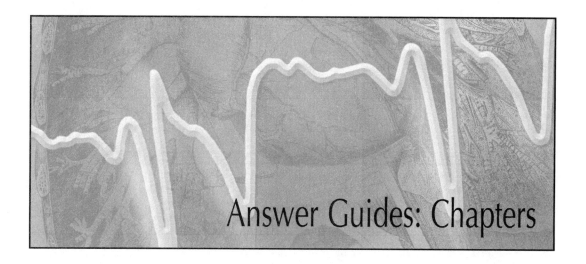

CHAPTER

# 5    Arterial Blood Gas Interpretation

## EXERCISE

1. Examine an oxygen dissociation curve ($PaO_2$ versus $SaO_2$ plot, Figure 5-1) carefully and complete Table 5-6.

Table 5-6

*Matching Values of Oxygen Saturation and Arterial Partial Pressure of Oxygen*

Complete the table using the oxygen-dissociation curve in Figure 5-1. These are the values one would expect with a normal body temperature and pH. If the temperature were higher and the pH were lower, the $SaO_2$ would be lower for a given $PaO_2$.
Note: $SaO_2 \neq PaO_2$

| $SaO_2$ (%) | $PaO_2$ (mmHg) |
|---|---|
| 75 | 40 |
| 83 | 50 |
| 85 | 55 |
| 89 | 60 |
| 93 | 70 |

CHAPTER

# 7

# Pulmonary Function Testing

## EXERCISES

1. Figure 7-1 shows a spirometric tracing for a healthy man. Draw in a tracing for a similar-sized man with severe obstructive lung disease and a tracing for a man with severe restrictive lung disease.

   • See Figure 7-1 below for tracings of men with obstructive or restrictive lung disease.

2. Label the different lung volumes and lung capacities on Figure 7-2.

   • See Figure 7-2 below for lung volumes and lung capacities.

**Figure 7-1.** Spirometric tracings of a healthy man, and men with restrictive and obstructive lung disease. Tracings were based on men of 52 years of age and 6 ft tall. Dashed line: healthy person; dotted line: restrictive lung disease; solid line: obstructive lung disease.

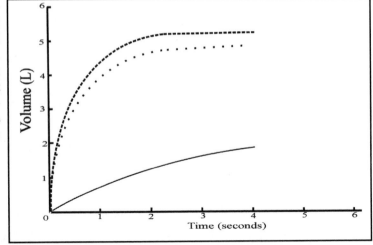

**Figure 7-2.** Lung volumes and capacities. ERV: expiratory reserve volume; FRC: functional residual capacity; IC: inspiratory capacity; IRV: inspiratory reserve volume; RV: residual volume; TLC: total lung capacity; TV: tidal volume; VC: vital capacity.

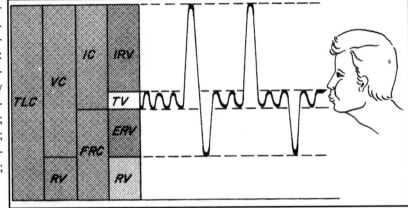

CHAPTER

# 13

# Positioning

1. Where is the most common site of atelectasis in surgical patients?
   - The dependent lung zone
2. Why?
   - See Chapter 13, Figure 13-1, Distribution of ventilation at FRC and low lung volumes
3. How do you position these patients to improve ventilation and gas exchange?
   - Position patients upright or with the atelectatic area uppermost

CHAPTER

# 18

# Respiratory Conditions

## QUESTION

1. What components are reversible by physical therapy?
   - Components of different respiratory conditions reversible by physical therapy:

| Condition | Pathophysiology That is Reversible by Physical Therapy |
|---|---|
| Pneumonia | None. Physical therapy can facilitate clearance of secretions if present. |
| Atelectasis | Can facilitate expansion of atelectasis. |
| Chest trauma | Can facilitate expansion of atelectasis. |
| Pleuritis and pleural effusion | None |
| Lung abscess | None unless communicating with airway. In this case, physical therapy can facilitate clearance of secretions if present. |
| Pulmonary edema | None |
| Acute respiratory distress syndrome | None |

| Restrictive chest wall disorders | Can increase flexibility of chest wall and design exercise program to reverse some of the skeletal muscle dysfunction depending on the disorder. |
|---|---|
| Restrictive lung diseases | Cannot affect the underlying lung disease but can design exercise program to reverse some of the skeletal muscle dysfunction. |
| Asthma | Cannot affect the underlying lung disease but can work with patient to avoid triggers especially in response to designing an appropriate exercise program if exercise-induced asthma is present. |
| COPD | Cannot affect the underlying lung disease but can design exercise program to reverse some of the skeletal muscle dysfunction. |
| Bronchiectasis | Physical therapy can facilitate clearance of secretions if present and design exercise program to reverse some of the skeletal muscle dysfunction. |
| Cystic fibrosis | Physical therapy can facilitate clearance of secretions if present and design exercise program to reverse some of the skeletal muscle dysfunction. |
| Lung cancer | None |
| Aging | Can facilitate maintenance of strength, range-of-motion, mobility, and fitness that is associated with inactivity but cannot affect the underlying aging process. |
| Smoking | Can actively encourage and increase awareness of smoking cessation programs available in community. |
| Obesity | Can design a fitness program to facilitate weight loss. |

It is important to note that physical therapy is not directed towards reversing the underlying pathophysiology of lung disease in many respiratory conditions. The focus of treatment is often directed toward optimizing lung and cardiovascular function, preventing complications, modifying risk factors, promoting overall function, and discharge planning.

# EXERCISE

Photocopy Table 18-3, Problems and Associated Outcome Measures, and complete 1 table for acute respiratory conditions and 1 table for chronic respiratory conditions by identifying outcome measures that could be used by a physical therapist to evaluate whether improvement has occurred after treatment for a specific problem. The problems are grouped because often outcome measures do not distinctly reflect 1 problem but may reflect similar or related problems.

## Problems and Associated Outcome Measures (Acute Respiratory Disease)

| Problem | Outcome Measure |
|---|---|
| • Poor gas exchange in affected regions especially at low lung volumes ($\uparrow PaCO_2$ and $\downarrow PaO_2$)<br>• May desaturate with exercise/mobility | $SpO_2$, arterial blood gas values, auscultation, chest wall movement, chest x-ray, cyanosis, drowsy, coherence |
| • Poor cardiovascular function<br>• Myocardial ischemia<br>• Decreased cardiac output<br>• Decreased oxygen transport/circulation to periphery | Do not routinely monitor unless coexisting cardiac disease. See Table on page 228 for details. Routinely examine temperature and cyanosis of periphery. |
| • Pain—incisional or trauma<br>• Chest or musculoskeletal or peripheral vascular | Visual analogue scale, facial expression, ease of movement, type of medication and mode of delivery. |
| • Decreased mobility/poor exercise tolerance<br>• Decreased fitness<br>• Decreased strength and endurance | Bed and dressing mobility, progressing in ambulation regarding distance and independence as expected. |
| • Retained/increased secretions<br>• Recurrent infections | Expectorated sputum, auscultation, cough, temperature, chest x-ray, interview patient |
| • Dyspnea<br>• Increased work of breathing<br>• Increased use of accessory muscles | Respiratory rate, pursed lip breathing, nostril flaring, indrawing, asynchronous chest wall movement. |
| • Deep vein thrombosis | Warmth & swelling of calf, Homan's sign |
| • Altered cognitive status | Interview patient |
| • Altered coordination and/or balance | Observation of movement |
| • Ileus | Listening for bowel sound and questioning |
| • Urinary retention | Observation |
| • Poor posture | Observation |
| • Decreased ROM of shoulder and other related joints<br>• Sternal limitations | Observation of general movement but goniometer not often used. |
| • Poor nutrition | Observation, chart, nutritional consult |
| • Poor understanding of condition, care of condition, and self-management | Questioning and discussion with patient |
| • Decreased sense of well-being/depression | Interview, consult by other professionals |
| • Discharge planning needs | Interview with patients, caregivers, staff |

## Problems and Associated Outcome Measures (Chronic Respiratory Disease)

| Problem | Outcome Measure |
|---|---|
| • Poor gas exchange in affected regions especially at low lung volumes ($\uparrow PaCO_2$ and $\downarrow PaO_2$)<br>• May desaturate with exercise/mobility | $SpO_2$, auscultation, chest wall movement, cyanosis, coherence. Arterial blood gases and chest x-ray not done routinely. |
| • Poor cardiovascular function<br>• Myocardial ischemia<br>• Decreased cardiac output<br>• Decreased oxygen transport/circulation to periphery | Performance with exercise. Signs and symptoms associated with exercise such as HR, BP, dyspnea or lightheadedness, intermittent claudication. See Chapter 9 for details. |
| • Pain—incisional or trauma<br>• Chest or musculoskeletal or peripheral vascular | Interview for chest, musculoskeletal or peripheral vascular pain |
| • Decreased mobility/poor exercise tolerance<br>• Decreased fitness<br>• Decreased strength and endurance | Formalized exercise testing on treadmill, cycle ergometers and/or 6-minute walk test distance. Performance on exercise modalities, range-of-motion and strengthening activities |
| • Retained/increased secretions<br>• Recurrent infections | Expectorated sputum, auscultation, cough, interview patient |
| • Dyspnea<br>• Increased work of breathing<br>• Increased use of accessory muscles | Observation, respiratory rate of 20 to 30/min, pursed lip breathing, nostril flaring, indrawing (intercostal, diaphragmatic, supraclavicular), observation of accessory muscle recruitment, facial expression, asynchronous chest wall movement |
| • Deep vein thrombosis | Warmth & swelling of calf, Homan's sign |
| • Altered cognitive status | Interview |
| • Altered coordination and/or balance | Observation |
| • Poor posture | Observation |
| • Decreased ROM of shoulder and other related joints<br>• Sternal limitations | Observation and interview; may refer to orthopedic physical therapy or do detailed assessment dependent on severity of problem |
| • Poor nutrition | Interview, observation, nutritional consult |
| • Poor understanding of condition, care of condition, and self-management | Interview and discussion, knowledge test |
| • Decreased sense of well-being/depression | Interview, formal questionnaires such as health related quality of life or depression questionnaires |

CHAPTER
# 19

# Cardiovascular Conditions

## EXERCISE

1. Photocopy Table 18-3, Problems and Associated Outcome Measures, and complete a table for cardiac conditions by identifying outcome measures that could be used by a physical therapist to evaluate whether improvement has occurred after treatment for a specific problem.

## Problems and Associated Outcome Measures (Cardiovascular Disease)

| Problem | Outcome Measure |
|---|---|
| • Poor gas exchange in affected regions especially at low lung volumes ($\uparrow PaCO_2$ and $\downarrow PaO_2$) <br> • May desaturate with exercise/mobility | SpO$_2$, arterial blood gas values, auscultation, chest wall movement, chest x-ray, cyanosis, drowsy, coherence |
| • Poor cardiovascular function <br> • Myocardial ischemia <br> • Decreased cardiac output <br> • Decreased oxygen transport/circulation to periphery | Hemodynamic measures (eg, BP, HR, and cardiac output), EKG, troponin I, echocardiogram, and other diagnostic tests. Routinely examine temperature, peripheral pulse, and cyanosis of periphery |
| • Pain—incisional or trauma <br> • Chest or musculoskeletal or peripheral vascular | Visual analogue scale, angina scale, facial expression, ease of movement, distance walked before onset of pain, type of medication and mode of delivery |
| • Decreased mobility/poor exercise tolerance <br> • Decreased fitness <br> • Decreased strength and endurance | Bed mobility, ability to transfer self, muscle strength testing, progressing in ambulation regarding distance, and independence as expected |
| • Retained/increased secretions <br> • Recurrent infections | Sputum weight or volume, auscultation, cough, temperature, chest x-ray, and ask patient |
| • Dyspnea <br> • Increased work of breathing <br> • Increased use of accessory muscles | RR, pursed lip breathing, nostril flaring, indrawing, asynchronous chest wall movement, and objective scales (eg, Borg scale of perceived breathlessness) |
| • Deep vein thrombosis | Warmth & swelling of calf, Homan's sign, passive dorsiflexion elicits pain |
| • Altered cognitive status | Interview |
| • Altered coordination and/or balance | Observation, assess functional status, and use objective balance scales |
| • Poor posture | Observation |
| • Decreased ROM of shoulder and other related joints <br> • Sternal limitations | Observation, measure ROM, assess functional status, and interview |
| • Poor nutrition | Interview, observation, weight and dietary changes |
| • Poor understanding of condition, care of condition, and self-management | Interview and discussion, and knowledge test |
| • Decreased sense of well-being/depression | Interview, formal questionnaires such as health-related quality of life or depression questionnaires |

Case 15 ¢

16 ①

Myocardial ischemia ?

Decreased cardiac output → ↓BP

②

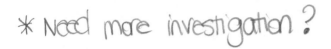

✱ Need more investigation ?

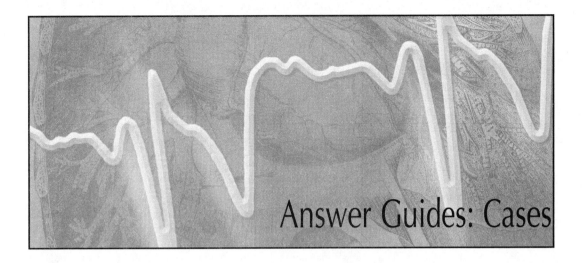

# CASE
# 1

# Atelectasis Postoperatively in an Older Patient

## HISTORY/CHART NOTES

*Several factors which place this patient at high risk for postoperative cardiopulmonary complications are:*
- Related to patient
  - o Age
  - o 47-year history of smoking
  - o Poor breathing pattern with high respiratory rate
- Related to procedure
  - o Site of surgery and size of incision
  - o 3 hours supine on operating table, 2 hours of anaesthetic
  - o Epidural morphine infusion

## CHEST X-RAY

*Chest x-ray findings consistent with atelectasis are:*
- A shift in structures towards the RLL atelectasis—ie, the trachea, heart, and mediastinum are shifted to the right
- The right oblique fissure is apparent with increased opacity inferior and medial to this fissure
- The right costophrenic angle is not sharply defined

*Other features of interest are:*
- The heart is enlarged with a corresponding large cardiothoracic index
- A breast shadow is apparent on the right below the right hemidiaphragm
- The patient's shoulder girdle is elevated

# PULMONARY FUNCTION RESULTS

1. *Do these values indicate any pathology in the lungs?*

   Normal pulmonary function results are usually within 5% to 20% of predicted values. The variability of the $FEV_1$ and FVC is fairly small—about 5% to 8%. The FVC is normal but the $FEV_1$ is slightly abnormal for someone of this age. The slightly lower $FEV_1$ might be indicative of some minor pathological changes or might be a reflection of the normal variation of the aging process.

2. *How do the values compare to someone of similar height but much younger age?*

   The $FEV_1$, FVC and the $FEV_1$/FVC ratio are lower in someone older. This reflects the increased airways obstruction due to the loss of lung elastic recoil leading to dynamic compression in the elderly.

3. *How are the predicted values determined?*

   Predicted values are determined by collecting pulmonary function data from large numbers of individuals who have a healthy respiratory system. These data are then examined to determine which factors help predict values in someone of similar sex and age. Also the average values for someone of a given age are determined. Regression equations and nomograms are derived from the data obtained in these studies of large populations of people. Usually sex, age, and height are the major factors that assist in predicting mean normal values.

4. *How are the percent predicted values calculated?*

   Percent predicted values are calculated by taking the best or average value that the patient obtained on the test (in the case of $FEV_1$ and FVC, the best values

   $$\% \text{ predicted} = \frac{\text{Best result from patient}}{\text{Mean value from healthy sample}} \times 100$$

   are taken) and dividing by the mean value from a large sample of healthy individuals of similar age, sex, and height.

## Other Questions

5. *What is some of the other information that can be derived from this Pulmonary Function Report regarding patient characteristics and test information?*

   Other information that can be obtained from the pulmonary function report includes:
   - Patient Characteristics—name, age, sex, height, weight, race (weight and race can influence pulmonary function although less so than age, sex, and height).
   - Test Information—Date and time of test. Name of technician. Sometimes this report contains the time of the last medication. This is especially important if bronchodilators were taken.

6. *What do the 2 sets of tracings in Case 1, Figure 1-2 show?*
   - The tracing on the left is a typical spirometric tracing with time on the horizontal axis and volume on the vertical axis. The dotted line shows the test result expected from a healthy person of similar age, sex , and height and the solid line shows the patient's performance. The patients $FEV_1$ and FVC can be determined from a spirometric tracing.
   - The tracings on the right are flow-volume loops; similarly, the dotted line shows the test result expected from a healthy person of similar age, sex, and height and the solid line shows the patient's performance. The flow-volume loop is derived from the same forced expiratory manoeuvre as the spirometry tracings, however, the information is plotted differently. Rather than being a volume-time tracing, it is a volume-flow tracing where flow is derived from volume ÷ time. The flow-volume loop can show specific shapes characteristic of certain pathologies when there is intrathoracic or extrathoracic obstruction.

# ARTERIAL BLOOD GASES

pH 7.51        $PaCO_2$ 27        $PaO_2$ 146        $HCO_3^-$ 21

The arterial blood gas values are consistent with a respiratory alkalosis with some compensation.

*Rule of Thumb 1 (Chapter 5, Table 5-5):* $HCO_3^-$ is decreased by 4 mEq/L. The directional change in $HCO_3^-$ is consistent with a respiratory alkalosis; however, the shift is 4 mEq/L which is greater than that expected for an acute respiratory alkalosis (which would be ~2.6 mEq/L). The greater decrease of 4 mEq/L is consistent with renal/metabolic compensation in response to the respiratory alkalosis.

- The expected $PaO_2$ of a healthy person on 35% oxygen would be ~220 mm Hg, however, this person's $PaO_2$ is much lower consistent with some lung pathology.

$$PaO_2 \leq [35\% \times (P_{atm} - P_{H20})] - PaCO_2$$
$$PaO_2 \leq [35\% \times (760 - 47)] - 27$$

*Rule of Thumb 2* (Chapter 5, Table 5-5) is not applicable because the patient has a respiratory alkalosis and is on supplemental oxygen. This patient is on oxygen via a facemask that is contributing to a $PaO_2$ greater than that attainable if this patient were breathing room air.

# PHYSICAL THERAPY MANAGEMENT

*Develop a physiotherapy problem list and treatment plan for this patient. Can you identify any treatment outcomes to use for reassessment of the effectiveness of your treatment plan?*

| Problem | Outcomes |
|---|---|
| Pain | Timing of treatment; patient response to treatment; amount and type of pain medication |
| Poor gas exchange, atelectasis compounded by ineffective breathing pattern—rapid and shallow | $SpO_2$ and arterial blood gas values <br> Auscultation findings <br> Respiratory rate <br> Temperature <br> $FiO_2$ |
| Decreased mobility | Level of mobility |

## Treatment Plan

*Problems 1 and 2.* Deep breathing exercises (diaphragmatic, lateral costal, and maximum inspiratory hold), positioning for comfort and optimizing gas exchange.

*Problem 3.* Thoracic mobility exercises, relaxation techniques, review bed mobility techniques with patient (including rolling and moving from lying to sitting using a supportive pillow). Dangle at bedside in the morning, up to chair in the afternoon, initiate ambulation tomorrow. Review postoperative lower extremity exercises. Ensure administration of pain medication is coordinated with physical therapy treatment.

# CASE 2

# Atelectasis Postoperatively in a Smoker

## HISTORY/CHART NOTES

1. *Briefly describe the pertinent features related to her smoking history.*
   - Smokes 2 to 3 packs/day for over 30 years
   - Has a chronic cough and expectorates yellowish, sometimes brownish sputum every morning
   - Has bronchitis diagnosed by a physician and probably has chronic bronchitis
2. *List the clinical signs of a chest infection and atelectasis in this patient.*
   - Signs of a chest infection are the patient is febrile, has rapid shallow breathing, and has a loose congested cough. May have bronchial breath sounds on auscultation. Chest x-ray findings consistent with a chest infection are increased opacity that can appear in different distributions depending on the type of pneumonia.
   - Atelectasis is not synonymous with a chest infection but it can lead to a chest infection. Signs of atelectasis are: poor breathing pattern, may have mid-onset or end inspiratory crackles and/or bronchial breathing on auscultation. The chest x-ray findings (see below) are indicative of atelectasis.

## CHEST X-RAY

Chest x-ray findings consistent with atelectasis are :
- A shift in structures toward the lower left lobe (LLL) atelectasis—ie, the trachea, heart, and mediastinum are shifted to the left
- The left oblique fissure is apparent behind the shadow of the heart and the collapsed LLL has obliterated the medial shadow of the left hemidiaphragm
- The left hemidiaphragm is elevated

Another feature of interest is:
- Breast shadows are apparent bilaterally

## AUSCULTATION

In a patient with left lower lobe atelectasis and some congestion, one would expect to hear:
- Bronchial breathing/bronchial breath sounds over LLL, or may have decreased air entry/breath sounds over left base
- May have fine (medium to high-pitched) mid-onset or end-inspiratory crackles over affected area consistent with atelectasis
- May have low-pitched wheezes or coarse crackles throughout lung fields secondary due to loose congestion

## ARTERIAL BLOOD GASES

pH 7.50        $PaCO_2$ 32        $PaO_2$ 85        $HCO_3^-$ 24.0

*Rule of Thumb 1* (Chapter 5, Table 5-5): The $HCO_3^-$ is 1.0 mEq/L lower than the mean value and within the normal range. All these are consistent with an acute respiratory alkalosis.

The lower $PaCO_2$ is indicative of increased ventilation. One would expect a higher $PaO_2$ if this person's lungs had no pathology.

*Rule of Thumb 2* (Chapter 5, Table 5-5) is not applicable because the patient has a respiratory alkalosis.

## PHYSICAL THERAPY MANAGEMENT

*Formulate a problem list and treatment plan for this patient.*

### Problem List

1.  Secretion retention
2.  Pain
3.  Shallow breathing pattern
4.  Poor gas exchange and atelectasis
5   Decreased mobility

### Treatment Plan

*Problem 1.* Secretion removal techniques such as ACBT (see Chapter 15 for details)

*Problem 2 through 4.* Deep breathing exercises (diaphragmatic, lateral costal, and maximum inspiratory hold), positioning for comfort and optimizing gas exchange. Ensure administration of pain medication is coordinated with physical therapy treatment.

*Problem 5.* Mobilize to tolerance; however, if chest is infected, aggressive mobilization is not recommended until the chest infection and general malaise of the patient is improving.

# CASE
# 3

# Aspiration Pneumonia—Elderly

## HISTORY/CHART NOTES

1.  *List sequence of events leading to gastric aspiration.*
    -   Wife recently died → depression → suicide attempt
    -   Uncooperative in emergency room → unable to establish patency of the airway → vomited during nasogastric tube insertion → aspiration of gastric contents into right upper and lower lobes
2.  *List the physical findings related to respiratory compromise.*
    -   Febrile
    -   Drowsy but rousable
    -   Respiratory rate is 26/min and on oxygen
    -   Using accessory muscles to breathe
    -   Tactile fremitus and loose congestion present
    -   Will have abnormal auscultatory and chest x-ray findings. See below.

# AUSCULTATION

In a patient with extensive aspiration pneumonia and being mechanically ventilated, one would expect to hear:
- Very coarse breath sounds
- Bronchial breathing/bronchial breath sounds over consolidated areas
- Possibly coarse/ low-pitched crackles and wheezes heard over several lung regions if secretion retention is problematic
- Possibly decreased breath sounds over the area of pneumonia

Once this patient was extubated, auscultatory findings will be similar except for the coarse breath sounds characteristically heard during mechanical ventilation.

# CHEST X-RAY

Chest x-ray findings consistent with aspiration pneumonia are:
- Increased opacity with a fluffy distribution over the left mid-lung, and upper and lower right lung fields

Atelectasis and consolidation of the right upper lobe (RUL) and right lower lobe (RLL) is apparent as shown by:
- Outline of the horizontal and right oblique fissures, which have increased opacity above and below, respectively
- Increased opacity above the horizontal fissure and below the right oblique fissure
- Marked shift of the trachea, mediastinum, and heart toward the right
- Loss of the silhouette of the right hemidiaphragm, and costophrenic angle

Other features of interest are:
- An EKG wire on an EKG electrode
- Outline of the endotracheal tube
- Outline of the nasogastric tube

# ARTERIAL BLOOD GASES

pH 7.2          $PaCO_2$ 40          $PaO_2$ 60          $HCO_3^-$ 15

The arterial blood gas values are consistent with a metabolic acidosis and likely a respiratory acidosis.

*Rule of Thumb 1* (Chapter 5, Table 5-5): The $HCO_3^-$ is decreased 10 mEq/L combined with a decreased pH that is consistent with a metabolic acidosis. With a metabolic acidosis, one expects respiratory compensation to occur relatively quickly (approximately 1 to 2 hours). The $PaCO_2$ is within the normal range and does not show a tendency to decrease as would be expected with a respiratory compensation in response to a metabolic acidosis. Therefore, there must be an underlying respiratory disorder contributing to a respiratory acidosis. In this case of the patient being mechanically ventilated, the mechanical ventilator settings could be the major cause of inducing a respiratory acidosis.

*Rule of Thumb 2* (Chapter 5, Table 5-5): is not applicable because the patient is on the mechanical ventilator and the $FiO_2$ is greater than room air.

# PHYSICAL THERAPY MANAGEMENT

*1. List the problems and treatment plan for this patient.*

## Problem List

1. Poor gas exchange and atelectasis
2  Secretion retention
3. Decreased mobility
4. Possibly some pain and discomfort
5. Depressed and recent change in home situation

## Treatment Plan

*Problem 1.* Deep breathing exercises (diaphragmatic, lateral costal, and maximum inspiratory hold), positioning for comfort and optimizing gas exchange.

*Problem 2.* Secretion removal techniques such as modified postural drainage and manual or mechanical vibrations (see Chapter 15 for details). Patient status may require use of airway clearance techniques that require less cooperation and participation.

*Problem 3.* Mobilize as tolerated. Determine if an aid is required. Educate regarding the importance of mobilization and try to motivate patient.

*Problem 4.* Monitor pain and discomfort during treatment and inform physician if patient feels significant pain.

*Problem 5.* Be sensitive to recent changes in patient's life. Examine patient's support network with friends and family. Refer patient to social worker, or other health professional for counselling. Begin planning for discharge—ie, determining where the patient is able to live upon discharge.

2. *What aspects of the patient need to be considered when positioning him? How would you position him and how often would you recommend a position change?*

Positioning the patient should be based on:
- How airway clearance is promoted
- Optimisation of $SpO_2$
- How patient comfort is optimized—ie, pain, dyspnea

Positioning would likely be a combination of
- Side lying in positions that optimize airway clearance and $SpO_2$
- Sitting
- Ambulation as tolerated—ie, initially to chair and bathroom and then later to outside room

The patient's position should change as frequently as tolerated, preferably every couple of hours.

# CASE
# 4
# Chest Trauma— Pneumothorax/Fractured Ribs

# HISTORY/CHART NOTES

1. *Briefly describe the mechanism of injury and the medical management.*

   The patient injured himself.
   - Possibly while drunk, tripped and fell over his headboard and landed on left chest
   - He sustained multiple fractures of ribs on the left side

   Medical management included:
   - Insertion of chest tube
   - Frequent pain medication including bupivacaine injection into the pleural space

2. *Describe the physical findings of this patient related to respiratory compromise.*

   Physical findings of this patient related to respiratory compromise include:
   - Nicotine stains on his fingers indicative of a heavy smoking history

- Mildly drowsy but oriented in all spheres
- Marked discomfort with movement or taking a big breath
- Subcutaneous emphysema on left chest with mild bruising
- Abnormal auscultatory findings. See below for details.

# PHYSICAL EXAM—PICTURES OF CHEST TUBE

1. *List the precautions and considerations when assessing the mobility of a patient with a chest tube.*
   - Pain
     o Ensure that patient receives sufficient pain medication prior to assessment and treatment
     o Provide support to the chest tube insertion site as required
     o Select appropriate positioning and transfer technique
   - Maintain the patency of the chest tubing
   - Inquire if the patient can be disconnected from the wall suction during ambulation
2. *List the structures that the chest tube pierces.*
   - Skin and connective tissues
   - Intercostal muscles
   - Parietal pleura

# AUSCULTATION

*In a patient with multiple rib fractures and a pneumothorax, one would expect to hear:*
- Decreased air entry/ breath sounds over pneumothorax and affected lung regions that might be collapsed or contused
- Possibly coarse crackles due to movement of subcutaneous air making it difficult to hear other sounds
- Possibly a coarse pleural rub with a few inspiratory crackles on the left chest

# CHEST X-RAY

*Chest x-ray findings consistent with a pneumothorax shown in this x-ray are:*
- A shift in the mediastinum away from the side of the pneumothorax—in this case toward the right
- Loss of lung markings over left lung field
- Outline of lung not directly apposed against the chest wall. In this case, the outline of the left lung is apparent in the middle of the left lung field. This is a very large pneumothorax.

*Other features of interest are:*
- Distinct rib shadows anteriorly. The eighth, ninth, and tenth ribs can be seen intersecting the lateral half of the right hemidiaphragm shadow.

# ARTERIAL BLOOD GASES

pH 7.21        $PaCO_2$ 70        $PaO_2$ 55        $HCO_3^-$ 27

These arterial blood gas values are consistent with a respiratory acidosis.

*Rule of Thumb 1* (Chapter 5, Table 5-5): The $HCO_3^-$ is just at the high end of the normal range and has increased 2 mEq/L from the mean value relative to an increase in 30 mmHg of $PaCO_2$, which is consistent with an acute respiratory acidosis.

*Rule of Thumb 2* (Chapter 5, Table 5-5): The patient has a low $PaO_2$. The $PaO_2$ and $PaCO_2$ show reciprocal changes ($PaO_2$ decreased 25 to 45 mmHg and $PaCO_2$ increased 30) consistent with hypoventilation being the primary cause contributing to a lower $PaO_2$.

# PHYSICAL THERAPY MANAGEMENT

1. *List the problems and treatment plan.*

## Problem List

1. Poor gas exchange in affected lung regions
2. Pain
3. Retention of secretions may occur
4. Decreased mobility

## Treatment Goals

*Problem 1.* Encourage deep breathing exercises with inspiratory hold. Position to optimize $SpO_2$.

*Problem 2.* Ensure pain medication is adequate to carry out effective deep breathing and mobilization

*Problem 3.* Monitor carefully by auscultation, reviewing chart, and checking with team members including patient. Treat as indicated. Ensure cough or huff is effective.

*Problem 4.* Instruct in bed exercises and mobilize early to tolerance. Ensure adequate precautions are taken when handling the chest tube drainage system. Assess shoulder range of motion and instruct in shoulder mobility exercises as required.

2. *What aspects of medical care need to be carefully coordinated with the physical therapy treatment?*

The main consideration is to ensure pain management is adequate and maintained so that patient can carry out effective deep breathing and mobilization.

# CASE

# 5

# Restrictive Lung Disease

# HISTORY

1. *What are some key features of his medical history that may have contributed to his lung disease?*

Two major factors that could have contributed to his present lung condition include:

- Smoking for a prolonged period of time—104 pack-years (52 years x 2 ppd)
- Working in a grain elevator for prolonged periods of time exposing him to inhalation of grain dust

# AUSCULTATION

In a patient with restrictive lung disease, one would expect to hear:

- Decreased air entry/breath sounds due to decreased ventilation of fibrotic alveoli
- Possibly, fine end-inspiratory high-pitched crackles (similar to the sound heard when pulling apart Velcro [Velcro USA, Manchester, NH])

# CHEST X-RAY

Chest x-ray findings consistent with restrictive lung disease are:

- Small lung volumes

- Interstitial pattern on lung field

Other features of interest are:
- Poorly defined cardiophrenic angles bilaterally
- Small cardiothoracic index

# ARTERIAL BLOOD GASES

pH 7.32        $PaCO_2$ 60        $PaO_2$ 47        $HCO_3^-$ 30

*Rule of Thumb 1* (Chapter 5, Table 5-5): The $PaCO_2$ has increased 20 for an increase in $HCO_3^-$ of 5 mEq/L from the mean values. The $HCO_3^-$ has increased more than expected for the change associated with an acute respiratory acidosis that is consistent with a compensated or chronic respiratory acidosis

*Rule of Thumb 2* (Chapter 5, Table 5-5): The $PaCO_2$ has increased 20 relative to a decrease in the $PaO_2$ of 33 to 53 mmHg. Thus, the decrease in $PaO_2$ was disproportionately higher than the increase in $PaCO_2$, which is consistent with hypoventilation and other causes contributing to hypoxemia. The main contributing causes of a lower $PaO_2$ in restrictive lung disease are ventilation-perfusion mismatch followed by diffusion impairment.

# PULMONARY FUNCTION TESTS

1. *Examine the spirometric values. Are these values abnormal? Is so, what major category of chronic lung disease are they consistent with?*

   Both the $FEV_1$ and the FVC are somewhat reduced (the normal range is ±5%) but the $FEV_1$/FVC ratio is almost normal. This pattern is consistent with restrictive lung disease.

2. *With the exception of the ERV, all the lung volumes exhibit changes consistent with what major category of lung disease?*

   All lung volumes are reduced with the exception of the ERV. The normal range for lung volumes is ± 20% of the mean values. The decreased lung volumes are consistent with restrictive lung disease.

3. *Are the inspiratory or expiratory flows low, high, or normal? What would you expect in this patient? Is the (vital capacity) horizontal dimension in this patient low, high, or normal? What would you expect in this patient?*

   The inspiratory and expiratory flows are normal on vertical axis but the horizontal dimension on the flow-volume plot is decreased which is what one would expect in this patient. There is no airway obstruction, which would decrease flow rates, but the lungs are small, which would decrease lung volumes as shown on the horizontal axis of the flow-volume loop.

# PHYSICAL THERAPY MANAGEMENT

*What are some of his major complaints that might be addressed by physical therapy and pulmonary rehabilitation?*
- Increasing fatigue and inability to do daily activities

  During and after adequate medical management (medications, oxygen therapy) is obtained, physiotherapy techniques can improve exercise tolerance and the ability to perform daily activities. These include techniques such as breathing control, exercise training, energy conservation techniques, relaxation positions, and other aspects of patient education.

- Dyspnea

  Techniques such as breathing control, and relaxation positions may help diminish the perception of dyspnea in the short term. Exercise training, energy conservation techniques, and patient education may have more long-term benefits to help diminish the perception of dyspnea.

CASE

# 6

# Stable Chronic Obstructive Pulmonary Disease

## HISTORY/CHART NOTES

1. *Describe the functional history of this patient.*
   - Developed progressive shortness of breath over the last few years
   - At present, she has difficulty walking the 2 blocks to the community centre
   - She cannot manage stairs at all and rarely gets out of her house
   - She has a homemaker to help with her laundry and with some of the heavier housework
2. *Describe the smoking history of this patient.*
   - Smokes 2 packs of cigarettes per day for 44 years, which is equivalent to 88 pack-years
   - Quit smoking 6 years ago

## AUSCULTATION

*In a patient with stable COPD, one would expect to hear:*
- Most often very decreased air entry/ breath sounds throughout
- Less frequently, may have some medium or high-pitched wheezes
- May have early inspiratory crackles if diffuse airway obstruction

## CHEST X-RAY

*Chest x-ray findings consistent with severe COPD are:*
- Large lung fields
- An elongated mediastinum with a small cardiothoracic index
- Flattened diaphragm
- Horizontal ribs
- Increased vascular markings

*Another feature of interest is:*
- The presence of breast shadows bilaterally

## ARTERIAL BLOOD GASES

pH 7.32        $PaCO_2$ 60        $PaO_2$ 51        $HCO_3^-$ 31

*Rule of Thumb 1* (Chapter 5, Table 5-5): The $PaCO_2$ has increased 20 mm Hg for an increase in $HCO_3^-$ mEq/L of 6 from the mean values. The $HCO_3^-$ has increased more than expected for an acute respiratory acidosis consistent with a compensated or chronic respiratory acidosis. In addition, the $HCO_3^-$ is greater than 30 mEq/L, which is usually indicative of a chronic respiratory acidosis.

*Rule of Thumb 2* (Chapter 5, Table 5-5): The $PaCO_2$ has increased 20 mmHg for a decrease in $PaO_2$ of 29 to 49 mmHg. Thus, the decrease in $PaO_2$ was disproportionately higher than the increase in $PaCO_2$, which is consistent with hypoventilation and other causes contributing to hypoxemia. Contributing causes of a lower $PaO_2$ in COPD are ventilation-perfusion mismatch and alveolar hypoventilation.

# PULMONARY FUNCTION RESULTS

1. *Look at the FEV$_1$, FVC and FEV$_1$/FVC ratio. Of what pattern of disease are these results suggestive?*

   These results are suggestive of chronic obstructive pulmonary disease.

   *Why?*

   Because both the FEV$_1$ and the FVC are decreased very markedly and the FEV$_1$ is affected to a much greater degree.

   *Is there a significant bronchodilator response? How do you know?*

   Yes, there is a significant bronchodilator response. A 14% to 15% increase in the FEV$_1$ is indicative of a clinically significant improvement. This is shown by the improved value of FEV$_1$ under the post and % change headings.

2. *Look at the lung volumes. Of what pattern of lung disease are these results suggestive?*

   These results are suggestive of chronic obstructive pulmonary disease.

   *What pathophysiologic factors contribute to such large lung volumes?*

   Increased airways resistance results in dynamic compression leading to gas trapping and larger lung volumes.

Anything <80 or >120% of predicted = abnormal

# PHYSICAL THERAPY MANAGEMENT

1. *List the problem list and treatment plan for this patient.*

## Problem List

1. Dyspnea
2. Decreased exercise tolerance
3. Possibly poor understanding of condition and how to self-manage

## Treatment Plan

*Problem 1.* Techniques such as breathing control, and relaxation positions may help diminish the perception of dyspnea in the short-term. Exercise training, energy conservation techniques, and patient education may have more long-term benefits to help diminish the perception of dyspnea.

*Problem 2.* Instruct patient in breathing control, exercise training, and energy conservation techniques.

*Problem 3.* Determine patients needs and instruct in areas of patient education from which the patient will benefit.

2. *What challenges or obstacles do you think this woman will need to overcome to regularly attend a respiratory rehabilitation program? What support would facilitate her ability to attend the rehabilitation program?*

   Obstacles and challenges include: living on her own, cannot drive, and fatigue. The therapist would want to know about support from friends and family, attitude towards attending rehabilitation program, and literacy level.

   The therapist could facilitate her ability to attend the rehabilitation program by ensuring that the patient is aware of public transport for disabled and ensuring that attendance to program is manageable in terms of time commitment and scheduling for the time of day that coincides with patient's optimal wellness.

CASE

# 7

# Cystic Fibrosis

## History/Chart Notes

1. *What other information besides that shown for this case would you want on your initial assessment?*

### History of Present Illness

*Hemoptysis:* How much/amount? Ie, streaking of sputum; Color of blood? Last episode?

Percussion and postural drainage may be contraindicated dependent on the nature of the hemoptysis because of the possibility of initiating another episode. The physical therapist should clarify this issue with the respirologist before initiating this treatment.

*Sputum:* How much does the patient usually cough up? What is the consistency? What is the usual color?

This is important to determine if the patient is in an acute exacerbation and to provide a reference point to assess the patient's progress.

*Fever:* Cystic fibrosis patients are usually not exercised until their fever has passed.

### Previous Medical History

*Last hospital stay:* Frequency of hospital admissions? Usual length of hospital admission?

*Usual treatment (physical therapy) received in hospital:* Does patient know which are his "worse" lung zones?

*Other medical conditions:* Diabetes? Is there a pancreatic component of cystic fibrosis?

*Activity level:* What type and how much? Is this used as an adjunct for airway clearance?

*Bronchial hygiene:* What routine for airway clearance does the patient usually follow?

*Social history:* Does this patient live alone? Does he have a strong support system of friends or family? What social activities does he enjoy?

2. *Examine Case 7, Figure 7-1 to observe some of the features of a 22-year-old man with cystic fibrosis. List the features of this man that are consistent with respiratory compromise and cystic fibrosis.*

General appearance:
- Small frame, malnourished, muscle wasting

Chest wall:
- Raised shoulder girdle and increased prominence of accessory muscles
- Intercostal indrawing
- Barrel chest apparent on lateral view

Monitoring and lines:
- On supplemental oxygen by nasal cannula
- Central line for administration of medication

Periphery:
- Finger clubbing

*Other features that can be observed in these individuals not apparent in these photographs are:*

Breathing pattern and chest wall movement:
- Nasal flaring/pursed lip breathing
- Dyspnea

- Increased accessory muscle use
- Reduced chest expansion

# AUSCULTATION

*In a patient with cystic fibrosis, one would expect to hear:*
- Decreased air entry/ breath sounds over affected lung regions
- Possibly medium and low pitched wheezes and crackles if there is mucus partially obstructing the airways
- Possibly high-pitched wheezes if there is an asthmatic component

# CHEST X-RAY

*Chest x-ray findings consistent with cystic fibrosis are:*
- Abnormalities of the bony skeleton. Note the asymmetry of the ribs
- Flattening of hemidiaphragms
- Elongated mediastinum and small cardiothoracic index
- Increased interstitial markings that are consistent with scarring

# ARTERIAL BLOOD GASES

pH 7.30          $PaCO_2$ 110          $HCO_3^-$ 52          $PaO_2$ 45

*Rule of Thumb 1* (Chapter 5, Table 5-5): The $PaCO_2$ has increased 70 mmHg for an increase in $HCO_3^-$ of 27 mEq/L. The $HCO_3^-$ has increased more than expected for an acute respiratory acidosis consistent with a compensated or chronic respiratory acidosis. Clinical Note: A $HCO_3^-$ of 52.5 is beyond normal compensation. This person likely has a metabolic alkalosis as well.

*Rule of Thumb 2* (Chapter 5, Table 5-5): The $PaCO_2$ has increased 70 mmHg for a decrease in $PaO_2$ of 35 to 55 mmHg. This person is on $O_2$ so this rule of thumb does not apply. The patient was critically ill and put on mechanical ventilation.

# PULMONARY FUNCTION

1. *What kind of lung disease pattern is shown by the $FEV_1$, FVC, and $FEV_1$/FVC ratio?*

   The $FEV_1$, FVC, and $FEV_1$/FVC are all reduced well below normal, consistent with an obstructive pattern of lung disease.

2. *What characteristic shape is shown on the flow-volume loop? Which curve is the flow-volume loop?*

   The flow-volume loop is the curve on the left. The top half shows the expiratory flows and the bottom half shows inspiratory flows. The top half shows a characteristic scalloped shape that is consistent with obstructive lung disease.

3. *Look at the flow-time curve on the bottom right. Why do you think the flow-time curve terminated between 9 and 10 seconds?*

   The forced expiratory manoeuvre is often terminated in patients with moderate to severe disease because the patient feels breathless and needs to take another breath in.

# PHYSICAL THERAPY MANAGEMENT

1. *What other health professionals would you expect to be involved with this patient?*
   - *Respirologist and residents:* act as case managers for the patient; order tests, investigations, procedures, drug therapy, refer to other health professionals
   - *Social worker:* handles some government and third-party funding issues; act as counselors
   - *Psychiatrist:* often involved with patients as disease process worsens
   - *Dietician:* involved with patients dietary needs, advises respirologists on feeding tube options

- Nursing: day-to-day care of patient
- Clinic coordinator: if the patient is at the hospital that houses the CF clinic, often the clinic coordinator will be involved in the patient's concerns
- Respiratory therapist: handles pulmonary function tests, arterial blood tests, monitors $SaO_2$, handles inpatient and outpatient oxygen requirements

2. *List the problem list and treatment plan.*

## Problem List

1. Increased secretions and chest infection
2. Poor exercise tolerance
3. Education to ensure airway clearance and exercise will be performed well at home

## Treatment Plan

*Problem 1.* Airway clearance techniques to manage acute exacerbation followed by instruction using techniques that patient will self-manage upon discharge (see Chapter 15 for details).

*Problem 2.* Aerobic component to improve exercise tolerance. An increased emphasis is being placed on higher impact or heavy resistance training to minimize osteoporosis is this group of patients.

*Problem 3.* Focused patient education on airway clearance and exercise techniques to be performed at home. May have to arrange for home care physical therapy if unable to manage airway clearance independently upon discharge.

CASE

# 8

# Asthma—Acute Exacerbation

# HISTORY/CHART NOTES

1. *What assessment parameters would you monitor?*
   - Vitals: HR, RR, BP, $SpO_2$ if oximeter available but this device is not usually available in this situation
   - Cyanosis
   - Dyspnea; difficulty with speaking because of shortness of breath; indrawing (supraclavicular, intercostal, diaphragmatic)
   - Posture
   - Is the patient barrel chested?
   - Accessory muscle use
   - Abnormal auscultatory findings
   - PEFR but unlikely to have peak flow meter
2. *What factors would be indicative of worsening or improvement of her respiratory and cardiovascular status?*
   - Worsening of condition would include vitals moving further away from normal range, increased cyanosis, increased dyspnea, increased indrawing, worsening of auscultatory findings

- Improvement would include vitals moving toward the normal range, and the patient attaining some level of composure, decreased dyspnea, and improved auscultatory findings

# AUSCULTATION

*In a patient with acute asthma, one would expect to hear:*
- Most commonly, high- or medium-pitched wheezes in both inspiratory and expiratory phases. The wheezes may also be polyphonic.

# CHEST X-RAY

*Chest x-ray findings consistent with acute asthma are:*
- Large lung fields
- Horizontal ribs
- Elongated mediastinum and small cardiothoracic index
- Flattening of hemidiaphragms

Other features of interest are:
- EKG electrodes
- Breast shadows bilaterally

Often, the chest x-ray of people with asthma can appear normal when they are not having an acute exacerbation.

# ARTERIAL BLOOD GASES

pH 7.25        $PaCO_2$ 59        $HCO_3^-$ 25        $PaO_2$ 60

$PaCO_2$ and pH indicate a respiratory acidosis.

*Rule of Thumb 1* (Chapter 5, Table 5-5): The $PaCO_2$ has increased 19 and no large change in $HCO_3^-$ has occurred. The $HCO_3^-$ may have increased 2 mEq/L if the patient's $HCO_3^-$ was usually 23 mEq/L. Regardless, the $HCO_3^-$ is well within the normal range and is consistent with an acute respiratory acidosis.

*Rule of Thumb 2* (Chapter 5, Table 5-5): The $PaCO_2$ has an increased 19 for a decrease in $PaO_2$ of 20 to 40 mmHg consistent with hypoventilation and other causes contributing to hypoxemia.

# SPIROMETRY AND PEAK EXPIRATORY FLOW RATES

*Interpret the spirometric values.*

This person's $FEV_1$, FVC, and the PEFR are reduced compared to the predicated values provided for a sample of healthy people of similar age, gender, and height. A more precise estimate of how abnormal these results are can be determined by calculating the percent-predicted values (see below).

*What pattern of lung pathology is shown?*

The pattern is consistent with an obstructive pattern because both the $FEV_1$ and FVC are reduced.

*Complete the table and calculate the % Predicted values and the % improvement after bronchodilator administration.*
The % predicted values are calculated from:  patient's result ÷ predicted value × 100 = % predicted

There is a significant bronchodilator response as shown by large improvement in the $FEV_1$. The percent change postbronchodilator for the $FEV_1$ can be calculated from:    = (Post − Pre) ÷ Pre × 100
= (3.0 − 1.8) ÷ 1.8 × 100 = 67% change

A change in the $FEV_1$ after a bronchodilator of 14% to 15% or more is considered to be clinically significant.

Calculated values for spirometry and peak expiratory flow rate for Case 8:

|            | Pre BD (L) | Pred | % Predicted | Post BD(L) | % Improvement |
|------------|------------|------|-------------|------------|---------------|
| $FEV_1$    | 1.8        | 3.8  | 47          | 3.0        | 67            |
| FVC        | 3.2        | 4.7  | 68          | 4.2        |               |
| $FEV_1/FVC$| 56%        | 80%  | 70          | 71%        |               |
| PEFR       | 3.81       | 8.87 | 43          |            |               |

Abbreviations: Pre BD: before bronchodilator; Pred: predicted; Post BD: after bronchodilator.

## PHYSICAL THERAPY MANAGEMENT

*What health professionals would you advise this woman to see?*

The women should see a physician so that her asthma can be specifically diagnosed and managed optimally from a medical perspective. This could be a general practitioner, pulmonologist, and/or sports medicine physician. The patient may need specific advice on the medications that she is able to take to manage her asthma while she is competing. Some prescription drugs register positively when the athletes are drug tested.

# CASE 9
# Chronic Obstructive Pulmonary Disease And Pneumonia

## HISTORY/CHART NOTES

1. *List the relevant features pertinent to the history of his acute exacerbation.*
   - Complained of feeling feverish, increased shortness of breath and general weakness
   - Prescribed antibiotics 2 days ago
   - Breathing no better and having diarrhea
   - Not coughing up much mucus
   - This morning felt more shortness of breath and had to be admitted to hospital

2. *List the pertinent physical findings related to worsening of his respiratory status.*
   - Face is flushed and diaphoretic
   - Predominately a mouth breather and use of accessory muscles
   - Pauses every sentence to catch his breath
   - Prefers to sit up rather than lie down
   - Increased AP diameter of chest or barrel chested
   - Decreased lateral costal excursions
   - Indrawing of intercostals
   - Obvious nicotine stains on his fingers

## PHYSICAL FEATURES

*The physical features of this gentleman shown in Case 9, Figure 9-1 consistent with respiratory compromise and COPD are:*
   - Prominent accessory muscles—ie, trapezius, sternocleidomastoid
   - Elevated shoulder girdle
   - Barrel chested—especially apparent on lateral view

- Flared lower ribs apparent on frontal and side views
- Some muscle wasting

# AUSCULTATION

*In a patient with COPD and pneumonia one would expect to hear:*
- Very decreased air entry/ breath sounds throughout due to the COPD
- Possibly medium and high-pitched wheezes if the pneumonia has caused bronchospasm
- Possibly coarse (medium or low-pitched) crackles if the pneumonia has resulted in increased secretions
- Possibly bronchial breathing over a consolidated region of the lung; however, the pneumonia in this individual is more diffuse (see chest x-ray)

# CHEST X-RAY

*Chest x-ray findings consistent with:*
- Pneumonia:
  - Increased diffuse fluffy opacity on lung fields especially on RML and RLL
  - Obscuring of cardiophrenic angles and less distinct costophrenic angles.
- COPD:
  - Large lung fields
  - Elongation of mediastinum and small cardiothoracic index
  - Horizontal ribs
- The tubing crossing the patient's chest is the tubing the supplies oxygen to his nasal prongs

# ARTERIAL BLOOD GASES

pH 7.22          $PaCO_2$ 50          $HCO_3^-$ 20          $PaO_2$ 50

The $PaCO_2$ and pH indicate a respiratory acidosis.

*Rule of Thumb 1* (Chapter 5, Table 5-5): The $PaCO_2$ has increased 10 mmHg and $HCO_3^-$ has decreased by 5 mEq/L. The $HCO_3^-$ has decreased which is the opposite direction to that expected for compensation to a respiratory acidosis. These changes in $HCO_3^-$, pH, and $PaCO_2$ are consistent with a respiratory and metabolic acidosis.

*Rule of Thumb 2* (Chapter 5, Table 5-5): The $PaCO_2$ has increased 10 mmHg for a decrease in $PaO_2$ of 30 to 50 mmHg consistent with hypoventilation and other causes contributing to hypoxemia.

# PHYSICAL THERAPY MANAGEMENT

1. *List the problem list and treatment plan for this patient.*

## Problem List

1. Poor gas exchange
2. Possibly secretion retention
3. Decreased mobility and exercise tolerance
4. Possibly poor understanding of condition and ability to self-manage

## Treatment Plan

*Problem 1.* Breathing control and pursed lip breathing, positioning to decrease dyspnea and optimize gas exchange. Ensure patient is using supplemental oxygen as prescribed.

*Problem 2.* Carefully assess and continue to monitor. The pneumonia may not result in excessive secretions or it may progress to a stage when the patient may require airway clearance techniques.

*Problem 3.* Mobilize and progress as tolerated. Determine if an aid is required. Educate regarding the importance of mobilization and improving exercise tolerance. Discuss the possibility of entering a pulmonary rehabilitation program.

*Problem 4.* Do a needs assessment and provide focused patient education as required. Explore possibility of patient doing pulmonary rehabilitation upon discharge. Determine details of home situation including support and social activities. Begin discharge planning.

2. *Would your treatment plan be different for this patient compared to a young adult with a similar pneumonia? Why or why not?*

   Yes, the treatment plan for this person would be different than a young person with a similar pneumonia. This patient would:

   - Be a higher priority because a pneumonia compromises a person with COPD to a greater extent and there is a much greater risk of mortality.
   - Require more specific instruction and careful monitoring of breathing techniques and position(s) to optimize gas exchange and minimize dyspnea.
   - Require more careful monitoring to determine if secretion retention is a problem and airway clearance techniques are indicated.

# CASE 10

# Left-Sided Congestive Heart Failure—Pulmonary Edema

## HISTORY

1. *Why does mitral valve prolapse lead to regurgitation? What are some of the causes of mitral valve prolapse leading to regurgitation? What are some of the signs and symptoms of mitral valve prolapse?*

   Mitral valve prolapse is elongation of the valve such that it becomes incompetent and regurgitation occurs. In the majority of cases, the cause is unknown. Mitral valve prolapse can be caused from rheumatic fever, ischemic heart disease and cardiomyopathies. The person can be asymptomatic. As the valve becomes more incompetent, signs and symptoms include arrhythmias, palpitations, lightheadedness, syncope, transient ischemic attacks, fatigue, dyspnea, and hemoptysis.

2. *Examine Starling's equation (under section titled Pulmonary Edema in Chapter 18, Respiratory Conditions) and the description of the factors that contribute to capillary exchange and the net outflow of fluid from the capillaries. Which is the primary factor that increases the interstitial fluid level in left-sided heart failure? Incorporate the factors outlined in this equation in Case 10, Figure 10-1. Use different-sized arrows to indicate the relative contribution of each factor.*

   The primary factor that increases the interstitial fluid level in left-sided heart failure is the hydrostatic pressure within the capillaries. Factors that contribute to pulmonary edema in left-sided heart failure for are shown on page 248, Figure 10-1.

3. *Has the patient improved or deteriorated? On what information do you base your answer?*

   The patient has improved based on the following changes:

   - $SpO_2$ is higher on a lower flow delivery system of supplemental oxygen (40% oxygen by face mask to 2L/min by nasal prongs)
   - Blood pressure and heart rate are lower in supine
   - Temperature has decreased slightly
   - Pain is lower
   - Hemoglobin has almost doubled
   - The skin is warm and dry rather than cool and clammy
   - Decreased air entry is in the left lower lobe rather than in both lower lobes bilaterally

**Figure 10-1.** Factors that contribute to pulmonary edema in left-sided heart failure.

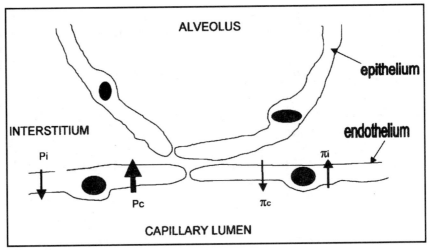

# CHEST X-RAY

*Chest x-ray findings consistent with left-sided congestive heart failure and pulmonary edema shown in this x-ray are:*
- A very large heart with a corresponding large cardiothoracic index
- Increased vascular markings that are most prominent near the mediastinum and radiate outward toward the periphery of the lungs
- Increased interstitial lung markings
- Outlining of the horizontal fissure

EKG electrodes are also features of interest that can be observed in people with cardiac problems.

# PHYSICAL THERAPY MANAGEMENT

*How will your treatment approach change? How will you progress your treatment as the patient improves?*

The treatment approach will change in 4 main problems areas:
- Poor gas exchange: will be targeted until it reaches normal values. Breathing exercises with coughing or huffing only as required will be promoted. Positioning into the upright position as much as possible and increasing mobilization will be promoted.
- Decreased mobility:
  - o Because of postural hypotension, slow movements with pauses after each position change will be instructed. There will be a shift in focus from bed mobility to sitting in chair to ambulation in room then to hallway. The duration and level of independence will be increased.
  - o Upper extremity range-of-motion exercises will be promoted within the limitations of a median sternotomy (see the table in Answer Guide Case 12).
  - o Functional activities, such as dressing and stair-climbing, will be addressed as tolerated
  - o Progress will be within the pain and fatigue limits of the patient
- Pain will be less but still significant. The physical therapist needs to ensure that pain medication is adequate. Supportive coughing or huffing should be encouraged.
- Discharge planning—will include assessment of functional ability required for current home and ensuring patient is capable of returning home without or without additional assistance—ie, home care.

CASE

# 11

# Acute Myocardial Infarction—Good Recovery

## HISTORY/CHART NOTES

1. *Assess the cardiac risk factors for this patient and outline your plan for secondary prevention.*

Advise the patient to modify the lifestyle to decrease the risk of a future myocardial infarct. Provide links to local support groups, Web sites, the local heart association, reading materials, and videotapes. Smoking cessation is paramount for this patient. Dietary changes and consultation are needed. Encourage the patient to increase his or her activity level in a walking program, in an air-conditioned indoor shopping mall, or outdoor walking.

*↳ doesn't like to sweat*

Contraindications for exercising cardiac patients:

- o Unstable angina
- o Resting systolic BP >200 mmHg or diastolic >110 mmHg
- o Symptomatic drop of BP >20 mmHg during exercise
- o Moderate to severe aortic stenosis
- o Other acute illness or fever
- o Uncontrolled atrial or ventricular arrthymias
- o Uncontrolled tachycardia or third degree heart block
- o Uncontrolled CHF, diabetes
- o Active pericarditis, myocarditis, recent embolism, or thrombophlebitis
- o Resting ST segment changes >2 mm
- o Clinical signs such as pallor, cold sweats, dizziness, severe dyspnea

*↳ swelling of limb from clot (like DVT but more chronic)*

## ELECTROCARDIOGRAM

*Review the V2 and V3 lead EKG of this patient. What are the main features consistent with an MI shown by these leads?*

The main features of the EKG consistent with an MI are ST segment depressions in leads V2, and V3 and that it is a non Q-wave infarct. The findings are indicative of an anterior myocardial infarct. See Chapter 19, Table 19-5 for the site of myocardial infarct, diagnosis, and clinical significance.

## PHYSICAL THERAPY MANAGEMENT

1. *On day 2 post-MI, the patient is stable and transferred to step down cardiac unit. You were asked to see Mr. G for rehabilitation. Outline your in-patient rehabilitation plan for this patient.*

Details of the contraindications to exercise and phases of exercise during cardiac rehabilitation in these patients are outlined under "History/Chart Notes" above, and phases of cardiac rehabilitation are:

- Phase I—Acute/In-patient Phase

  Start once patient is deemed medically stable

  - o Level 1 (1 METs)

    Bed rest but allow gentle upper and lower extremities active range-of-motion exercises. However, those patients who have sternotomy following open-heart surgery need to follow sternal precautions

- o Level 2 (2 METs)

  Allow sitting up in a chair for meals and walking to the bathroom or inside the room (up to 50 ft) a few times a day. Allow performing activities of daily living. Increase repetitions of active range-of-motion exercises

- o Level 3 (3 METs)

  Allow a sitting shower. Ambulate up to 250 ft 3 to 4 times per day

- o Level 4 (4 METs)

  Perform activities of daily living independently and ambulate up to 1000 ft 3 to 4 times per day. Allow climbing 1 flight of stairs

- *Phase II—Subacute/Post-Discharge Conditioning Phase*

  Usually begins after the discharge from the hospital during the first 6 weeks. Conditioning exercises are done with close cardiac monitoring. Start education on risk factor reduction if not already initiated.

- *Phase III—Intensive Rehabilitation*

  After completion of phase II, patient proceeds to exercise in large groups. Resistance training is often initiated during this phase.

- *Phase IV—Maintenance Phase*

  Ongoing exercise training in a group setting or self-monitored program.

See Chapter 9 for more details.


In general:

- Familiarize yourselves with the patient's resting vital signs including the EKG.
- During activity, watch the bedside monitor or alert the cardiac nurse if the patient is on telemetry for any unusual EKG changes.
- Explain the purpose of the visit, benefits and risks of rehabilitation. Reassure patient that the rehabilitation program is done in a safe environment with close supervision and medical help is readily available if needed.
- Take into account of the patient's previous functional level and customize the rehabilitation program to the patient's ability.
- Watch for signs of activity intolerance.
- Provide details of the rehabilitation program for the patient to do.  Include type, frequency, intensity, and duration.
- During exercise, other than the heart rate and EKG, use additional objective measures such as an angina pain scale, a dyspnea scale, pulse oximetry, and blood pressure level as indicated.
- Liaison with the health care team to provide outpatient cardiac rehabilitation.

# BIBLIOGRAPHY

American College of Sports Medicine. *Guidelines for Exercise Testing and Prescription.* 5th ed. Philadelphia: Lea & Febiger; 1995.

# CASE
# 12

# Acute Myocardial Infarction—
# Coronary Artery Bypass Graft

## HISTORY/CHART NOTES

1. *After CABG, what are the wound and sternal precautions taught to patients and why are these instructions provided?*

Wound and sternal care:

- Showers (10 minutes or less) are allowed if incisions are dry and healing.
- Avoid extreme water temperatures.
- Gentle soap and water are permitted, but do not scrub hard until the skin is healed.
- Lotions, ointments or dressings are not recommended.
- Slight itching, numbness or tightness of the incision area is normal.
- The sternum takes 6 to 8 weeks to heal. Avoid lifting objects greater than 10 lbs or any activity that causes clicking of the sternum. Occasional clicking is normal.
- Use a pillow to splint the sternum during cough or sneeze.
- Perform neck, limbs (including shoulder girdle) and trunk ROM exercises.
- Symmetrical and proper posture is essential.
- Do not use arms to push when getting in and out of the bed or chair.
- Avoid lying on the stomach while in bed.
- If leg vein was used for the graft, keep the affected leg elevated or wear a supportive stocking.

Notify the physician if the patient experiences the following signs of infection:

- Increased drainage or opening of the incision
- Increased redness or warmth around the incision
- Fever ≥38°C or 100°F

Sternal precautions are taught to patients to avoid damage to the sternotomy site, for pain control, and to allow the wound to heal properly.

## ELECTROCARDIOGRAM

1. *Identify the acute EKG changes.*

The patient suffered a ST segment elevation *anterior* infarct. It is transmural. The patient has had a left anterior descending coronary artery occlusion. During the *hyperacute* phase, ST segment elevation is often noted.

In the *acute* phase, EKG changes are shown in Case 12, Figure 12-1. Well-defined Q-waves are shown with no RS deflection. Q-waves are indicative of necrosis. There is persistent ST elevation and the T wave are upright, which are typical signs of this phase.

Later in the *subacute* phase, the ST segment elevation is less than in the acute phase, the T waves will invert and the QRS complex will widen. In the *chronic phase*, ST segment change is minimal or reverted back to normal. The Q-wave persists with larger infarcts (resolves with small infarct), the QRS complex remains wide, and T-wave reverts back to the usual upright configuration.

# PHYSICAL THERAPY MANAGEMENT

1. *On day 2 post-CABG, the patient is stable and transferred to the step down cardiac unit. You were asked to see Mr. G for rehabilitation. Outline your in-patient rehabilitation plan for this patient.*

   Familiarize yourselves with the contraindications for exercising cardiac patients and the phases of cardiac rehabilitation in Answer Guide for Case 11, and wound and sternal care reviewed above before starting in-patient rehabilitation. The patient should:

   - Follow the sternal precautions
   - Refrain from using the arms for any lifting
   - Practice transferring in and out of the bed and to the chair, and stair climbing without using arms
   - Perform deep breathing exercises, cough with a pillow to support the sternum, and up for meals. The therapist should gradually increase the level of self-care and ambulation of the patients

   The patient should attend post-CABG in-patient exercise class. The exercise program usually consists of:

   - Warm-up exercises: deep breathing, relaxation, and gentle circulatory exercises
   - Core exercise program: neck, shoulder girdle, bilateral upper extremity exercise, trunk, and lower extremity ROM exercises
   - Cool-down period: deep breathing, relaxation, and gentle circulatory exercises
   - Exercises done on a chair
   - Allows patients to achieve ROM that they can tolerate (ie, without undue discomfort and clicking of the sternum).
   - Allow patients to exercise at their own rate. Because patients from different days post CABG are attending the same class, encourage patients to listen to their bodies. They do not necessarily have to do what the other patients in the class do

   Note: Sternotomy is usually less painful and better tolerated by patients than a thoracotomy. Pulmonary complication rate and average length of stay after open heart surgery is shorter than after upper abdominal and thoracic surgeries.

# BIBLIOGRAPHY

Charlson ME, Isom OW. Care after coronary-artery bypass surgery. *N Engl J Med.* 2003;348:1456-1463.

Eagle KA, Guyton RA. ACC/AHA Guidelines for SABG surgery. *JACC.* 1999;34:1262-1347. Available from: http://www.acc/org/clinical/guidelines/bypass/dirIndex.htm

CASE
# 13

# Chronic Heart Failure— Cardiomyopathy

# HISTORY/CHART NOTES

1. *What are the differentiating features of acute coronary syndrome from this form of heart failure?*

   This patient had no cardiac history apart from hypertension and low CAD risk. He had no complaints of chest pain. Further laboratory tests, such as Troponin I levels and ECGs on admission and on serial testings, were negative.

However, the signs and symptoms that Mr. C is experiencing are consistent with heart failure. Review Chapter 19 under the section titled Congestive Heart Failure for details.

2. *From the clinical information given, what is his preadmission cardiac function?*

The patient could manage stairs slowly, work in the garden, and go for walks on better days. The patient has minimal to mild symptoms and is likely at class I/II on the New York Heart Association Functional Classification of Cardiovascular Disability and Specific Activity Scale:

| Class | Severity | Characteristics | Activity Scale |
|-------|----------|-----------------|----------------|
| I | Minimal | Have cardiac disease No limitations of physical activity | Can perform activities up to 7 METs |
| II | Mild | Slight limitation of physical activity Comfortable at rest Ordinary activity results in fatigue, palpitations, dyspnea, or angina pain | Can perform activities to completion >5 METs but cannot complete >7 METs |
| III | Moderate | Marked limitation of physical activity Comfortable at rest Less than ordinary activity results in fatigue, palpitations, dyspnea, or angina pain | Can perform activities to completion >2 METs but cannot complete >5 METs |
| IV | Severe | Inability to carry on any physical activity without discomfort Symptoms of cardiac insufficiency may be present at rest | Cannot perform activities to completion >2 METs |

# AUSCULTATION

*What breath sounds and adventitious sounds would you expect to hear from this patient?*

The patient is likely to have inspiratory crackles when symptomatic. These adventitious sounds would not clear after taking some deep breaths.

# PHYSICAL THERAPY MANAGEMENT

*After the patient's medical condition is optimized and given the patient's functional history, what advice would you give to the patient in terms of activity and exercise?*

The patient may gradually increase exercise and activity level to his tolerance:

- General overview of an exercise program:

  Exercise can improve the quality of life and health of heart failure patients. Even short periods of bed rest can weaken the body. Exercise can strengthen the heart and the cardiovascular system and aerobic exercise trains the heart to beat more efficiently. With training, resting, and exercise, heart rate decreases, and the heart pumps out more blood per beat. The physical therapist or the doctor should outline an exercise routine and activities to avoid prior to discharge. To chart the progress and to track the cardiac condition, a daily record of exercise duration, intensity, and response is recommended for patients to record.

- Recommended activities:

  Recommend resuming activities that the patient enjoys. Include walking as part of the program. Cycling and swimming can be considered if the patient was previously physically active. Advise the patient to start slowly and increase the length or the intensity of the activity when the patient feels up to it. Teach the patient to listen to the body and stop exercising if shortness of breath, dizziness, chest pain, nausea, or a cold sweat is experienced. Instruct the patient to give the body rest days to recharge from exercising.

- Some useful exercise tips for patients:

  o Warm up with stretching exercises at the beginning of the exercise session

- o  Exercise with a buddy
- o  Avoid exercises that require quick bursts of energy
- o  Avoid exercises that cause shortness of breath, chest pain, or dizziness
- o  Don't exercise if haven't eaten for a long time
- o  Exercise 1 to 2 hours after a light meal
- o  Avoid exercising in extreme weather
- o  Monitor the pulse and perceived level of exertion
- o  Exercise at the level recommended by the therapist or doctor

Approximate metabolic cost of activities:

| Energy Expenditure | Activities of Daily Living | Recreation & Training |
|---|---|---|
| 1.5 to 2 METs | Washing, shaving, deskwork, writing, washing dishes, sewing, knitting, and driving. | Shuffleboard, billiards, archery, walking 1 mph, and stationary bike with very low resistance. |
| 2 to 5 METs | Carry up to 30 lbs, cleaning windows, raking leaves, weeding, stacking light objects, light welding, light carpentry, auto repair, and painting. | Golf, sailing, tennis (doubles), walking up to 4 mph, bicycling up to 8 mph, table tennis, and dancing (fox-trot) |
| 5 to 7 METs | Carry up to 60 lbs, climbing stairs slowly, easy digging in garden, carpentry and using pneumatic tools. | Badminton, tennis (single), downhill skiing, skating, walking up to 5 mph, bicycling up to 10 mph, swimming breast stroke, and square dancing. |
| 7 to 8 METs | Carry up to 80 lbs, climbing stairs at moderate speed, shovel snow, and dig ditches. | Skiing, basketball, squash, jog/walk 5 mph, bicycling 12 mph, ice hockey, mountain climbing, and swimming crawl stroke. |

## REFERENCE

Goldman L, Hashimoto B, Cook EF, et al. Comparative reproducibility and validity of systems for assessing cardiovascular functional class: advantages of a new specific activity scale. *Circulation*. 1981; 64:1227-34.

## CASE 14

# Chronic Heart Failure—Post Myocardial Infarct

## HISTORY/CHART NOTES

1. *What are the differentiating features between pneumonia and acute heart failure?*

   Pneumonia is an infection. Common clinical signs that distinguish it from heart failure are:

   - Increased temperature
   - Cough usually productive of purulent sputum
   - Common physical findings of the involved area may include inspiratory crackles, bronchial breath sounds, dullness on percussion, or bronchophony
   - Positive sputum culture

- Laboratory findings such as increased white blood cells and particular types of white cells
- Localized chest x-ray findings in a particular lung segment and/or lobe

2. *From the clinical information given, what was her preadmission cardiac function level?*

The patient had a large anterior infarct, which frequently results in left heart failure. The patient has moderate to severe symptoms and is likely at class III/IV New York Heart Association Functional Classification of Cardiovascular Disability (see the Answer Guide for Case 13).

The patient shows signs of left systolic dysfunction in terms of decreased ejection fraction and peripheral perfusion. In addition, the clinical signs of biventricular failure were also present. Echocardiography or radionuclide ventriculography are frequently used to evaluate left ventricular performance in patients.

In diseases such as hypertension, blocked aortic valve, or underlying genetics abnormalities, the ventricular wall thickens in concentric circles without dilatation. As a result, the filling of the heart is impaired and the heart works less effectively, resulting in a decreased ejection fraction.

# ARTERIAL BLOOD GASES

1. Is there a primary acid-base disturbance? Is there hypoxemia?

pH 7.38        $PaCO_2$ 40 mmHg        $PaO_2$ 64 mmHg        $HCO_3^-$ 23 mmol/L

*Rule of Thumb 1* (Chapter 5, Table 5-5): The $PaCO_2$, pH, $HCO_3^-$ are within the normal limits for this patient. The carbon dioxide level and bicarbonate level were appropriate with respect to each other, indicating no mixed disorder has occurred.

However, the $PaO_2$ level is low especially considering that the patient was receiving 50% oxygen. Because the level of ventilation ($PaCO_2$) is normal, her hypoxemia is caused by gas exchange disorders (ventilation-perfusion mismatch and shunting).

# PHYSICAL THERAPY MANAGEMENT

*Once the patient medical condition is optimized and given the patient's functional history, what advice can you give to the patient in terms of activity and exercise?*

The patient could manage at home but needs help with heavy housework. Her activities outside the house are also very limited. Because her clinical and functional history shows that she has moderate to severe chronic heart failure, a slow gradual activity program is required. See details in the Answer Guide for Case 13. Upon discharge from the hospital, the patient might benefit from increased homemaker help and home care physical therapy involvement with her activity and exercise program.

CASE
# 15
# Exercising Outpatient— Arrhythmia and Hypotension

## HISTORY/CHART NOTES

*What should the therapist do?*

1. *What should the therapist's instructions be to the patient?*

   The patient should be instructed to begin her cool-down immediately. The therapist should reduce the speed of the treadmill to its slowest speed or to approximately 1 mph.

2. *What should be monitored?*

   The therapist should continuously monitor the well-being of the patient. The therapist should converse with the patient in a calming manner that enables the therapist to ascertain whether the patient is not becoming increasingly more lightheaded. The therapist should monitor vitals including HR and BP.

3. *What should be communicated to nearby colleagues?*

   A nearby colleague could be informed that the patient is feeling lightheaded so that the colleague will be ready to offer additional assistance if need be.

## ELECTROCARDIOGRAM

An EKG monitor is in the department, and the therapist immediately connects the patient to the monitor. The tracing from a modified V5 is shown in Case 15, Figure 15-1.

1. What are the rate, rhythm, and aberrant conduction shown?

   *Rate:* 82 BPM    *✱Didn't count abnormal QRS*

   *Rhythm:* regularly-irregular

   *Aberrant conduction:* Normal sinus rhythm is interspersed with broad bizarre QRS configurations, which are premature ventricular contractions (PVCs). The pause after the PVC is compensatory— ie, the distance between the normal beat, PVC, and the next normal beat is 2 RR intervals. Every third beat is a PVC, which is known as trigeminy.

2. *What should be done at this point in time before the patient leaves the department?*

   The therapist needs to determine that the patient is stable and the EKG has returned to a sinus rhythm. The patient should be questioned regarding previous episodes of palpitations and dizziness precipitated by exercise or other cardiovascular stresses.

3. *Will you refer the patient to another health professional before exercising her again in the physical therapy department?*

   Depending on the relationship of the department with referring physicians, the patient may be referred immediately to a physician if available. Otherwise the patient should see a physician as soon as possible and before returning to the exercise program.

*✱PVC's generally not cause for alarm but always concerned about*

CASE
# 16

# Atelectasis—Postoperatively in an Older Patient—Hypotensive and Atrial Fibrillation

## HISTORY/CHART NOTES

*What are common clinical findings of patients with atrial fibrillation?*
   Common findings are:
   • Palpitations, arrhythmia, dyspnea, chest discomfort, and dizziness
   • Feelings of weakness caused by decreased cardiac output
   • Anxiety from the awareness of a rapid and/or irregular heart beat
   • Patients with underlying heart disease are generally less able to tolerate AF without complications

Symptomatic AF is indicative of poor overall cardiac function, whereas AF can be well tolerated by some patients. However, some patients with impaired ventricular function need coordinated atrial pumping. Otherwise they develop a drop in both stroke volume and in cardiac output. These types of patients tend to suffer the effects of AF.

## ELECTROCARDIOGRAM

*Identify the acute EKG changes.*
   The upper panel is an example of a normal EKG tracing. The lower panel is an example of an atrial fibrillation EKG tracing. In the lower tracing, there are multiple P waves preceding the QRS complex. They are irregular in shape (looks like an irregular baseline) and in frequency. This differs from atrial flutter when the multiple P waves are similar in shape and regular in frequency.

## PHYSICAL THERAPY MANAGEMENT

   *By day 2 postoperative, patient was able to mobilize with an IV pole and your assistance for 80 feet. On day 3 after surgery, however, your patient complains of feeling tired and dizzy while in bed and has had palpitations. What cardiopulmonary assessment procedures will you perform?*
   Check for regularity of the pulse, blood pressure, oximetry, and auscultate the patient. Ask if the patient felt any irregular heartbeats or palpitations.

# CASE 17
# Atelectasis—Postoperatively in an Obese Patient—Pulmonary Embolus and Acute Arterial Insufficiency

## HISTORY/CHART NOTES

1. *What are the most common causes and presentations of pulmonary emboli?*

   The most common cause of PE is a DVT. See Chapter 19 under section Peripheral Vascular Disease for the clinical signs of DVT. However, not all patients that show the typical clinical signs will have a DVT and the reverse is also true. PE frequently develops 4 to 6 days after surgery. Patients tend to be mobilizing well by this point postoperatively; they commonly present with a sudden onset of symptoms after an activity.

2. *How would you differentiate between an arterial insufficiency and venous insufficiency? What signs and/or symptoms would you examine for? Are there any tests that you would perform?*

   Arterial insufficiency in the limbs, especially if complete, needs urgent medical or surgical intervention. Ischemic pain worsens after activity. Venous insufficiency tends to be more chronic with edema and skin changes. See below for more details regarding distinguishing features of peripheral vascular diseases:

| Characteristics | Partial Arterial Occlusion | Complete Arterial Occlusion | Chronic Venous Insufficiency |
|---|---|---|---|
| Type of pain | Ischemic | Ischemic, very severe pain | None or minimal pain |
| Aggravating factor | Increased metabolic demand such as ambulation | Constant and nonrelenting | Hanging down the affected limb |
| Relieved by | Rest | None | Elevation and compression stocking. More comfortable in the morning. |
| Pulse in affected areas | Weak | None | Normal or might be difficult to palpate due to swelling |
| Skin color and temperature | Pale, white, and cold. Skin tends to be shiny, smooth and hairless. Ulceration, decreased wound healing and fungal / bacteria infections are common. | Mottling, blue, purplish, and cold. Can progress to black and gangrenous over time. | Slight redness initially but becomes discolored (brownish). Skin may become thick and rubbery. Serous drainage is common in severe cases. |
| Edema | None or minimal | None or minimal | Prominent and in some cases may be massive. Worse in the evening or after keeping the limb in a dependent position. |
| Neurological function | Motor strength is limited by pain | Rapid onset of weakness, and paraesthesia | Mild changes in motor and sensory function |

## PHYSICAL EXAMINATION

1. *Relate the physical appearance of the patient to possible respiratory impairments.*

   Extreme obesity will result in:

   - Restricted chest wall movement

- Increased work of breathing
- Prone to atelectasis
- Decreased lung volumes due to chest wall restriction from obesity
- May not tolerate head-down positions

2. *List possible postoperative problems amenable to physiotherapy.*

- Decreased bed mobility, transfer, and ambulation. (See Table 19-7 for details about an outpatient program)
- Decreased inspiratory effort and cough due to pain and/or weakness
- Decreased circulation secondary to decreased mobility
- More prone to have general weakness from immobility and its consequences are more profound than in an average-sized patient

CASE

# 18     Lobar Pneumonia With Angina

## HISTORY/CHART NOTES

1. *What is the common clinical presentation of angina?*

Chest pain is the most common sign. Check with the patient if the pain she has now is angina and if the angina is any different from her usual pain pattern. See Chapter 19, Table 19-3 for distinguishing features of angina and other types of pain localized to the chest.

Patients with angina should learn the pattern of their angina. In particular:

- What causes their angina attack?
- What does it feel like?
- How long do episodes usually last?
- Does medication relieve the attack?
- If the pattern changes drastically, patients should receive immediate medical attention.

## CHEST X-RAY

*This woman was diagnosed as having pneumococcal pneumonia. Look at the chest x-ray. What lobe is affected? What are the key features of pneumonia shown in this chest x-ray?*

Chest x-ray findings consistent with lobar pneumonia shown in the PA view:

- Increased fluffy opacity over left lung fields
- Elevation of left hemidiaphragm and shift of the mediastinum toward the left lung, indicative of volume loss on the left side
- Outline of left hemidiaphragm is clearly apparent, which indicates that the pathology is in the left upper lung fields
- Increased radiolucency of right lung field, which may in part be due to overexposure of chest x-ray

  The lateral view clearly shows that the increased opacity is located in an upper lobe.

# AUSCULTATION

*What breath sounds and adventitious sounds would you expect to hear on auscultation?*

In lobar pneumonia, bronchial breathing/ breath sounds or decreased air entry/ breath sounds are heard over the affected lobe. Medium-pitched crackles can be heard during resolution of the pneumonia.

# PHYSICAL THERAPY MANAGEMENT

1. *What advice will you give this patient to facilitate coughing and mobilization?*

   Instruct the patient to perform active cycle breathing techniques (see Chapter 15). The patient might require longer breathing control periods to avoid overstressing her cardiopulmonary system. Start activity when cleared by the physician. Gradually increase activity (review Case 14 and Answer Guide for Case 13) and advise the patient to carry her nitroglycerin with her.

2. *List the outcome measures you would use to reassess the treatment effectiveness.*

   Think of objective outcome measures such as the ease of transfer, sitting duration, walking distance, heart rate, respiratory rate, oxygenation saturation, Borg scales of perceived exertion, use of nitroglycerin, and pain scales.

3. *The patient was in head-down position and you were percussing the patient. The patient had a coughing spell earlier and is now complaining of chest pain. How would you manage this patient?*

   Stop treatment! Reposition the patient to the upright sitting position and allow the patient to rest. Give supplementary oxygen and nitroglycerin if the patient has already been prescribed these drugs. Alert the nurse and the physician. Check pulse, oximetry, blood pressure, and auscultate patient. If patient has a coughing spell, encourage relaxation and breathing control exercises.

4. *How would you modify your subsequent treatment for this patient?*

   If the patient did not have angina before, speak to the physician before resuming physiotherapy interventions. Once the patient is medically cleared to resume physiotherapy for lobar pneumonia, the benefit of applying airway clearance techniques versus the risks should be carefully weighed. With close monitoring, ACBT in sitting with longer breathing control periods might be safe. Ensure proper oxygenation during treatment. If needed, modified postural drainage can be used. Percussion especially to the left chest in patients with arrhythmias or susceptible to developing arrhythmia should be avoided. Mobilization is important, but should not be done concurrently with other physical therapy treatments in order to allow patient time to recuperate. If copious expectoration and secretion retention are not a concern, breathing exercises and mobilization may be the only required treatments.

CASE

# 19

# Pleural Effusion Complicated by Cardiac Effusion and Cardiac Tamponade

# HISTORY/CHART NOTES

1. *What are the common signs and symptoms of cardiac effusion and tamponade?*

   The usual symptoms of pain, dyspnea, and pericardial friction rub are frequently present first. As the condition progresses, signs and symptoms of cardiac tamponade may present such as:

- Jugular venous distension, hypotension, and muffled heart sounds.
- *Pulsus paradoxus*. The first sphygmomanometer reading is recorded at the point when beats are audible during expiration and disappear with inspiration. The second reading is taken when each beat is audible during the respiratory cycle. A difference of more than 10 mmHg defines pulsus paradoxus.
- Cyanosis, decreased level of consciousness, and shock.

# CHEST X-RAY

*Review the chest x-ray. What are the features consistent with pulmonary edema shown by the chest x-ray in Case 19, Figure 19-1?*

In patients with slow fluid accumulation >200 mL, the chest x-ray may show an enlarged cardiac silhouette. However with rapid fluid accumulation, the cardiac silhouette may be normal. In the chest x-ray shown in Case 19, Figure 19-1, the most prominent feature is increased opacity in the basal lung fields which has obliterated the shadows of:

- The hemidiaphragms
- Cardiophrenic and costophrenic angles

# AUSCULTATION

*Describe the breath sounds you would expect to hear in patients with pleural effusion. How are the auscultatory findings of a pericardial rub different from a pleural rub?*

The breath sounds are diminished or absent in the lung region with the effusion. The pericardial rub is similar in quality to that of pleural rub (2 pieces of leather rubbing together). The distinguishing features are their locations and dependency on respiration. A pleural rub occurs during breathing while a pericardial rub occurs when the heart beats.

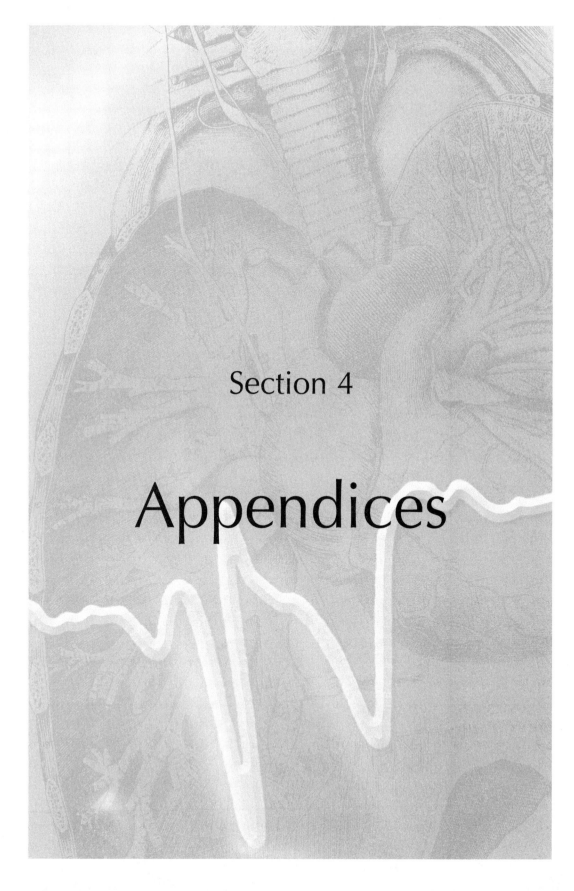

Section 4

Appendices

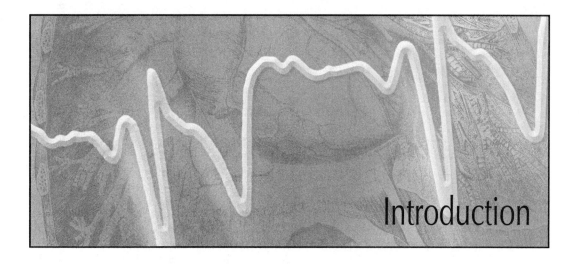

# Introduction

*Clinicians today are in a bind. Increasing demands on their time are squeezing out opportunities to stay abreast of the literature, much less read it critically. Results of several studies indicate an inverse relation between knowledge of contemporary care and time since graduation from medical school.[1,2] In many jurisdictions, attendance at a specified number of hours of continuing medical education courses is mandatory to maintain a license to practice. However, the failure of these courses to improve patient care[3,4] emphasizes the importance of self-directed learning through reading. Many clinicians in practice, though, report that they feel unqualified to read the medical literature critically.[5] Scientific illiteracy is a major failing of medical education.[6]*

Lancet. 2002;359: 57-617.[7]

Clinicians frequently fall into the scenario described above. One of the purposes of this book is to fill in the void and meet the clinical needs of physical therapists. We all hope that a textbook or journal article will provide us with all the clinical information and practice guidelines we need for our clinical practice. However, the reality may be a long way from our expectation. The recent narrative reviews by Chung and Reid[8,9] point out that:

- Statistical significance, determined mathematically, is essential but not synonymous to clinical importance
- Determination of clinical importance will vary depending on the outcome measure and its specific context
- Data presented in clinical trials are not always valid
- Narrative reviews and systematic reviews may contain erroneous information
- The authors concluded that clinicians should avoid scanning research papers or reviews and accepting the conclusions at face value

Not only is the validity of published clinical trials, practice guidelines, narrative and systematic reviews in question,[8-10] but the authenticity of authorship also remains an issue.[11,12] The Cochrane Database of Systematic Reviews used a substantial number of honorary and ghost authors in their reviews.[12] Newspaper headlines have frequently reported new medical discoveries that sometimes are based on unpublished abstracts from scientific meetings.[13] At the same time, an author may not be able to input or publish unfavorable or unpopular ideas.[14,15] The editor of the *Lancet* found evidence of censored criticism, obscured meanings, confused assessment of implications, and that research papers rarely represent the opinions of all contributors to the research.[15] In order to obtain a large sample size to increase the probability of significant results, researchers recruit different centers across the country or continents into their study. The potential heterogeneity, bias, confounding factors and effect modification among involved centers need to be addressed.[16] How long will the truth in scientific literature remain true? The half-life of truth in scientific literature was 45 years.[17,18] The 20-year survival of conclusions derived from a meta-analysis was lower (57%) than that from nonrandomized studies or randomized trials (87% and 85%, respectively). In randomized trials, the 50-year survival rate was higher for negative conclusions

(68%) than positive conclusions (14%).[17] Conclusions based on recognized, good methodology had no clear survival advantage. Also, quality measures are not reliably associated with the strength of treatment effect.[17,19]

> *The hypothetico-deductive model of Karl Popper contends that "An assertion is true if it corresponds to, or agrees with, the facts".[20] Because "the facts" change over time, truth is relative. In this view of events, science progresses via a series of theories (paradigms) that are held to be true until they are replaced by a better approximation of reality.[21]*

> *Lancet.* 1997;350:175-218.[18]

It appears then that "the truth" or "the facts" are moving targets. Despite these problems, most of the contents in this book are based on recent clinical trials and the authors have made every attempt to review and critique references quoted in this book. In the process, we identified and explained some of the limitations associated with different studies. The reality is that research in physical therapy as a whole is still in its early stages. Relatively few randomized control trials exist in the field of cardiopulmonary physical therapy. In those few trials, the sample sizes per groups tended to be very small (<50 subjects). Underpowered clinical trials have limited clinical value and are considered unethical except in research on rare diseases or pilot studies.[22]

Despite of these shortcomings in the literature, in order to provide treatment rationale based on research, information from recent clinical randomized control trials, nonrandomized trials and repeated measures trials were included in this book. The authors are aware that even though the results of randomized and nonrandomized trials were well correlated, nonrandomized trials tend to exaggerate the treatment effects and sometimes provide conflicting results when compared to randomized trials.[23] Due to the uncertainty principle, reader discretion is encouraged when reading any published material.

# REFERENCES

1.  Ramsey PG, Carline JD, Inui TS, et al. Changes over time in the knowledge base of practicing internists. JAMA. 1991;266:1103-1107.

2.  Evans CE, Haynes RB, Birkett NJ, et al. Does a mailed continuing education program improve physician performance? Results of a randomized trial in antihypertensive care. JAMA. 1986;255:501-504.

3.  Davis DA, Thomson MA, Oxman AD, Haynes RB. Changing physician performance: a systematic review of the effect of continuing medical education strategies. JAMA. 1995;274:700-705.

4.  Sibley JC, Sackett DL, Neufeld V, et al. A randomized trial of continuing medical education. N Engl J Med. 1982;306:511-515.

5.  Olatunbosun OA, Edouard L, Pierson RA. Physicians' attitudes toward evidence based obstetric practice: a questionnaire survey. BMJ. 1998;316:365-366.

6.  Grimes DA, Bachicha JA, Learman LA. Teaching critical appraisal to medical students in obstetrics and gynecology. Obstet Gynecol. 1998;92:877-882.

7.  Grimes DA, Schulz KF. An overview of clinical research: the lay of the land. Lancet. 2002;359:57-61.

8.  Chung F, Reid WD. Evidence based practice: assess the quality of the evidence part I: applied statistics. Cardiopul Phys Ther. 2001;12:112-116.

9.  Chung F, Reid WD. Evidence based practice: assess the quality of the evidence part II: grading the evidence. Cardiopul Phys Ther. 2001;12:117-122.

10. Hopayian K. The need for caution in interpreting high quality systematic reviews. BMJ. 2001;323:681-684.

11. Davidoff F, DeAngelis CD, Drazen JM, et al. Sponsorship, authorship, and accountability. JAMA. 2001;286:1232-1233.

12. Mowatt G, Shirran L, Grimshaw JM, et al. Prevalence of honorary and ghost authorships in Cochrane Reviews. JAMA. 2002;287:2769-2771.

13. Schwartz LM, Woloshin S, Baczek L. Media coverage of scientific meetings. Too much, too soon? JAMA. 2002;287:2859-2863.

14. Blumenthal D, Campbell EG, Anderson MS, et al. Withholding research results in academic life science: evidence from a national survey of faculty. JAMA. 1997;277:1224-1228.

15. Horton R. The hidden research paper. JAMA. 2002;287:2775-2778.

16. Localio R, Berlin JA, Ten Have TR, et al. Adjustments for center in multicenter studies: An overview. *Ann Intern Med.* 2001;135:112-123.

17. Poynard T, Munteanu M, Ratziu V, et al. Truth survival in clinical research: an evidence-based requiem? *Ann Intern Med.* 2002;136:888-895.

18. Hall JC, Platell C. Half-life of truth in surgical literature. *Lancet.* 1997;350:1752.

19. Balk EM, Bonis PA, Moskowitz H, et al. Correlation of quality measures with estimates of treatment effect in meta-analyses of randomized controlled trials. JAMA. 2002; 287:2973-2982.

20. Popper KR. *The Myth of Framework: In Defence of Science and Rationality.* London & New York: Routledge; 1994:174.

21. Polanyi M. *Science, Faith and Society.* Chicago and London: The University of Chicago Press; 1946.

22. Halpern SD, Karlawish JHT, Berlin JA. The continuing unethical conduct of underpowered clinical trials. JAMA. 2002; 288:358-362.

23. Ioannidis JPA, Haidich AB, Pappa M, et al. Comparison of evidence of treatment effects in randomized and nonrandomized studies. JAMA. 2001;286:821-830.

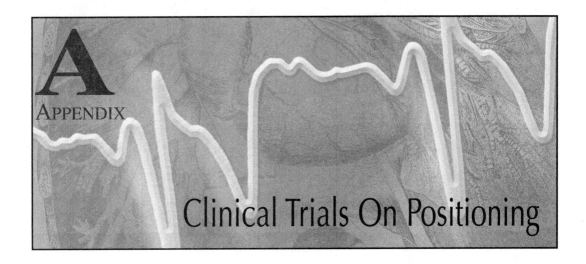

## APPENDIX

# Clinical Trials On Positioning

The objective of this appendix is to provide a review of clinical trials on positioning. The level of evidence and summary on positioning in Chapter 13 was made based on this review and other systematic reviews.

Table A-1

### Clinical Trials on Supine and Upright Positions

| References | Sample Size | RCT | Subjects | Results |
|---|---|---|---|---|
| | | | Effects on Oxygenation | |
| *Am J Respir Crit Care Med.* 1999; 159: 1070-1073[1] | 28 | No | Eisenmenger's syndrome | A significant decrease in $PaO_2$ and $SaO_2$ was reported when patients changed from the sitting to the supine position. |
| Anaesthesia 1996; 51:225-227[2] | 12 | No | Post laparotomy | $SaO_2$ was significantly higher during sitting and standing on days 1 and 4 after operation compared with the supine position. |
| *Anaesthesia.* 1997; 52:589-592[3] | 13 | No | Post major abdominal surgery | Individual mean $SaO_2$ decreased postoperatively but without a difference between the supine and side lying positions. Episodic desaturations were significantly more frequent in the supine position than on the side before surgery only. |
| *J Gerontol A Biol Sci Med Sci.* 2000; 55:M239-244[4] | 12 to 17 | No | First 72 hours following mild to moderately severe stroke | Mean $SaO_2$ for all patients were >90% for the hour spent in each test position. There were no changes in $SaO_2$ across the hour spent in the test positions (alternate side lying with head of bed at 45 degrees sitting with head of bed at 70 degrees and sitting in an armchair). |

Table A-1, continued

## *Clinical Trials on Supine and Upright Positions*

| References | Sample Size | RCT | Subjects | Results |
|---|---|---|---|---|
| | | | Effects on Oxygenation | |
| *Respiration.* 2002; 69:123-128[5] | 46 | No | Healthy elderly | A higher $PaO_2$ (5 mmHg) was observed in sitting than supine. |
| *Zhonghua Yi Xue Za Zhi (Taipei).* 1993; 51:183-192[6] | 15 | No | Obese patients post upper abdominal surgery | No clinically significant desaturation was seen in, 15 degrees of Trendelenburg, lateral decubitus, and bed-flat lateral decubitus following surgery. |
| | | | Other Effects | |
| *Blood Press.* 1999; 8:220-226[7] | 163 | NA | Healthy 30, 50, and 60 year old men | A transient decrease in systolic BP upon standing from supine in men aged 50 and 60 years and a transient increase in the 30-year-olds were reported. The diastolic BP increased in all age groups, but less in the older compared to the younger men. The HR increased to a similar extent upon standing from supine in all age groups. |
| *Gerontology.* 1996; 42:46-53[8] | 17 | No | Nursing home residents (mean age is 80) | Significant decreases in $FEV_1$, FVC, and PEF were reported in supine when compared to the sitting position. |

Table A-2

## Clinical Trials on Lateral Positions in Patients With Unilateral Lung Disease

| References | Sample Size | RCT | Subjects | Results |
|---|---|---|---|---|
| *Am J Crit Care.* 2002;11:65-75[9] | 15 | No | Single-lung transplant | No single position (supine, lateral with allograft lung down, and lateral with native lung down) in single-lung transplant maximizes oxygenation in the immediate postoperative period in these patients. |
| *Am J Respir Crit Care Med.* 2000; 161:1957-62[10] | 44 | No | Unilateral lung disease | In 26 patients, $PaO_2$ was higher with the normal lung in the dependent position than that with the diseased lung; the opposite was true for 18 patients. In 16 patients with full data available, 5/16 of them had the highest $PaO_2$ in the supine position. |
| *Chest.* 1993; 103: 787-791[11] | 35 | No | Unilateral lung disease | No difference in the alveolar—arterial $O_2$ difference was reported in the comparison of whether the affected or unaffected lung was dependent. |
| *Respir Med.* 1995; 89:297-301[12] | 30 | No | Unilateral pleural effusion | No difference in $PaO_2$ between normal-side down and the effusion-side down was reported. $PaO_2$ with normal-side down was higher than effusion-side down in 22 of 30 patients (conventional), and lower in 8 patients (paradoxical). |

Table A-3

## Clinical Trials on Positioning in Patients on a Mechanical Ventilator

| References | Sample Size | RCT | Subjects | Results |
|---|---|---|---|---|
| Am J Crit Care. 1996;5:121-126[13] | 120 | No | CABG | The mean $PaO_2$ in the left lateral position was lower than the values in the right lateral or supine positions. No significant effects for position and pH, $PaCO_2$, $PvO_2$, $PvCO_2$, or bicarbonate were detected. |
| Am J Crit Care. 1997;6:132-40[14] | 57 | No | Critically ill men | Turning to the left side decreases mixed venous oxygen saturation more than turning to the ride side. Oxygen saturation returns to clinically acceptable ranges within 5 minutes of turn. |
| Am Surg. 1996; 62:1038-1041[15] | 16 | No | Acute lung injury | Oxygenation was not improved and compliance was adversely affected by upright body positioning when compared to supine. |
| Anesth Analg. 1995;80:955-960[16] | 17 | No | Under GA | The prone position during did not negatively affect respiratory mechanics and improved lung volumes and oxygenation. |
| Anesth Analg. 1996;83:578-583[17] | 10 | No | Under GA | In anesthetized and paralyzed obese subjects, the prone position improved pulmonary function, increased FRC, lung compliance, and oxygenation. |
| Ann Emerg Med. 1994;23:564-567[18] | 8 | No | Hypovolemia postoperation | Increase in mean arterial BP, pulmonary artery wedge pressure, and the systemic vascular resistance were reported when patients were positioned from supine to the Trendelenburg position. However, there were no significant changes in cardiac index, oxygen delivery, oxygen consumption, or oxygen extraction ratio. |
| Heart Lung. 2001; 30:269-276[19] | 12 | No | Critically ill patients | Position change (right and left 45 degrees lateral and supine) did not result in changes of cardiac function, oxygenation, or lactate level. |
| Heart Lung. 1992; 21:448-456[20] | 30 | No | CABG | No difference in $PaO_2$ and pulmonary shunt were reported between supine and left and right side lying with 30 degrees of elevation. |
| J Clin Anesth. 1996; 8:236-244[21] | 15 | No | Under GA | Total respiratory E&R (elastance and resistance) increased in the head-down posture compared with supine due to increases in lung E&R; but chest wall E&R did not change. Lung and chest wall E&R were not affected by shifting from supine to head-up. |

## Table A-3, continued

### *Clinical Trials on Positioning in Patients on a Mechanical Ventilator*

| References | Sample Size | RCT | Subjects | Results |
|---|---|---|---|---|
| Lancet 1999; 354: 1851-1858[22] | 86 | Yes | Ventilated patients | The frequency of clinically suspected nosocomial pneumonia was lower in the semirecumbent group than in the supine group (3 of 39 [8%] vs 16 of 47 [34%]). Supine body position and enteral nutrition were independent risk factors and the risk is increased by long-duration mechanical ventilation and decreased LOC. |

Abbreviations: GA: general anesthesia; LOC: level of consciousness; $PvCO_2$: mixed venous carbon dioxide partial pressure; $PvO_2$: mixed venous carbon dioxide partial pressure.

Table A-4

## Clinical Trials on Continuous Rotation in Patients on a Mechanical Ventilator

| References | Sample Size | RCT | Subjects | Results |
|---|---|---|---|---|
| *Arch Surg.* 1989; 124:352-355[23] | 10 | No | Acute lung disease (on ventilator) | There were no significant hemodynamic or ventilatory differences among the four positions (supine, right side down, left side down, and rotating). In 5 out of 6 patients, differences in $PaO_2$ between sides were reported. Continuous rotation did not significantly alter the $PaO_2$ from the supine values in these patients. |
| *Chest.* 1999; 115: 1658-66[24] | 24 | Yes | Mixed non-ventilated and ventilated patients | KT (rotation of a patient > 40 degrees to each side continuously) and mechanical percussion therapy resulted in significantly greater partial or complete resolution of atelectasis as compared with conventional therapy (turn and manual percussion every 2 hr). There was a generalized trend toward statistical significance in the improvement of oxygenation. (See discussion in the section below.) |
| *Crit Care.* 2001; 5:81-87[25] | 19 | No | ARDS (on ventilator) | Turning and secretion management regimens for 6 hr each over a period of 24 hr were studied: (1) routine turning every 2 hr from the left to right lateral position; (2) routine turning every 2 hr from the left to right lateral position including a 15 min P&PD; (3) Continuous lateral rotation (CLR) from left to right lateral position, pausing at each position for 2 min; and (4) CLR and a 15 min period of mechanical P provided by the bed every 2 hr. Sputum productions were higher with (3) & (4) than (1). However, in the 4 patients producing more than 40 ml of sputum per day, P&PD increased sputum volume significantly. |
| *Crit Care Med.* 2001; 29:51-56[26] | 26 | Yes | ARDS (on ventilator) | In severe lung injury, continuous rotational therapy (maximum angle of 124 degrees) seems to exert effects comparable to prone positioning and could serve as alternative when prone positioning seems inadvisable. |
| *Intensive Care Med.* 1998;24:132-137[27] | 10 | No | Acute lung injury (on ventilator) | Continuous axial rotation reduced intrapulmonary shunt and general V/Q mismatch but improved arterial oxygenation as compared to the supine position. Continuous axial rotation is not effective in late or progressive ARDS. |

Table A-4, continued

## Clinical Trials on Continuous Rotation in Patients on a Mechanical Ventilator

| References | Sample Size | RCT | Subjects | Results |
|---|---|---|---|---|
| J Crit Care. 1998; 13:119-125[28] | 13 | No | Ventilated patients | Continuous lateral rotational therapy (<40 degrees) did not appear to stimulate significant mucus removal from the lung in critically ill patients but also did not cause any adverse effects. |

Abbreviations: P&PD: percussion and postural drainage; V/Q: ventilation perfusion ration.

# CRITIQUE OF A RANDOMIZED CONTROL TRIAL ON THE EFFECT OF CONTINUOUS ROTATION

The study[24] that provides the strongest support for continuous rotation had some major methodological problems as outlined below:

- Physicians involved were not blinded and thus, decisions regarding treatment were biased, favoring the continuous rotation group
- The length of stay was longer in patients that were put on the rotating bed
- Sample sizes between groups were uneven and standard deviations in some instances were many times higher in the continuous rotation group. Appropriate statistical analysis was not used to consider these uneven sample sizes and variances

# REFERENCES

1. Sandoval J, Alvarado P, Martinez-Guerra ML, et al. Effect of body position changes on pulmonary gas exchange in Eisenmenger's syndrome. Am J Respir Crit Care Med. 1999;159:1070-1073.

2. Mynster T, Jensen LM, Jensen FG, et al. The effect of posture on late postoperative oxygenation. Anaesthesia. 1996;51:225-227.

3. Rosenberg-Adamsen S, Stausholm K, Edvardsen L, et al. Body position and late postoperative nocturnal hypoxaemia. Anaesthesia. 1997;52:589-592.

4. Chatterton HJ, Pomeroy VM, Connolly MJ, et al. The effect of body position on arterial oxygen saturation in acute stroke. J Gerontol A Biol Sci Med Sci. 2000;55:M239-244.

5. Hardie JA, Morkve O, Ellingsen I. Effect of body position on arterial oxygen tension in the elderly. Respiration. 2002;69:123-128.

6. Bien MY, Zadai CC, Kigin CM, et al. The effect of selective drainage positions on oxygen saturation in obese patients after upper abdominal surgery. Zhonghua Yi Xue Za Zhi (Taipei). 1993;51:183-192.

7. Hofsten A, Elmfeldt D, Svardsudd K. Age-related differences in blood pressure and heart rate responses to changes in body position: results from a study with serial measurements in the supine and standing positions in 30-, 50- and 60-year-old men. Blood Press. 1999;8:220-226.

8. Vitacca M, Clini E, Spassini W, et al. Does the supine position worsen respiratory function in elderly subjects? Gerontology. 1996;42:46-53.

9. George EL, Hoffman LA, Boujoukos A, et al. Effect of positioning on oxygenation in single-lung transplant recipients. *Am J Crit Care.* 2002;11:65-75.

10. Choe KH, Kim YT, Shim TS, et al. Closing volume influences the postural effect on oxygenation in unilateral lung disease. *Am J Respir Crit Care Med.* 2000;161:1957-1962.

11. Chang SC, Chang HI, Shiao GM, et al. Effect of body position on gas exchange in patients with unilateral central airway lesions. Down with the good lung? *Chest.* 1993;103:787-791.

12. Romero S, Martin C, Hernandez L. Effect of body position on gas exchange in patients with unilateral pleural effusion: influence of effusion volume. *Respir Med.* 1995;89:297-301.

13. Banasik JL, Emerson RJ. Effect of lateral position on arterial and venous blood gases in postoperative cardiac surgery patients. *Am J Crit Care.* 1996;5:121-126.

14. Lewis P, Nichols E, Mackey G, et al. The effect of turning and backrub on mixed venous oxygen saturation in critically ill patients. *Am J Crit Care.* 1997;6:132-140.

15. Bittner E, Chendrasekhar A, Pillai S, et al. Changes in oxygenation and compliance as related to body position in acute lung injury. *Am Surg.* 1996;62:1038-1041.

16. Pelosi P, Croci M, Calappi E, et al. The prone positioning during general anesthesia minimally affects respiratory mechanics while improving functional residual capacity and increasing oxygen tension. *Anesth Analg.* 1995;80:955-960.

17. Pelosi P, Croci M, Calappi E, et al. Prone positioning improves pulmonary function in obese patients during general anesthesia. *Anesth Analg.* 1996;83:578-583.

18. Sing RF, O'Hara D, Sawyer MA, et al. Trendelenburg position and oxygen transport in hypovolemic adults. *Ann Emerg Med.* 1994;23:564-567.

19. Banasik JL, Emerson RJ. Effect of lateral positions on tissue oxygenation in the critically ill. *Heart Lung.* 2001;30:269-276.

20. Chan M, Jensen L. Positioning effects on arterial oxygen and relative pulmonary shunt in patients receiving mechanical ventilation after CABG. *Heart Lung.* 1992;21:448-456.

21. Fahy BG, Barnas GM, Nagle SE, et al. Effects of Trendelenburg and reverse Trendelenburg postures on lung and chest wall mechanics. *J Clin Anesth.* 1996;8:236-244.

22. Drakulovic MB, Torres A, Bauer TT. Supine body position as a risk factor for nosocomial pneumonia in mechanically ventilated patients: a randomised trial. *Lancet.* 1999;354:1851-1858.

23. Nelson LD, Anderson HB. Physiologic effects of steep positioning in the surgical intensive care unit. *Arch Surg.* 1989;124:352-355.

24. Raoof S, Chowdhrey N, Raoof S, et al. Effect of combined kinetic therapy and percussion therapy on the resolution of atelectasis in critically ill patients. *Chest.* 1999;115:1658-66.

25. Davis K Jr, Johannigman JA, Campbell RS, et al. The acute effects of body position strategies and respiratory therapy in paralyzed patients with acute lung injury. *Crit Care.* 2001;5:81-87.

26. Staudinger T, Kofler J, Mullner M, et al. Comparison of prone positioning and continuous rotation of patients with adult respiratory distress syndrome: results of a pilot study. *Crit Care Med.* 2001;29:51-56.

27. Bein T, Reber A, Metz C, et al. Acute effects of continuous rotational therapy on ventilation-perfusion inequality in lung injury. *Intensive Care Med.* 1998;24:132-137.

28. Dolovich M, Rushbrook J, Churchill E, et al. Effect of continuous lateral rotational therapy on lung mucus transport in mechanically ventilated patients. *J Crit Care.* 1998;13:119-125.

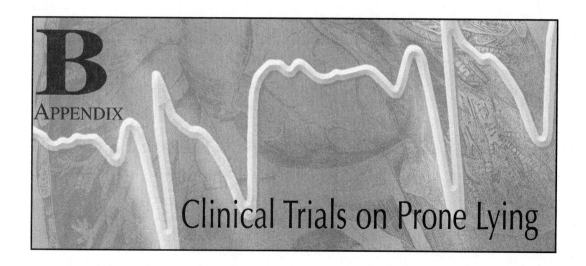

APPENDIX

# Clinical Trials on Prone Lying

The objective of this appendix is to provide a review of clinical trials on prone lying. The level of evidence and summary on prone lying in Chapter 13 was made based on this review and other systematic reviews.

Table B-1

### Clinical Trials on Prone Lying

| References | Sample Size | RCT | Subjects | Results |
|---|---|---|---|---|
| *Am J Respir Crit Care Med.* 1997; 155:473-478[1] | 32 | No | ARDS | $PaO_2$ increased when turned from supine to prone position. 78% of patients were responders to prone lying. |
| *Am J Respir Crit Care Med.* 1998; 157:580-585[2] | 14 | No | ARDS | In ARDS patients, inhalation of nitric oxide in the prone position significantly improved oxygenation compared with the prone position without nitric oxide, which in turn was better than nitric oxide inhalation in the supine position. |
| *Anesth Analg.* 1996; 83:1206-1211[3] | 20 | No | ARDS | $PaO_2$ and $(A-a)PO_2$ increased while intrapulmonary shunt decreased when turned from supine to prone position. Patients stayed prone for 20 hours. |
| *Anesthesiology.* 1998; 89:1401-1406[4] | 47 | No | ARDS | In ARDS patients, inhalation of nitric oxide in the prone position significantly improved oxygenation compared to prone position without nitric oxide, which in turn was better than nitric oxide inhalation in the supine position. |
| *Chest.* 1988;94: 103-107[5] | 13 | No | ARDS | $PaO_2$ increased when turned from supine to prone position. 62% of patients were responders to prone lying. |
| *Chest.* 1994;106: 1511-1516[6] | 12 | No | ARDS | $PaO_2$ increased when turned from supine to prone position. 67% of patients were responders to prone lying. |

Table B-1, continued

## Clinical Trials on Prone Lying

| References | Sample Size | RCT | Subjects | Results |
|---|---|---|---|---|
| Crit Care Med. 1997; 25:1539-1544[7] | 13 | No | Acute lung injury | $PaO_2/FiO_2$ and $(A-a)PO_2$ increased when turned from supine to prone position. 92% of patients were responders to prone lying. |
| Crit Care Med. 1998; 26:1977-1985[8] | 19 | No | ARDS | Among the responders, subsequent prone lying produces a 71% positive response. Among the nonresponders, subsequent prone lying produces a 25% positive response. $PaO_2/FiO_2$ ratio increased while venous admixture decreased when turned from supine to prone position. Patients stayed prone for 12 hours. |
| Intensive Care Med. 1996;22:1105-1111[9] | 15 | No | ARDS | $(A-a)PO_2$ increased when turned from supine to prone position. 60% of patients were responders to prone lying. |
| Intensive Care Med. 1997;23:1033-1039[10] | 23 | No | ARDS | $PaO_2/FiO_2$ ratio and respiratory system compliance increased while intrapulmonary shunt decreased when turned from supine to prone position. Cardiac output and other hemodynamic parameters were not affected. 70% of patients were responders to prone lying. The data suggest that prone positioning should be carried out early during the course of ARDS. |
| Intensive Care Med. 1999;25:29-36[11] | 14 | No | ARDS | $PaO_2/FiO_2$ ratio increased while venous admixture decreased when turned from supine to prone position. In the supine position, inhalation of nitric oxide improved $PaO_2/FiO_2$ and decreasing venous admixture to a lesser extent than prone lying alone. The combination of nitric oxide and prone positioning was additive in increasing $PaO_2/FiO_2$ and decreasing venous admixture. 71% of patients were responders to prone lying. |

Table B-1, continued

## Clinical Trials on Prone Lying

| References | Sample Size | RCT | Subjects | Results |
|---|---|---|---|---|
| Am J Respir Crit Care Med. 2000; 161:360-368[12] | 39 | Yes | Hydostatic pulmonary edema, ARDS, pulmonary fibrosis | $PaO_2/FiO_2$ increased when turned from supine to prone position in HPE (100% responder) and ARDS (75% responder) patients. No improvement in $PaO_2/FiO_2$ when turned from supine to prone position in PF patient was reported. The presence of pulmonary edema, as in early ARDS and HPE, predicts a beneficial effect of the prone position on gas exchange. In contrast, the presence of fibrosis, as in late ARDS and pulmonary fibrosis, predisposes to nonresponsiveness to prone positioning. |
| Intensive Care Med. 2002;28:564-569[13] | 51 | Yes | Ventilated comatose patients | The incidence of lung worsening was lower in the prone group (12%) than in the supine group (50%). There were no serious complications attributable to prone positioning; however, there was a significant increase of intracranial pressure in the prone group. |
| N Engl J Med. 2001; 345:568-573[14] | 304 | Yes | Acute lung injury and ARDS | $PaO_2/FiO_2$ increased when turned from supine to prone position. However, there is no difference in patient survival between supine and prone group. (See following section on critical review about this study.) |

Abbreviations: (A-a)$PO_2$: alveolar arterial oxygen partial pressure difference; HPE: hydrostatic pulmonary edema; PF; pulmonary fibrosis.

# CRITIQUE OF A RANDOMIZED CONTROL TRIAL ON THE EFFECT OF PRONE POSITIONING ON THE SURVIVAL OF PATIENTS WITH ACUTE RESPIRATORY FAILURE

The majority of ARDS patients die from multiple-organ failure but not from hypoxemia. The mechanisms leading to multiple-organ failure are probably multifactorial, but there is evidence that lung injury caused by mechanical ventilation can result in the release of several mediators including proinflammatory cytokines. These mediators, as well as endotoxin or bacteria can enter the systemic circulation leading to multiple-organ failure. Hence, prone positioning might decrease the severity of hypoxemia in patients but might not contribute significantly to a decrease in mortality in ARDS patients.[15-18]

Given the imprecision inherent in the diagnosis of the ARDS, the heterogeneity of the underlying diseases that confer a predisposition to the syndrome, and the lack of uniformity among other interventions used, the study[14] did not have adequate statistical power. Furthermore, the problem was further complicated by the fact that the study[14] was terminated early (before the predetermined sample size was reached) because of progressively slower rate of recruitment due largely to an increasing unwillingness among clinicians to forgo the use of prone positioning.

In the study,[14] patients were placed in the prone position for an average of only 7 hours per day. Thus, the patients were exposed to the potentially injurious effects of mechanical ventilation in the supine position for more than 70% of each day. In addition, the authors limited the use of the prone position to 10 days, which may have been too short a period for any significant long-term benefit to occur.[15]

Furthermore, despite randomization, 12 patients in the supine group used the prone position 43 times and 41 patients in the prone lying group missed a total of 91 turns. On day 1, 144/152 or 95% of patients were positioned prone. On day 5, 62 patients (or less than half), and day 10, 33 (or about one-quarter) of the patients were positioned prone. The compliance for turning patients to prone was low, which resulted in a lot of missing data, and a high likelihood of a type II error. The study results might have been different if they actually used the prone position as the methods outlined for the patients in the prone lying group. Alternate end-points such as the percentage of patients in the supine group that fit the criteria for prone on day 10 compared to that of the prone group might have been more meaningful.

In summary, better-planned and executed randomized controlled trials are needed on the prone position. The possible mechanisms by which the prone position improves oxygenation are likely related to improved ventilation and perfusion of the previously collapsed dorsal lung field.

# REFERENCES

1. Chatte G, Sab JM, Dubois, et al. Prone position in mechanically ventilated patients with acute respiratory failure. *Am J Respir Crit Care Med.* 1997;155:473-478.

2. Papazian L, Bregeon F, Gaillat F, et al. Respective and combined effects of prone posiition and inhaled nitric oxide in patients with acute respiratory distress syndrome. *Am J Respir Crit Care Med.* 1998;157:580-585.

3. Fridrich P, Krafft P, Hochleuthner H, et al. The effects of long-term prone positioning in patients with trauma-induced adult respiratory distress syndrome. *Anesth Analg.* 1996;83:1206-1211.

4. Germann P, Poschl G, Leitner C, et al. Additive effect of nitric oxide inhalation on the oxygenation benefit of the prone position in the adult respiratory distress syndrome. *Anaesthesiology.* 1998;89:1401-1406.

5. Langer M, Mascheroni D, Marcolin R, et al. The prone position in ARDS patients. A clinical study. *Chest.* 1988;94:103-107.

6. Pappert D, Rossaint R, Slama K, et al. Influence of positioning on ventilation-perfusion relationships in severe adult respiratory distress syndrome. *Chest.* 1994;106:1511-1516.

7. Mure M, Martling CR, Lindahl SG. Dramatic effect on oxygenation in patients with severe acute lung insufficiency treated in the prone position. *Crit Care Med.* 1997;25:1539-1544.

8. Jolliet P, Bulpa P, Chervolet JC. Effects of the prone position on gas exchange and hemodynamics in severe acute respiratory distress syndrome. *Crit Care Med.* 1998;26:1977-1985

9. Vollman KM, Bander JJ. Improved oxygenation utilizing a prone positioner in patients with acute respiratory distress syndrome. *Intensive Care Med.* 1996;22:1105-1111.

10. Blanch L, Mancebo J, Perez M. Short-term effects of prone position in critically ill patients with acute respiratory distress syndrome. *Intensive Care Med.* 1997;23:1033-1039.

11. Martinez M, Diaz E, Joseph D, et al. Improvement in oxygenation by prone position and nitric oxide in patients with acute respiratory distress syndrome. *Intensive Care Med.* 1999;25:29-36.

12. Nakos G, Tsangaris I, Kostanti E, et al. Effect of the prone position on patients with hydrostatic pulmonary edema compared with patients with acute respiratory distress syndrome and pulmonary fibrosis. *Am J Respir Crit Care Med.* 2000;161:360-368.

13. Beuret P, Carton MJ, Nourdine K, et al. Prone position as prevention of lung injury in comatose patients: a prospective, randomized, controlled study. *Intensive Care Med.* 2002;28:564-569.

14. Gattinoni L, Tognoni G, Pesenti A, et al. Effect of prone positioning on the survival of patients with acute respiratory failure. *N Engl J Med.* 2001;345:568-573.

15. Slutsky AS. The acute respiratory distress syndrome, mechanical ventilation, and the prone position. *N Engl J Med.* 2001;345:610-612.

16. Kraft P, Fridrich P, Pernerstorfer T, et al. The acute respiratory distress syndrome: definitions, severity and clinical outcome. An analysis of 101 clinical investigations. *Intensive Care Med.* 1996;22:1105-1111.

17. Albert RK. The prone position in acute respiratory distress syndrome: where we are, and where do we go from here. *Crit Care Med.* 1997;25:1453-1454.

18. Klein D. Prone positioning in patients with acute respiratory distress syndrome: Vollman prone positioner. *Crit Care Nurse.* 1999;19:66-71.

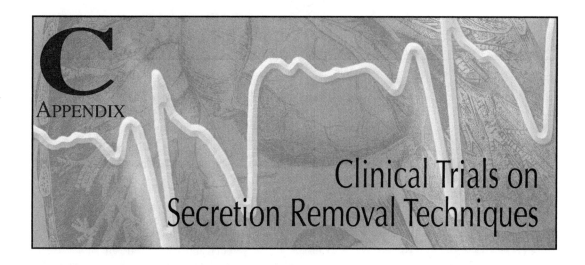

# Clinical Trials on Secretion Removal Techniques

The objective of this appendix is to provide a review of clinical trials on secretion removal techniques. The level of evidence and Summary of secretion removal techniques in Chapter 15 were determined based on this review and other published reviews.

Table C-1

## Clinical Trials on Secretion Removal Techniques

| References | Sample Size | RCT | Subjects | Results |
|---|---|---|---|---|
| Am J Resp Crit Care Med. 1994; 150:1154-1157[1] | 50 | Yes | Cystic fibrosis | The study reported similar improvement in spirometry after treatment with HFCWO and PDPV. |
| Chest. 1990;97: 645-650[2] | 43 | Yes | Chronic bronchitis | Treatment with PEP mask can reduce morbidity in patients with chronic bronchitis and may preserve lung function from a more rapid decline. |
| J Cardiopulm Rehabil. 2000;20: 37-43[3] | 30 | Yes | COPD | PEFR and $PaCO_2$ improved significantly with AD treatment more so than ACBT. $SaO_2$ was higher with ACBT than AD. It was concluded that AD is as effective as the ACBT in secretion removal and improving lung functions. (There is a contradiction in results section in the abstract and the results section in the text.) |
| J Pediatr. 1997; 131:570-574[4] | 40 | Yes | Cystic fibrosis | Improvement in spirometry with PEP mask group when compared to PDPV group. |
| J Pediatr. 2001; 138:845-850[5] | 40 | Yes | Cystic fibrosis | The flutter group demonstrated a mean annual rate of decline in FVC and in Huang scores (p=0.05) when compared with the PEP group. There was a significant decline in hospitalizations and antibiotic use in the Flutter group. |

---

## Table C-1, continued

### *Clinical Trials on Secretion Removal Techniques*

| References | Sample Size | RCT | Subjects | Results |
|---|---|---|---|---|
| *Pediatr Pulmonol.* 1999;28:255-260[6] | 23 | Yes | Cystic fibrosis | Patients using the Flutter device had better pulmonary function after 1 week of therapy than CPT group. However, both groups had similar improvement in pulmonary function and exercise tolerance after 2 weeks of therapy. |
| *Arch Phys Med Rehabil.* 2000;81: 558-60[7] | 10 | No | Chronic bronchitis | Flutter and ELTGOL (is an airway clearance technique that uses the lateral posture and different lung volumes to control expiratory flow rate to avoid airway compression) techniques were more effective than the PD method in secretion removal. |
| *Chest.* 1998;113: 1019-1027[8] | 14 | No | Cystic fibrosis | Two modes of oral airway oscillation and PDPV were compared. No difference between treatment modalities was reported. |
| *Chest.* 1998;114: 171-177[9] | 14 | No | Cystic fibrosis | No significant changes were noted for spirometry or sputum volume. Sputum viscoelasticity was lower after therapy with the Flutter in comparison with autogenic drainage. |
| *Chest.* 2000;118: 92-97[10] | 129 | No | Cystic fibrosis | The survey reported that Flutter had the highest total satisfaction and Flutter and HFCWO had higher overall satisfaction than PDPV. |
| *Chest.* 2002;121: 702-707[11] | 23 | No | COPD | Use of Flutter is associated with improvement of spirometry, 6-minute walk distance and dyspnea score when compared with the sham Flutter device. |
| *Clin Pediatr (Phila).* 1998;37:427-32[12] | 8 | No | Cystic fibrosis | PDPV, the intrapulmonary percussive ventilator (IPV) and Flutter were compared. There was no difference in sputum quantity produced with any method studied. Transiently lower $SaO_2$ was noted with PDPV compared with the IPV and Flutter. Inconsistent but significant improvements in flow rates were noted with the 2 devices compared to standard CPT. |
| *Del Med J.* 1999; 71:13-18[13] | 6 | No | Cystic fibrosis | No difference in spirometry and pulmonary mechanics between Flutter and PEP mask treatment. |
| *Eur Respir J.* 1992; 5:748-753[14] | 9 | No | Cystic fibrosis | No difference in mucous clearance between PD + ACBT, PEP mask breathing + FET, exercise on a bicycle ergometer + FET. All treatments had the same duration and FET was standardized. |

## Table C-1, continued

### *Clinical Trials on Secretion Removal Techniques*

| References | Sample Size | RCT | Subjects | Results |
|---|---|---|---|---|
| *Eur Respir J.* 1998; 2:143-147[15] | 22 | No | Cystic fibrosis | No difference in spirometry and sputum production was reported between Flutter and the PEP mask technique. |
| *Pediatr Pulmonol.* 1995;19:16-22[16] | 16 | No | Cystic fibrosis | Wet and dry weights of sputum collected during the sessions were greater for PD, PEP, and HFCWO regimens than no treatment. |
| *Pediatr Pulmonol.* 1996;22:271-274[17] | 29 | No | Cystic fibrosis | More sputum was expectorated during HFCWO than during PDPV as determined by both the wet and the dry measurements |
| *Respir Med.* 1994; 88:49-53[18] | 8 | No | Cystic fibrosis | Mean total sputum expectoration was lower on PDPV+ ACBT alone than on exercise and PDPV+ ACBT. |
| *Respirology.* 1998; 3:183-186[19] | 8 | No | Panbronchiolitis | The mean daily sputum weight, symptom score and peak expiratory flow rate increased significantly after treatment with Flutter compared to before treatment. |
| *Thorax.* 1995;50: 165-169[20] | 18 | No | Cystic fibrosis | AD cleared mucus from the lungs faster than ACBT over the whole day. More patients had an improved $FEF_{25\%-75\%}$ with AD, while more showed an improvement in FVC with ACBT. |
| *Thorax.* 2002;57: 446-448[21] | 17 | No | Bronchiectasis | No difference between ACBT and Flutter in health related quality of life (Chronic Respiratory Disease Questionnaire), ventilatory function, PEFR, breathlessness with either technique. |

Abbreviations: FET: forced expiration technique; $FEF_{25-75}$: forced expiratory flow between 25% and 75%; HFCWO: high frequency chest wall oscillation; PDPV: postural drainage, percussion, and vibration.

# CRITIQUE OF THE COPD PATIENTS' MANAGEMENT GUIDELINES BY THE AMERICAN COLLEGE OF CHEST PHYSICIANS AND AMERICAN COLLEGE OF PHYSICIANS—AMERICAN SOCIETY OF INTERNAL MEDICINE[22-25]

The ACCP guideline did not recommend chest physiotherapy. The rationale for their recommendation was seriously flawed.[26]

- The outcome measure against chest physiotherapy was based on spirometry ($FEV_1$ and FVC) only. However it also goes against recommendation 2 of their own practice guideline as quoted below:
  - o  "For patients hospitalized with an acute exacerbation of COPD, acute spirometry should not be used to diagnose an exacerbation or to assess its severity"
  - o  "... spirometric assessment at presentation or during treatment is not useful in judging severity or guiding management of patients with acute exacerbations of COPD"
  - o  "Despite this fact, many studies use changes in $FEV_1$ as the primary outcome rather than other, more pertinent clinical measures..."
- Their use of the term "Chest physiotherapy" was based on a single technique—manual percussion
  - o  Only 1 of the 3 reported randomized control trials (RCTs) that the authors based their recommendation against chest physiotherapy was an RCT
  - o  Both the internal and external validity scores of the 3 articles used were low
  - o  All 3 studies that the recommendation was based on were published from the 1970's to the mid 1980's
  - o  Outcomes measures favoring manual percussion were ignored from one of the studies

# REFERENCES

1.  Arens R, Gozal K, Omlin KJ, et al. Comparison of high frequency chest compression and conventional chest physiotherapy in hospitalized patients with cystic fibrosis. *Am J Resp Crit Care Med.* 1994;150:1154-1157.

2.  Christensen EF, Nedergaard T, Dahl R. Long-term treatment of chronic bronchitis with positive expiratory pressure mask and chest physiotherapy. *Chest.* 1990;97:645-650.

3.  Savci S, Ince DI, Arikan H. A comparison of autogenic drainage and the active cycle of breathing techniques in patients with chronic obstructive pulmonary diseases. *J Cardiopulm Rehabil.* 2000;20:37-43.

4.  McIlwaine PM, Wong LT, Peacock D, Davidson AG. Long-term comparative trial of conventional postural drainage and percussion versus positive expiratory pressure physiotherapy in the treatment of cystic fibrosis. *J Pediatr.* 1997;131:570-574.

5.  McIlwaine PM, Wong LT, Peacock D, et al. Long-term comparative trial of positive expiratory pressure versus oscillating positive expiratory pressure (Flutter) physiotherapy in the treatment of cystic fibrosis. *J Pediatr.* 2001;138:845-850.

6.  Gondor M, Nixon PA, Mutich R, et al. Comparison of Flutter device and chest physical therapy in the treatment of cystic fibrosis pulmonary exacerbation. *Pediatr Pulmonol.* 1999;28:255-260.

7.  Bellone A, Lascioli R, Raschi S, et al. Chest physical therapy in patients with acute exacerbation of chronic bronchitis: effectiveness of three methods. *Arch Phys Med Rehabil.* 2000;81:558-560.

8.  Scherer TA, Barandun J, Martinez E, et al. Effect of high-frequency oral airway and chest wall oscillation and conventional chest physical therapy on expectoration in patients with stable cystic fibrosis. *Chest.* 1998;113:1019-1027.

9.  App EM, Kieselmann R, Reinhardt D, et al. Sputum rheology changes in cystic fibrosis lung disease following two different types of physiotherapy: flutter vs autogenic drainage. *Chest.* 1998;114:171-177.

10. Oermann CM, Swank PR, Sockrider MM. Validation of an instrument measuring patient satisfaction with chest physiotherapy techniques in cystic fibrosis. *Chest.* 2000;118:92-97.

11. Wolkove N, Kamel H, Rotaple M, et al. Use of a mucus clearance device enhances the bronchodilator response in patients with stable COPD. *Chest.* 2002;121:702-707.

12. Newhouse PA, White F, Marks JH, et al. The intrapulmonary percussive ventilator and flutter device compared to standard chest physiotherapy in patients with cystic fibrosis. *Clin Pediatr (Phila).* 1998;37:427-432.

13. Padman R, Geouque DM, Engelhardt MT. Effects of the flutter device on pulmonary function studies among pediatric cystic fibrosis patients. *Del Med J.* 1999;71:13-18.

14. Lannefors L, Wollmer P. Mucus clearance with three chest physiotherapy regimes in cystic fibrosis: a comparison between postural drainage, PEP and physical exercise. *Eur Respir J.* 1992;5:748-753.

15. van Winden CM, Visser A, Hop W, et al. Effects of Flutter and PEP mask physiotherapy on symptoms and lung function in children with cystic fibrosis. *Eur Respir J.* 1998;12:143-147.

16. Braggion C, Cappelletti LM, Cornacchia M, et al. Short-term effects of three chest physiotherapy regimens in patients hospitalized for pulmonary exacerbations of cystic fibrosis: a cross-over randomized study. *Pediatr Pulmonol.* 1995;19:16-22.

17. Kluft J, Beker L, Castagnino M, et al. A comparison of bronchial drainage treatments in cystic fibrosis. *Pediatr Pulmonol.* 1996;22:271-274.

18. Baldwin DR, Hill AL, Peckham DG, et al. Effect of addition of exercise to chest physiotherapy on sputum expectoration and lung function in adults with cystic fibrosis. *Respir Med.* 1994;88:49-53.

19. Burioka N, Sugimoto Y, Suyama H, et al. Clinical efficacy of the FLUTTER device for airway mucus clearance in patients with diffuse panbronchiolitis. *Respirology.* 1998;3:183-186.

20. Miller S, Hall DO, Clayton CB, et al. Chest physiotherapy in cystic fibrosis: a comparative study of autogenic drainage and the active cycle of breathing techniques with postural drainage. *Thorax.* 1995;50:165-169.

21. Thompson CS, Harrison S, Ashley J, et al. Randomised crossover study of the Flutter device and the active cycle of breathing technique in non-cystic fibrosis bronchiectasis. *Thorax.* 2002;57:446-448.

22. McCrory DC, Brown C, Gelfand SE, Bach PB. Management of exacerbations of COPD: a summary and appraisal of the published evidence. *Chest.* 2001;119:1190-1209.

23. Bach PB, Brown C, Gelfand SE, McCrory DC. Management of exacerbations of chronic obstructive pulmonary disease: a summary and appraisal of published evidence. *Ann Intern Med.* 2001;134:600-620.

24. Snow V, Lascher S, Mottur-Pilson C, et al. The evidence base for management of acute exacerbations of COPD: clinical practice guideline, part 1. *Chest.* 2001;119:1185-1189.

25. Snow V, Lascher S, Mottur-Pilson C, et al. Evidence base for management of acute exacerbations of chronic obstructive pulmonary disease. *Ann Intern Med.* 2001;134:595-599.

26. Chung F, Johnson RL. Clinical practive guidelines in physiotherapy management of chronic obstructive pulmonary disease. Expert opinion versus clincian perspectives. *Gas Exchange.* 2003;11(2):11-13.

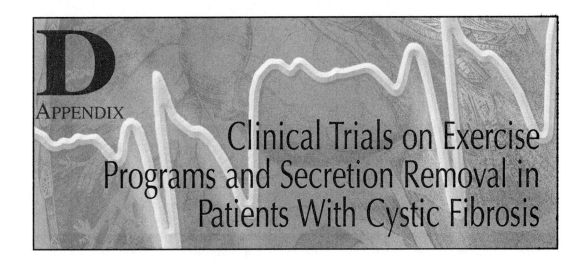

APPENDIX

# D

# Clinical Trials on Exercise Programs and Secretion Removal in Patients With Cystic Fibrosis

The objective of this appendix is to provide a review of clinical trials on exercise programs and secretion removal in patients with cystic fibrosis. The level of evidence and summary on exercise programs and secretion removal in patients with cystic fibrosis in Chapter 15 was made based on this review and other systematic reviews.

Table D-1

*Clinical Trials on Exercise Programs and Secretion Removal in Patients With Cystic Fibrosis*

| References | Sample Size | RCT | Results |
|---|---|---|---|
| *Acta Paediatr Scand.* 1987;76:70-75[1] | 7 | No | Patients were enrolled for 30 months in a daily exercise program. After 12 months conventional chest physiotherapy was withdrawn. Spirometric data and lung volumes showed improvement over the 30 months. |
| *Phys Ther.* 1989; 69:633-639[2] | 17 | Yes | Patients in Ex group had 2 cycle ergometer exercise sessions and 1 bronchial hygiene treatment session per day and PD group had 3 bronchial hygiene treatment sessions per day. Both groups showed the same degree of improvement. |
| *Lancet.* 1981; 2:1201-1203[3] | 10 | No | Patients participated in swimming training over 7 weeks. Ventilatory status assessed by spirometry had improved significantly after the swimming training. |
| *Thorax.* 1989; 44:1006-1008[4] | 22 | Yes | Patients in the exercise group reported higher maximum oxygen consumption and maximum minute ventilation while the increase in sputum weight was not significant. In the second study more sputum was expectorated during and after CPT than during and after exercise. Exercise may have a role in aiding sputum removal in but should not be considered as a replacement for CPT. |

Table D-1, continued

### Clinical Trials on Exercise Programs and Secretion Removal in Patients With Cystic Fibrosis

| References | Sample Size | RCT | Results |
|---|---|---|---|
| *Respir Med.* 1992; 86:507-511[5] | 18 | No | Ex alone was less effective than the other three modalities in clearing sputum (ACBT, ACBT+Ex, Ex+ACBT). The treatment option preferred by patients to continue at home was Ex+ACBT. <10% of patients preferred exercise alone. Note: The total treatment time for each group was identical. |
| *Respir Med.* 1994; 88:49-53[6] | 8 | No | On the exercise and physiotherapy (Ex+PT) day, subjects exercised 60 min before physiotherapy (PT). On the (PT) alone day, subjects rested for 60 min instead of exercising. PT was administered on both study days (PD+V, deep breathing, FET, and coughing). Mean total sputum expectoration was lower (14 g) after PT alone than after Ex+PT (21.5 g). Note: The Ex+PT day has an extra hour of treatment intervention than the PT alone day. |
| *Arch Dis Child.* 1982; 57:587-589[7] | 12 | No | After 17 days of vigorous physical exercise and sport, improvement in spirometry was reported. |

Abbreviations: ACBT: active cycle of breathing techniques; CPT: chest physical therapy which usually involves PD, percussion and vibration; Ex: exercise; FET: forced expiration technique; g: grams; PD: postural drainage; V: vibration.

# A BRIEF DISCUSSION ON THE RELATIVE EFFECT OF EXERCISE PROGRAMS AND AIRWAY CLEARANCE

Two studies provided some insight into the relative effects of exercise and airway clearance. A clinical trial[8] on healthy subjects showed that exercise can significantly increased bronchial clearance compared to quiet breathing exercises at rest. It is important to note that the healthy subjects exercised at 70% to 75% of their maximum heart rate continually for 30 minutes to induce an 8.7% higher increase in mucus clearance. A subsequent study from the same institution extended the trial to include postural drainage in left side lying with 15° head-down position and cough once every 5 minutes.[9] This study reported a similar difference in increased mucous clearance after exercise of 7.5% compared to the control group. However, coughing induced a 40% greater increase in mucous clearance than the control group. The most important clinical implication of these 2 studies[8,9] is that although statistically significant, exercise performed at a relatively high training intensity had only a small effect in mucous clearance especially when compared to coughing (8.7% or 7.5% compared to 40% greater than control values).

A systematic review[10] examined the effect of chest physical therapy management of patients with cystic fibrosis (CF). The modalities examined included PEP mask, forced expiratory technique (FET), exercise (Ex), autogenic drainage (AD), and standard physical therapy (STD), consisting of postural drainage, percussion, and vibration. In this review, seven separate meta-analyses comparing the independent techniques using the pooled effect size technique were performed. The review concluded that standard physical therapy resulted in a significantly greater sputum expectoration than no treatment. The combination of STD with EX was associated with a statistically significant increase in forced expiration in 1 second ($FEV_1$) over STD alone.

These conclusions provide helpful clinical guidance; however, it is important to realize that there were some inconsistencies in this review. Of the studies of STD with Ex included in the systematic review, two-thirds of the trials included in the meta-analysis were not randomized control trials. The only RCT included in the review, showed no difference in $FEV_1$ between the 2 groups. It was not apparent from reading about the 3 trials in the review, whether STD with Ex had a better outcome than STD alone especially since there was no STD group in two-thirds of the trials (these are the first 3 studies listed in the Table D-1).

Another concern was the presentation of the data in Table 4 of the systematic review.[10] The three trials used in meta-analysis are also the first 3 listed in Table D-1. However, the sample sizes reported in their systematic review and the original papers were quite different. In Table 4 of the review,[10] the first trial[1] had a sample size of 7 but was reported to be 14 and the third trial[3] had a sample size ten but was reported to be 22. The fourth trial[4] as Table D-1 had the same sample size as in the third trial in Table 4 of the review. It was an RCT but was excluded from the meta-analysis. Care review of this systematic review[10] illustrated limitations of systematic reviews and erroneous reporting of the data; however, the conclusions were interesting.

Furthermore, 2 other trials in this Appendix have shown that exercise alone was less effective in secretion removal than treatment ACBT with postural drainage.

Thus, as an airway clearance technique, exercise may be an useful adjunct. When used alone, it may not be the most effective airway clearance technique.

# REFERENCES

1. Andreasson B, Jonson B, Kornfalt R, et al. Long-term effects of physical exercise on working capacity and pulmonary function in cystic fibrosis. *Acta Paediatr Scand.* 1987;76:70-75.

2. Cerny FJ. Relative effects of bronchial drainage and exercise for in-hospital care of patients with cystic fibrosis. *Phys Ther.* 1989;69:633-639.

3. Zach MS, Purrer B, Oberwaldner B. Effect of swimming on forced expiration and sputum clearance in cystic fibrosis. *Lancet.* 1981;2:1201-1203.

4. Salh W, Bilton D, Dodd M, Webb AK. Effect of exercise and physiotherapy in aiding sputum expectoration in adults with cystic fibrosis. *Thorax.* 1989;44:1006-1008.

5. Bilton D, Dodd ME, Abbot JV, et al. The benefits of exercise combined with physiotherapy in the treatment of adults with cystic fibrosis. *Respir Med.* 1992;86:507-511.

6. Baldwin DR, Hill AL, Peckham DG, et al. Effect of addition of exercise to chest physiotherapy on sputum expectoration and lung function in adults with cystic fibrosis. *Respir Med.* 1994;88:49-53.

7. Zach M, Oberwaldner B, Hausler F. Cystic fibrosis: physical exercise versus chest physiotherapy. *Arch Dis Child.* 1982;57:587-589.

8. Wolff RK, Dolovich MB, Obminski G, et al. Effects of exercise and eucapnic hyperventilation on bronchial clearance in man. *J Appl Physiol.* 1977;43:46-50.

9. Oldenburg FA Jr, Dolovich MB, Montgomery JM, et al. Effects of postural drainage, exercise, and cough on mucus clearance in chronic bronchitis. *Am Rev Resp Dis.* 1979;120:739-745.

10. Thomas J, Cook DJ, Brooks D. Chest physical therapy management of patients with cystic fibrosis. A meta analysis. *Am J Respir Crit Care Med.* 1995;151:846-50.

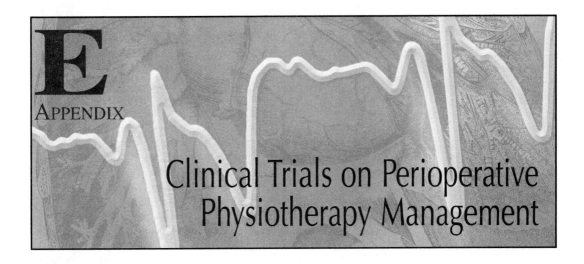

The objective of this appendix is to provide a review of clinical trials on perioperative physiotherapy management. The level of evidence and summary on perioperative physiotherapy management in Chapter 20 was made based on this review and other systematic reviews.

Table E-1

*Clinical Trials on Perioperative Physiotherapy Management*

| References | Sample Size | RCT | Subjects | Results |
|---|---|---|---|---|
| *Arch Phys Med Rehabil.* 1998;79:5-9[1] | 81 | Y | Abdominal surgery | The incidence of postoperative pulmonary complications was 7.5% in the breathing exercise group and 19.5% in the control group; the control group also had more radiologic alterations. Breathing exercise also protects against PPC and is more effective in moderate- and high-risk patients. |
| *BMJ.* 1996;312: 148-153[2] | 456 | Y | Abdominal surgery | No difference in respiratory complications between IS group and DB group was reported. Deep breathing exercises were recommended for low risk patients and incentive spirometry for high risk patients. |
| *Br J Surg.* 1997;84: 1535-1538[3] | 364 | Y | Abdominal surgery | Treatment consisted of preoperative teaching, pursed lip breathing, huffing/ cough, position change, and mobilization +/- PEP mask. Control group received no preoperative information but received EP mask treatment if pulmonary complications occurred postoperatively. Control group had a higher complication rate than the treatment group (27% versus 6%). |

Table E-1, continued

## Clinical Trials on Perioperative Physiotherapy Management

| References | Sample Size | RCT | Subjects | Results |
|---|---|---|---|---|
| Physiother Res Int. 2001;6:236-50[4] | 57 | Y | Abdominal surgery | The addition of periodic continuous positive airway pressure to a traditional physiotherapy postoperative treatment regimen after upper abdominal surgery did not significantly affect physiological or clinical outcomes. |
| Chest. 1994;105: 741-747[5] | 80 | Y | CABG | No difference in incidence or severity of fever, hypoxemia, chest roentgenologic abnormalities or postoperative pulmonary complications was reported between PT and no PT group. See following section on critique of this study. |
| Crit Care Med. 2000;28:679-83[6] | 67 | Y | Thoracic surgery | CPT plus IS was compared with CPT alone. The addition of IS to CPT did not further reduce pulmonary complications or hospital stay. |
| Intensive Care Med. 1995;21:469-74[7] | 97 | Y | Thoracic surgery | Routine CPT, PEP, and inspiratory resistance PEP were compared. No difference between the 3 groups was found except a tendency for decreased risk of having postoperative complications in the latter 2 groups. |
| J Rehabil Med. 2001;33:79-84[8] | 98 | Y | CABG | All patients performed DB, arm ROM, coughing, and mobilization. In addition, the blow bottle group exhaled against an expiratory peak pressure of 10 cm $H_2O$; IR-PEP group inhaled against a 5 cm $H_2O$ and exhaled against an expiratory peak pressure of 10 cm $H_2O$; deep breathing group breathed without the mechanical device. The blow bottle group had significantly less reduction in TLC compared to the deep breathing group, while the IR-EP group did not significantly differ from the other 2 groups. |

Abbreviations: cm $H_2O$: centimeters of water; CPT: breathing exercises, huffing, and coughing; DB: deep breathing; IR: inspiratory resistance; IS: incentive spirometry.

# CRITIQUE OF THE EFFECT OF MOBILIZATION ALONE IN CABG SURGERY

Two studies[5,9] reported that mobilization alone is as effective or more effective in reducing postoperative pulmonary complications. Both of these studies had limitations with their design and methodology.

The earlier study[9] lacks proper randomization. Patient assignment to mobilization and nonmobilization groups was based on medical and surgical considerations. Those who were surgically unwell or developed medical complications to the extent that they could not be mobilized were allocated to the nonmobilized group. The favorable outcomes in the mobilization group could be attributable to differences in the pre-existing health status that determined group assignment rather than to the treatment intervention of mobilization.

The second study[5] reported that a similar number of patients in the control and treatment groups developed cardiopulmonary complications. There were several limitations in this study:

- Firstly, all the patients that developed cardiopulmonary complications received "intensive chest physiotherapy" regardless of group assignment.

- The overall cardiopulmonary complication rate was 7.5% in this study, which means 3 of 40 individuals in each group had complications, which is similar to that reported in other open-heart surgery studies. Even if physical therapy could decrease the complication rate by half, the study did not have a large enough sample size to detect this kind of difference.

- Of those who developed cardiopulmonary complications, 3 patients in the control group had sputum retention whereas none had sputum retention in the treatment group. In addition, the control group showed an increased temperature in 12 subjects on day 1 and 4 subjects on day 4 whereas the treatment group showed an increase in temperature in 8 subjects on day 1 and 1 subject on day 4.

- With a low complication rate and an effect size of about 33%, a sample size of more than 170 subjects per group is required to have an 80% statistical power.

Results from underpowered clinical trials that show no significant differences do not imply clinical equivalency between control and treatment groups. Underpowered clinical trials have limited clinical values and have been considered to be unethical except in research on rare diseases or pilot studies.[10]

# REFERENCES

1. Chumillas S, Ponce JL, Delgado F. Prevention of postoperative pulmonary complications through respiratory rehabilitation: a controlled clinical study. *Arch Phys Med Rehabil.* 1998;79:5-9.

2. Hall JC, Tarala RA, Tapper J, et al. Prevention of respiratory complications after abdominal surgery: a radomised clinical trial. *BMJ.* 1996;312:148-153.

3. Olsen MF, Hahnn I, Nordgren S, et al. Randomized controlled trial of prophylactic chest physiotherapy in major abdominal surgery. *Br J Surg.* 1997;84:1535-1538.

4. Denehy L, Carroll S, Ntoumenopoulos G, et al. A randomized controlled trial comparing periodic mask CPAP with physiotherapy after abdominal surgery. *Physiother Res Int.* 2001;6:236-250.

5. Stiller K, Montarello J, Wallace M, et al. Efficacy of breathing and coughing exercises in the prevention of pulmonary complications after coronary artery surgery. *Chest.* 1994;105:741-747.

6. Gosselink R, Schrever K, Cops P, et al. Incentive spirometry does not enhance recovery after thoracic surgery. *Crit Care Med.* 2000;28:679-683.

7. Richter Larsen K, Ingwersen U, Thode S, et al. Mask physiotherapy in patients after heart surgery: a controlled study. *Intensive Care Med.* 1995;21:469-474.

8. Westerdahl E, Lindmark B, Almgren SO, et al. Chest physiotherapy after coronary artery bypass graft surgery—a comparison of three different deep breathing techniques. *J Rehabil Med.* 2001;33:79-84.

9. Scheidegger D, Bentz L, Piolino G, et al. Influence of early mobilisation on pulmonary function in surgical patients. *Eur J Int Care Med.* 1976;2:35-40.

10. Halpern SD, Karlawish JHT, Berlin JA. The continuing unethical conduct of underpowered clinical trials. *JAMA.* 2002;288:358-362.

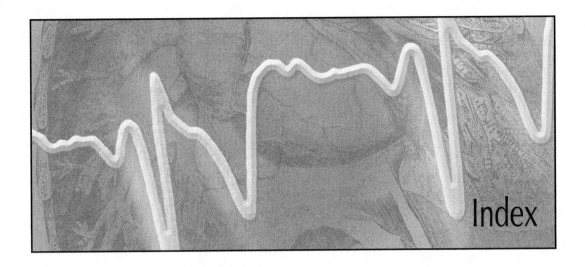

Index

# Build Your Library

Along with this title, we publish numerous products on a variety of topics. We are sure that you will find the below titles to be an essential addition to your library. Order your copies today or contact us for a copy of our latest catalog for additional product information.

## CLINICAL MANAGEMENT NOTES AND CASE HISTORIES IN CARDIOPULMONARY PHYSICAL THERAPY

*W. Darlene Reid, BMR(PT), PhD and Frank Chung, BSc(PT), MSc*

320 pp., Soft Cover, 2004, ISBN 1-55642-568-6, Order #45686, **$34.95**

*Clinical Management Notes and Case Histories in Cardiopulmonary Physical Therapy* is a succinct guide that facilitates a case-based learning approach to cardiopulmonary care. This one-of-a-kind text combines evidence-based assessment and management skills and well-thought-out cases of typical presentations of pulmonary and cardiovascular conditions. This combined approach helps students and clinicians learn meaningful skills in a clinically relevant manner.

## COMPREHENSIVE WOUND MANAGEMENT

*Glenn Irion, PhD, PT, CWS*

320 pp., Soft Cover, 2002, ISBN 1-55642-477-9, Order #44779, **$39.95**

*Comprehensive Wound Management* is written as a multilevel textbook on the management of wounds treated by clinicians. This unique book covers a wide spectrum of both chronic and acute wounds including pressure ulcers, neuropathic ulcers, vascular ulcers, and burn injuries. Full-color photographs of wounds, photographic descriptions of wound management, and line drawings illustrate and reinforce key concepts. These illustrations assist in creating a complete understanding of wound management. The author's seamless flow creates a user-friendly format that is suitable for both students and practicing clinicians of varying wound experience.

## Contact Us

*SLACK Incorporated, Professional Book Division*
*6900 Grove Road, Thorofare, NJ 08086*
*1-800-257-8290/1-856-848-1000, Fax: 1-856-853-5991*
*orders@slackinc.com or www.slackbooks.com*

# ORDER FORM

| QUANTITY | TITLE | ORDER # | PRICE |
|---|---|---|---|
| | Clinical Management Notes and Case Histories | 45686 | $ 34.95 |
| | Comprehensive Wound Management | 44779 | $ 39.95 |
| | | | |

| | |
|---|---|
| Subtotal | $ |
| Applicable state and local tax will be added to your purchase | $ |
| Handling | $ 5.00 |
| Total | $ |

Name: _____

Address: _____

City: _____ State:_____ Zip: _____

Phone:_____ Fax: _____

Email: _____

- Check enclosed (Payable to SLACK Incorporated)_____

- Charge my: ____ [AMEX] ____ [VISA] ____ [MasterCard]

Account #: _____

Exp. date: _____ Signature:_____

**CODE: 328**

NOTE: *Prices are subject to change without notice.*
*Shipping charges will apply.*
*Shipping and handling charges are non-refundable.*